USMLE Step 1

Biochemistry
Genetics

Lionel P. Raymon, Pharm. D., PhD
Director of Curriculum Integration
Chair of Biochemistry/Pharmacology

Iain McIntosh, PhD
National Instructor

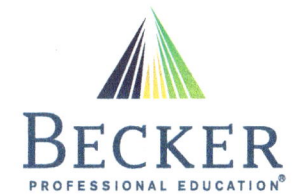

BECKER
PROFESSIONAL EDUCATION®

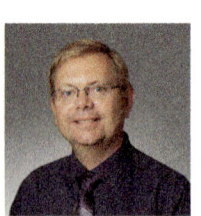

Lionel P. Raymon, Pharm. D., PhD
Director of Curriculum Integration
Chair of Biochemistry/Pharmacology

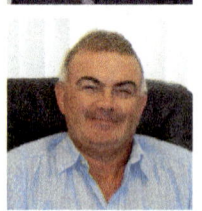

Iain McIntosh, PhD
President, Bendel Camus Medical Education, Inc.

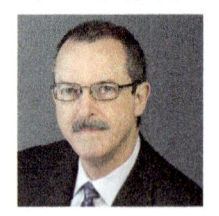

Steven R. Daugherty, PhD
Director, Faculty and Curriculum at Becker Professional Education
Chicago, IL

Disclaimer:

The authors have made reasonable efforts to provide information that is accurate and complete as of the date of publication. However, readers need to be aware that the field of pharmacology is constantly changing, and so recent changes and developments may not be reflected in the current edition. In addition, in view of the rapid changes occurring in medical science, as well as the possibility of human error, technical inaccuracies, typographical, or other errors may exist. The information contained herein is provide "as-is" without warranty of any kind, express or implied. The authors and publisher disclaim any liability or responsibility for any errors or omissions, or any actions taken, or results obtained from the use of the information contained in this publication.

In addition, no drug or other product should be administered without the direction and consultation of a qualified physician and consideration of the individual patient's health and physical condition. Always consult the product information provided by the manufacturer of each drug to be administered to verify the recommended dose, the method and duration of administration, and contraindications.

Cover Photo: Getty Images

The United States Medical Licensing Examination® (USMLE®) is a joint program of the Federation of State Medical Boards (FSMB) and National Board of Medical Examiners® (NBME®). United States Medical Licensing Examination, USMLE, National Board of Medical Examiners, and NBME are registered trademarks of the National Board of Medical Examiners. The National Board of Medical Examiners does not sponsor, endorse, or support Becker Professional Education in any manner.

ISBN: 978-1-94362-809-4

© 2016 by DeVry/Becker Educational Development Corp. All rights reserved.

No part of this work may be reproduced, translated, distributed, published or transmitted without the prior written permission of the copyright owner. Request for permission or further information should be addressed to the Permissions Department, DeVry/Becker Educational Development Corp.

Table of Contents

Biochemistry

Unit I General Principles of Biochemistry

Chapter 1 Enzyme Kinetics 1–1
    1 Overview 1–1
    2 Energy of Reaction ΔG 1–1
    3 Enzymes as Catalysts 1–3
    4 Enzyme Kinetics 1–4

Chapter 2 Signal Transduction 2–1
    1 Overview 2–1
    2 Insulin and Its Receptor 2–2
    3 Glucagon, Epinephrine, and G-Protein Coupled Receptors 2–3
    4 Cortisol 2–4

Chapter 3 Introduction to Metabolism 3–1
    1 Overview 3–1
    2 Dietary Fuels 3–2
    3 Approach to Metabolism 3–3

Unit II Metabolism: Making ATP

Chapter 4 Krebs Cycle (Tricarboxylic Acid Cycle) 4–1
    1 Overview 4–1
    2 Key Enzymes 4–3
    3 Krebs Cycle Intermediates 4–4
    4 Role of Key Intermediates Besides Krebs Cycle 4–5
    5 Clinical Significance of Krebs Cycle 4–6

Chapter 5 Electron Transport Chain 5–1
    1 Overview 5–1
    2 Important Sources of NADH and $FADH_2$ 5–2
    3 Electron Transport Chain 5–4
    4 Proton Gradient and ATP Synthesis 5–5
    5 Regulation 5–5
    6 Clinical Relevance 5–6

Table of Contents

Biochemistry

Unit III   Insulin World

Chapter 6   Carbohydrate Digestion and Glycolysis 6–1
    1   Overview 6–1
    2   Dietary Carbohydrates and Digestion 6–3
    3   Absorption and Cellular Transport 6–5
    4   Glycolysis 6–8
    5   Fructose and Galactose 6–13
    6   Polyol (Sorbitol) Pathway 6–15

Chapter 7   Pyruvate Metabolism 7–1
    1   Overview 7–1
    2   Pyruvate Dehydrogenase: Biochemistry 7–2
    3   Pyruvate Dehydrogenase: Clinical Relevance 7–3
    4   Pyruvate Carboxylase 7–4
    5   Pyruvate Carboxylase: Clinical Relevance 7–5

Chapter 8   Glycogen Synthesis and Fatty Acid Synthesis 8–1
    1   Overview 8–1
    2   Glycogen Synthesis 8–2
    3   Fatty Acid Synthesis 8–5
    4   Hexose-Monophosphate Shunt 8–7

Chapter 9   Lipid Digestion and Lipoprotein Metabolism 9–1
    1   Overview 9–1
    2   Lipid Digestion 9–2
    3   Lipoprotein Metabolism 9–3
    4   Storage of Dietary and Endogenous Triglycerides 9–7
    5   Hepatic Uptake of VLDL and Chylomicron Remnants 9–9
    6   IDL and LDL Production 9–10
    7   HDL Production and Role 9–10
    8   De Novo Synthesis of Cholesterol 9–12
    9   Hyperlipidemias 9–15
    10   Abetalipoproteinemia 9–17

Table of Contents

Biochemistry

Unit IV Glucagon World

Chapter 10 Lipid Catabolism and Ketone Bodies 10–1
    1 Overview 10–1
    2 Mobilization of Lipids 10–1
    3 β-Oxidation of Fatty Acids 10–2
    4 Clinical Relevance of Oxidation of Fatty Acids 10–6
    5 Ketogenesis and Ketogenolysis 10–8

Chapter 11 Gluconeogenesis and Glycogenolysis 11–1
    1 Overview 11–1
    2 Glycogenolysis 11–3
    3 Gluconeogenesis 11–5
    4 Cori and Alanine Cycles 11–8
    5 Clinical Relevance 11–8

Unit V Protein World

Chapter 12 Protein Digestion and Ammonia Detoxification 12–1
    1 Overview 12–1
    2 Dietary Protein Digestion and Absorption 12–2
    3 Detoxification of Amino Acid Nitrogen 12–3
    4 Urea Cycle 12–6
    5 Clinical Relevance: Urea Cycle Enzyme Deficiencies 12–7

Chapter 13 Amino Acid Metabolism and Special Products 13–1
    1 Overview 13–1
    2 Amino Acids 13–2
    3 Amino Acid Synthesis 13–5
    4 Amino Acid Degradation 13–6
    5 Special Products Derived From Amino Acids 13–13

Table of Contents

Biochemistry

Unit VI Molecular Biology

Chapter 14 Purines, Pyrimidines, and Nucleotides 14–1
    1   Overview 14–1
    2   Salvage Enzymes and Clinical Relevance 14–2
    3   De Novo Synthesis of Purines 14–4
    4   Purine Catabolism 14–6
    5   De Novo Pyrimidine Synthesis 14–8
    6   Nucleic Acid Chemistry 14–11

Chapter 15 DNA Replication 15–1
    1   Overview 15–1
    2   Cell Cycle Concepts 15–2
    3   DNA Replication 15–3
    4   DNA Proofreading 15–9
    5   DNA Polymerase Inhibitors 15–10
    6   DNA Repair 15–11

Chapter 16 Gene Expression: Transcription and Control 16–1
    1   Overview 16–1
    2   Gene Structure 16–2
    3   RNA Processing 16–7
    4   Types of RNA and RNA Polymerases 16–11
    5   Control of Gene Expression Through Epigenetic Modifications 16–14
    6   Control of Gene Expression Through Transcription Factors 16–16

Table of Contents

Biochemistry

Chapter 17 Gene Expression: Translation 17–1
    1   Overview 17–1
    2   The Genetic Code 17–1
    3   Ribosomes 17–5
    4   Transfer RNA (tRNA) 17–8
    5   Translation Factors 17–9
    6   Peptide Bond Formation 17–10
    7   Translation Process 17–11
    8   Protein Folding 17–15
    9   Protein Targeting 17–17
    10 Other Important Protein Modifications 17–20
    11 Example of Collagen 17–20

Chapter 18 Molecular Technologies 18–1
    1   Overview 18–1
    2   Restriction Enzymes and Palindromes 18–2
    3   Blotting Techniques 18–4
    4   DNA Polymorphisms 18–6
    5   Dot/Slot Blots and ASO Probes 18–10
    6   Northern Blots 18–11
    7   Western Blot 18–12
    8   Polymerase Chain Reaction 18–13

Chapter 19 Recombinant DNA Technologies 19–1
    1   Overview 19–1
    2   Sources of Human DNA 19–1
    3   Vectors and Cloning Strategy 19–2
    4   Cloning Applications 19–4

Table of Contents

Genetics

Chapter 1 Mendelian Inheritance 1–1
    1   Overview 1–1
    2   Patterns of Mendelian Inheritance 1–3

Chapter 2 Chromosomes 2–1
    1   Overview 2–1
    2   Mitosis 2–1
    3   Meiosis 2–2
    4   Karyotype 2–3
    5   Nomenclature 2–4
    6   Nondisjunction 2–4
    7   Translocation 2–8
    8   Inversions and Deletions 2–10

Chapter 3 Mutations and Disease 3–1
    1   Overview 3–1
    2   Residual Activity 3–5
    3   Promoter/Enhancer Mutations 3–6
    4   Contiguous Gene Syndromes 3–7
    5   Dynamic Mutations and Anticipation 3–8

Chapter 4 X-Inactivation and Epigenetics 4–1
    1   Overview 4–1
    2   Dosage Compensation 4–2
    3   Mechanism of X Inactivation 4–3
    4   "Nonrandom" or "Skewed" Inactivation 4–4
    5   Parent of Origin Effects 4–5
    6   Uniparental Disomy 4–7

Table of Contents

Genetics

Chapter 5 Genetic Testing and Gene Identification 5–1
    1   Overview 5–1
    2   Direct Testing 5–1
    3   Indirect Testing 5–3
    4   Gene Identification 5–5

Chapter 6 Population Genetics 6–1
    1   Overview 6–1
    2   Hardy-Weinberg Equilibrium 6–2

Chapter 7 Genetics of Multifactorial Diseases 7–1
    1   Overview 7–1
    2   Multifactorial Inheritance 7–1
    3   Identification of Genes Involved in Multifactorial Disease 7–4

Index

Biochemistry

General Principles of Biochemistry

Unit 1

CHAPTER 1 — Enzyme Kinetics

1 Overview

- Thermodynamics concerns the energy needed to drive reactions:
  - Enzymes do not alter energy of reaction ΔG
- Kinetics describe the rate of reactions:
  - Enzymes decrease the energy of activation ΔG‡
  - Two parameters describe reactions catalyzed by enzymes:
    — V_{max}
    — K_M
- Graphic representations are classic and used in many disciplines

USMLE® Key Concepts

For Step 1, you must be able to:

- Differentiate spontaneous, non-spontaneous, and reversible reactions based on ΔG.
- Define the role of catalysts in biochemistry.
- Describe K_M and V_{max}.
- Explain the graphical representations of enzyme kinetics.

2 Energy of Reaction ΔG

- $\Delta G = G_{product} - G_{substrate} = G_B - G_A$
- Predicts whether or not a reaction happens

Table 1--2.0 — ΔG Values and Reaction Characteristics

ΔG	Reaction	Remarks
ΔG < 0	Spontaneous	• Reaction will happen • Energy is released – Exergonic • Frequently irreversible
ΔG > 0	Non-spontaneous	• Reaction will NOT happen • Energy is required – Endergonic • Has to be coupled with exergonic reaction
ΔG = 0	Reversible	• Reaction is at equilibrium

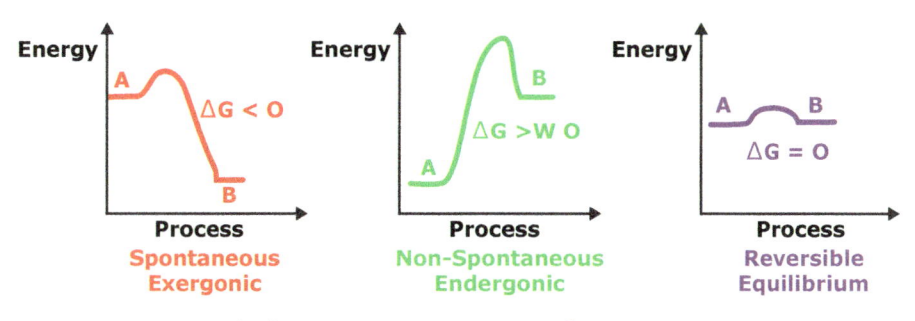

▲ Figure 1–2.0A Energy of Reaction

Spontaneous / Exergonic — ΔG < 0
Non-Spontaneous / Endergonic — ΔG > 0
Reversible / Equilibrium — ΔG = 0

- **ATP-coupled reactions:**
  - Endergonic reactions require energy:

ATP $\longrightarrow$ AMP + PPi	$\Delta G < 0$ releases energy
Amino Acid 1 + Amino Acid 2 $\xrightarrow{\text{Peptidyl transferase}}$ AA$_1$ – AA$_2$	$\Delta G > 0$ requires energy

  - ΔGs are additive

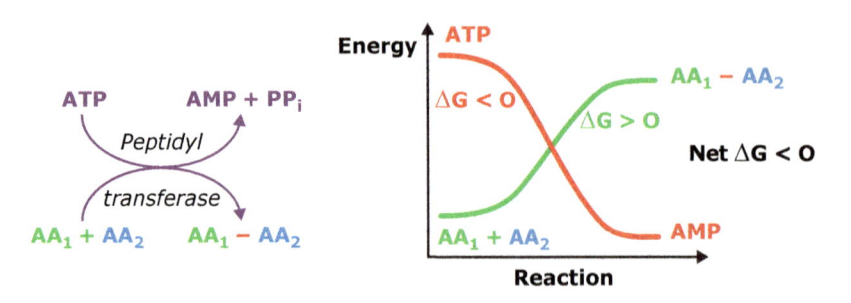

  ▲ **Figure 1–2.0B** ATP-Coupled Reactions

- **ΔG and substrate concentrations:**

  $$\Delta G = \Delta G° + R \times T \times \ln \frac{[B]}{[A]}$$

  - If B > A, $\frac{B}{A} > 1$ then ln is positive
  - If B < A, $\frac{B}{A} < 1$ then ln is negative

  - $\Delta G°$: Standard free energy change
  - R is the gas constant (1.987 cal/mol)
  - T is the temperature in Kelvin
  - As substrate A exceeds product B initially, reaction is spontaneous: A → B
  - As product B increases, A decreases and the ratio B/A increases, reaction reaches equilibrium: A ⇌ B

3 Enzymes as Catalysts

- **Transition state:**
  - Conversion of A → B requires an intermediate form A − B
  - This intermediate has higher free energy than substrate A
  - Energy required to reach transition must be reached before product B is made:
    —Known as energy of activation, ΔG‡
  - ΔG‡ affects the rate of reaction
  - Enzymes decrease ΔG‡ :
    —Accelerate the conversion of A → B

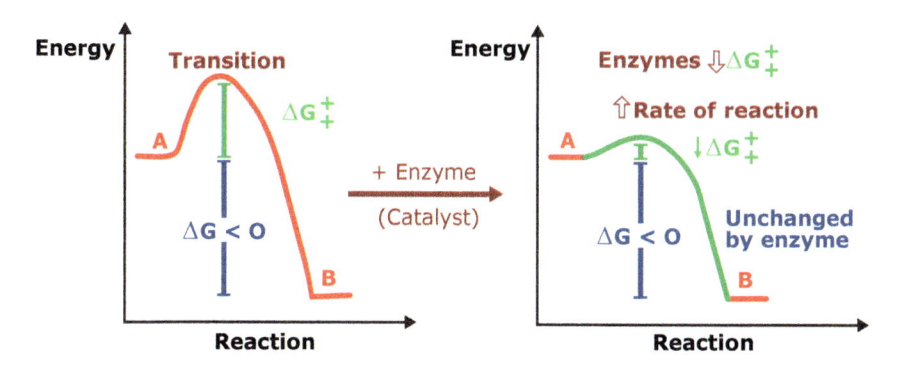

▲ **Figure 1-3.0** Effects of Enzyme on Energy Activation

4 Enzyme Kinetics

- Enzymes have specificity for substrates:
  - Affinity
  - Assessed as K_M
- Maximum rate is linked to number of enzymes available:
  - V_{max}
- Enzymes can be altered:
  - ↑ or ↓ number will alter V_{max}
  - ↑ or ↓ affinity (shape) will alter K_M
- Enzymes are not consumed by reaction
- Active site: Where substrates bind and are converted to products
- Cofactor: Metal ions, organic molecules (BH_4), or vitamins that associate with enzyme during catalysis
- Coenzyme: Loosely bound cofactor
- Prosthetic group: Tightly bound cofactor
- Apoenzyme: Inactive enzyme without cofactor
- Holoenzyme: Active enzyme with bound cofactor

4.1 Kinetic Analysis

- Two graphic representations:
  - Michaelis-Menten graph
  - Lineweaver-Burk (double reciprocal) plot

4.1.1 Michaelis-Menten Graph

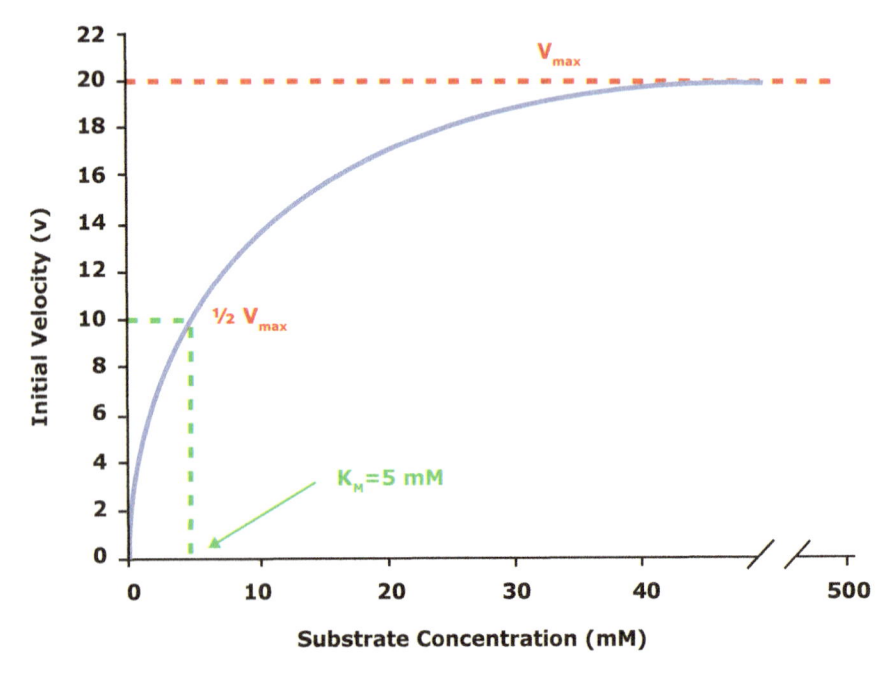

▲ Figure 1–4.1A Michaelis-Menten Graph

Chapter 1 • Enzyme Kinetics

- V_{max} is directly proportional to the number of enzymes
- K_M is the substrate concentration at ½ V_{max}
  - Inversely related to affinity
- Relationship for one substrate (first order reaction):

$$V = V_{max} \times \left(\frac{[S]}{[S] + K_M} \right)$$

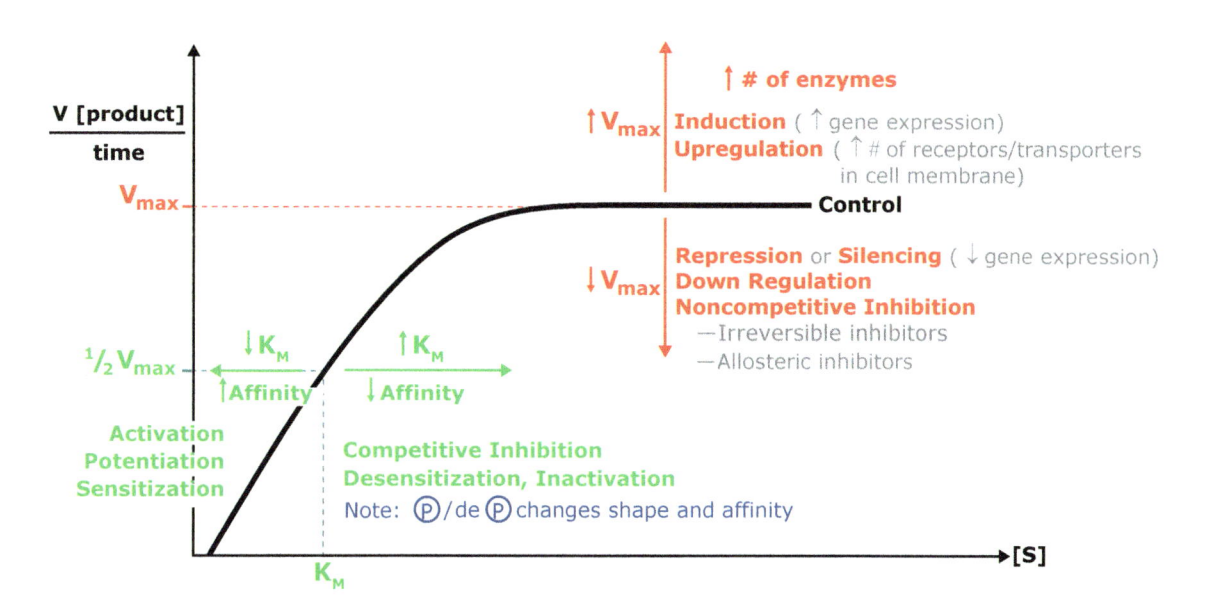

▲ Figure 1-4.1B Mechanisms Changing V_{max} or K_M on Michaelis-Menten Graph

4.1.2 Lineweaver-Burk Plot

- Writing the Michaelis-Menten equation as a double reciprocal gives a straight line relationship:

$$\frac{1}{V} = \frac{K_M}{V_{max}} \times \frac{1}{[S]} + \frac{1}{V_{max}}$$

- One must recognize K_M and V_{max} on the plot and the changes affecting them

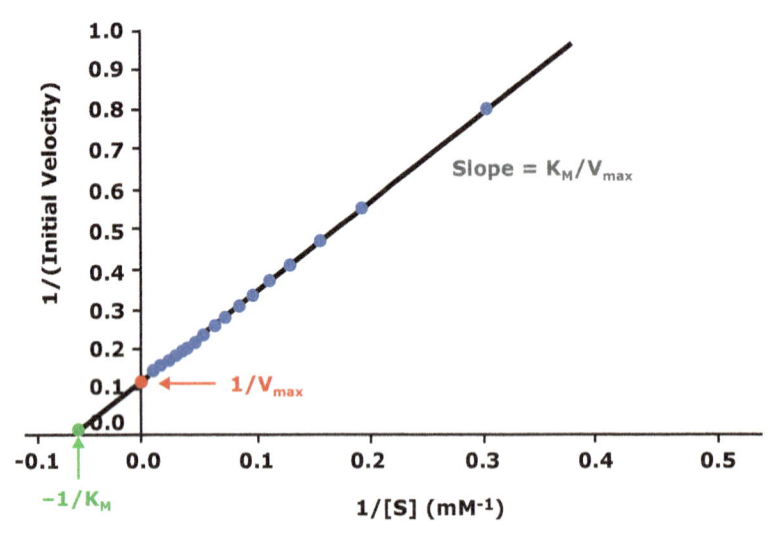

▲ Figure 1-4.1C Lineweaver-Burk Plot

- On this plot:
  - Y intercept is $1/V_{max}$
  - X intercept is $-1/K_M$
  - Slope is K_M/V_{max}

▼ Figure 1-4.1D Mechanisms Changing V_{max} or K_M on Lineweaver-Burk Plot

4.2 Regulation of Enzymes

Metabolites may ↑ or ↓ activity of enzymes (ΔK_M)

Transcription may ↑ or ↓ number of enzymes (ΔV_{max})

- K_M is not altered
- V_{max} is changed

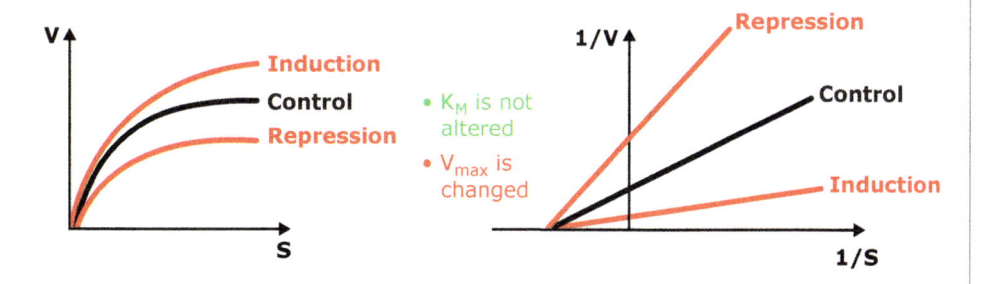

▲ Figure 1-4.2A Effects of Changes in Gene Expression

℗/de℗ can change affinity of enzyme

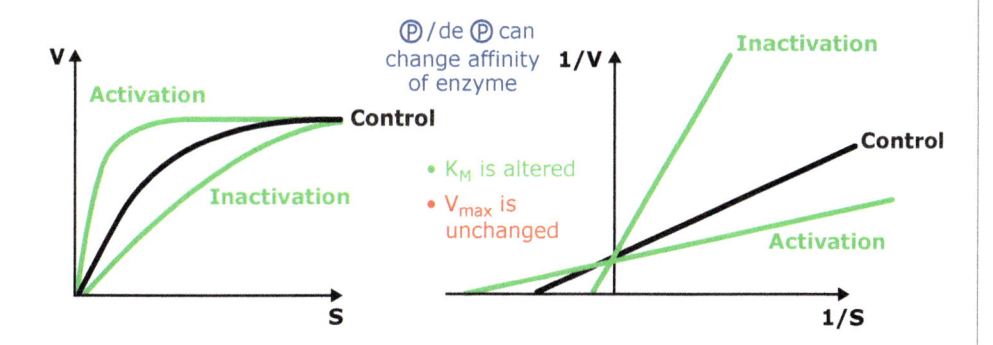

- K_M is altered
- V_{max} is unchanged

▲ Figure 1-4.2B Effects of Phosphorylation/Dephosphorylation

+ Competitive inhibitor: ↑K_M

+ Noncompetitive inhibitor: ↓V_{max}

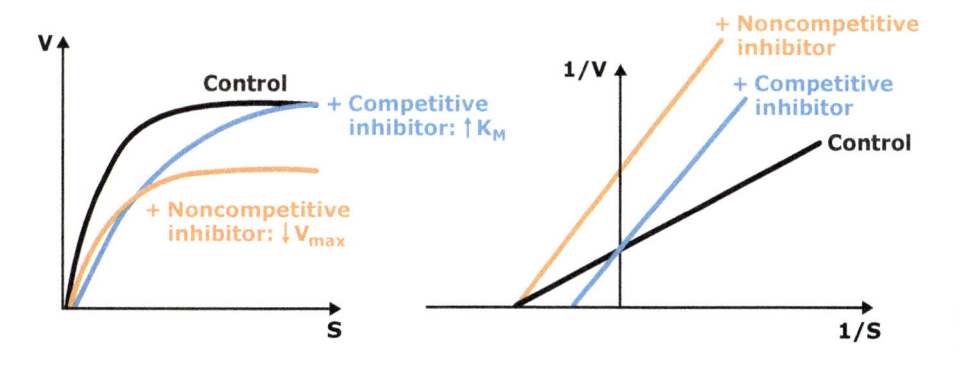

▲ Figure 1-4.2C Effects of Inhibitors

- Competitive inhibitors:
  - Bind active site reversibly
  - ↑ Substrate concentration displaces inhibitor
  - ↑ K_M but no change in V_{max}
- Noncompetitive inhibitors:
  - Bind active site irreversibly, or,
  - Bind reversibly, but allosterically
  - ↑ Substrate concentration cannot displace inhibitor
  - Similar to a loss of enzyme
  - ↓ V_{max} but no change in K_M
- Rate-limiting steps are regulated:
  - Often sigmoid rather than hyperbolic curve
  - Regulation can be local by metabolites or global through hormones and signal transduction

Table 1-4.2 — Competitive vs. Noncompetitive Inhibition

	Competitive	Noncompetitive
Slope (K_M/V_{max})	↑	↑
Y Intercept ($1/V_{max}$)	—	↑
X Intercept ($-1/K_M$)	↑	—

CHAPTER 2 Signal Transduction

1 Overview

- Control of metabolism involves hormone and receptor interaction
- Signal transduction through the receptor alters enzyme activity or gene expression
- Insulin opposes itself to stress hormones, such as glucagon, epinephrine, and cortisol:
  - Insulin dephosphorylates rate-limiting enzymes
  - Glucagon, epinephrine, phosphorylate rate-limiting enzymes
  - Cortisol alters gene expression

USMLE® Key Concepts

For Step 1, you must be able to:

- Describe the signal transduction steps from hormone binding to receptors to molecular changes inside the cell.
- Oppose the molecular effects of insulin to those of stress hormones.
- Contrast alterations in existing enzyme activities with changes in gene expression.

Insulin and Its Receptor

- Produced by β cells of the pancreas
- Secreted in response to rising blood glucose
- Main signal after a meal

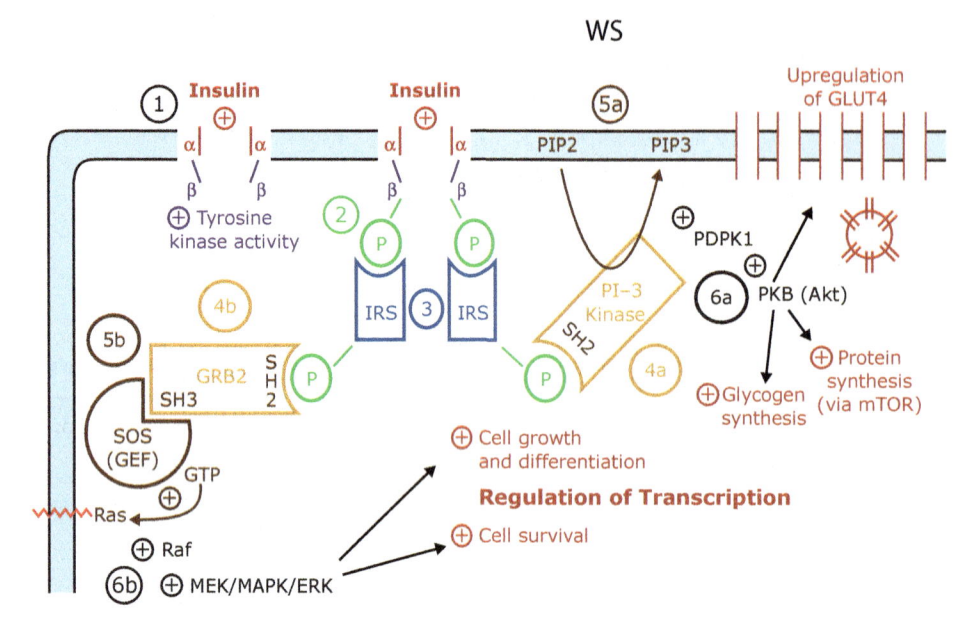

① **Insulin stimulates receptor**
  - Receptor is heterotetramer: 2α, 2β subunits
  - α subunits ⊖ intrinsic β subunit tyr kinase
  - Insulin binding disinhibits β subunits

② Transphosphorylation of receptor

③ Docking of insulin receptor substrate and their phosphorylation (ex: IRS1)

④ SH2 domain proteins bind to phosphorylated IRS (SH2 domains recognize phosphotyrosines)

④a PI-3 Kinase pathway

⑤a PIP2 in membrane is phosphorylated to PIP3

⑥a PIP3 activates PDPK1
  PDPK1 activates PKB (or Akt)
  resulting in:
  - Upregulation of GLUT4 in adipocytes and skeletal muscle
  - ⊕ glycogen synthesis
  - ⊕ protein synthesis

④b GRB2 to MAPK pathway

⑤b SH3 domain of GRB2 binds SOS, a guanine nucleotide exchange factor (GEF)
  SOS allows Ras activation by exchanging GDP to GTP

⑥b Active Ras stimulates Raf
  Raf activates MEK
  MEK turns on MAPK
  MAPK activates ERK
  resulting in:

Abbreviations

SH2:	Src Homology 2 domain; src is short for sarcoma
SH3:	Src Homology 3 domain
PI-3 kinase:	Phosphoinositide-3 kinase
GRB2:	Growth factor receptor bound protein-2
PIP2:	Phosphatidylinositol bisPhosphate, membrane phospholipid
PIP3:	Phosphatidylinositol trisPhosphate, second messenger, docking site for pleckstrin homology domains proteins (PH domains)
SOS:	Son Of Sevenless, a guanine nucleotide exchange factor (GEF)
Ras:	From "Rat Sarcoma"; A family of monomeric G-proteins
PDPK1:	Phosphoinositide dependent protein kinase-1, a PH domain kinase
PKB:	Protein kinase B, a ser/thr kinase; also known as Akt
Raf:	A member of the Raf kinase proteins (ser/thr kinases); from rapidly accelerated fibrosarcoma
MEK:	Mitogen/extracellular signal regulated kinase
MAPK:	Mitogen activated protein kinase
ERK:	Extracellular signal regulated

▲ **Figure 2-2.0** Insulin Receptor Signaling

- Insulin has many targets:
  - Activates protein phosphatases:
    - PP1: Protein phosphatase 1
    - Essentially reverses protein kinase A
  - Activates cAMP phosphodiesterases:
    - Degrade cAMP to inactivate 5' AMP
    - Opposes G_s-coupling of β_2 and glucagon receptors

3 Glucagon, Epinephrine, and G-Protein Coupled Receptors

- Glucagon is produced by α cells of pancreas
- Epinephrine is released by adrenal medulla
- Secreted in response to low blood glucose
- Main signal in between meals
- β_2 receptors and glucagon receptors are G_s-coupled

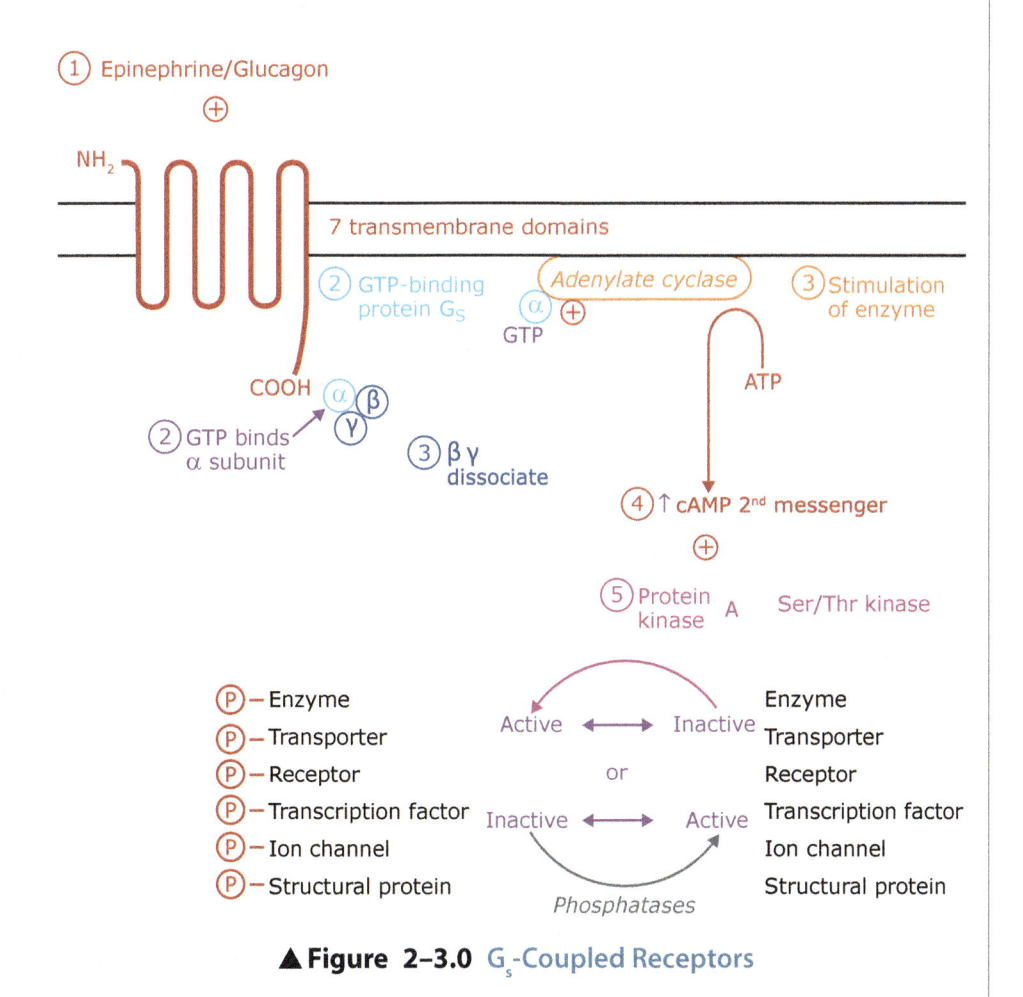

▲ Figure 2-3.0 G_s-Coupled Receptors

- All G-protein coupled receptors have seven transmembrane domains
- G-proteins have three subunits:
  - α subunit has GTPase activity

$$\alpha\text{-GTP (active)} \leftrightarrow \alpha\text{-GDP (inactive)}$$

  - βγ subunits dissociate on GTP-binding to α
    —Reassociate with α-GDP (inactive form)
  - G_s stimulates adenylate cyclase
  - G_i inhibits adenylate cyclase
  - Other G-proteins are reviewed in *Pharmacology* and *Physiology*

- General pattern of signal transduction:
  1. Receptor binding by first messenger:
     —Drug, hormone, neurotransmitter
  2. Activation of G-protein
  3. Activation or inhibition of enzyme
  4. ↑ or ↓ in second messengers
  5. ↑ or ↓ in phosphorylation by kinases

4 Cortisol

- Binds intracellular receptor
- Receptor is a specific transcription factor:
  - Binding of cortisol activates zinc fingers
  - Receptor-hormone complex translocate to nucleus
- DNA-binding site is a hormone response element (HRE)
- Gene expression for specific proteins is altered
- Note that glucagon and epinephrine can also alter gene expression:
  - PKA can activate specific transcription factor CREB
- See Chapter 16, "Gene Expression: Transcription and Control"

CHAPTER 3: Introduction to Metabolism

1 Overview

- Each cell must ensure adequate energy levels to function:
  - ATP is energy currency
- Once ATP levels are adequate cells can "work":
  - Make forms of stored energy:
    - Glycogen
    - Fat
  - Build proteins
  - Express genes
  - Replicate
  - Perform physiological functions
- Two major worlds of biochemistry:
  - Insulin World:
    - During a meal and up to 60–90 minutes after
    - Absorptive phase
    - Tissues preferentially use glucose as a source of energy
  - Glucagon World:
    - In between meals
    - Postabsorptive phase
    - Most tissues use fat as a source of energy:
      - CNS and RBCs still use glucose
      - Alternate fuel sources, such as ketones, are available:
        - Produced by liver
        - Used by muscle, kidney
        - Used by brain in prolonged starvation

USMLE® Key Concepts

For Step 1, you must be able to:

- Identify the major energy sources from diet.
- Describe the two worlds of biochemistry, Insulin versus Glucagon, by having a clear understanding of where the ATP derives from, and what to do if the ATP is high.

2 Dietary Fuels

- Carbohydrates:
  - 4 kcal/g
  - Starch, lactose, and sucrose give rise to glucose, galactose, and fructose
  - 45%–65% of total calories
  - Include fibers
- Lipids:
  - 9 kcal/g from fat
  - Triglycerides (fat)
  - 20%–35% of total calories
  - Include also:
    —Cholesterol
    —Essential fatty acids
    —Lipid soluble vitamins A, D, E, and K
- Proteins:
  - 4 kcal/g
  - 10%–35% of total calories
  - Include essential amino acids
- Alcohol:
  - 7 kcal/g
  - Considerable calorie content primarily for the liver
- Diet also brings vitamins and essential minerals, as well as water

Chapter 3 • Introduction to Metabolism — Biochemistry

3 Approach to Metabolism

1. Are you in the Insulin World or Glucagon World?
2. Ensure adequate ATP levels:
   - How do I make ATP?
3. Only if ATP levels are adequate:
   - What do I do with ATP?

3.1 Insulin World of Biochemistry

- Absorptive phase, within 60–90 minutes of food intake:
  - Insulin dephosphorylates rate-limiting steps
- How do I make ATP?
  - Use glucose and four pathways:
    - Glycolysis:
      - Glucose to pyruvate
      - ATP by substrate level phosphorylations (SLP)
      - SLP does not require O_2
      - SLP does not require mitochondria
      - SLPs are critical for RBCs
      - SLPs are the only source of ATP in hypoxic tissue
    - Pyruvate dehydrogenase (PDH):
      - Converts pyruvate to acetyl-CoA
      - Mitochondrial enzyme
    - Krebs cycle:
      - Burns acetyl-CoA to CO_2
      - Contains many dehydrogenases
      - Produces electron-rich NADH and $FADH_2$
    - Electron transport chain (ETC):
      - Recycles NADH and $FADH_2$ to NAD and FAD
      - Requires O_2 as final acceptor of electrons
      - Electricity is used to generate ATP:
        - ATP is the result of oxidative phosphorylation
        - Main source of ATP

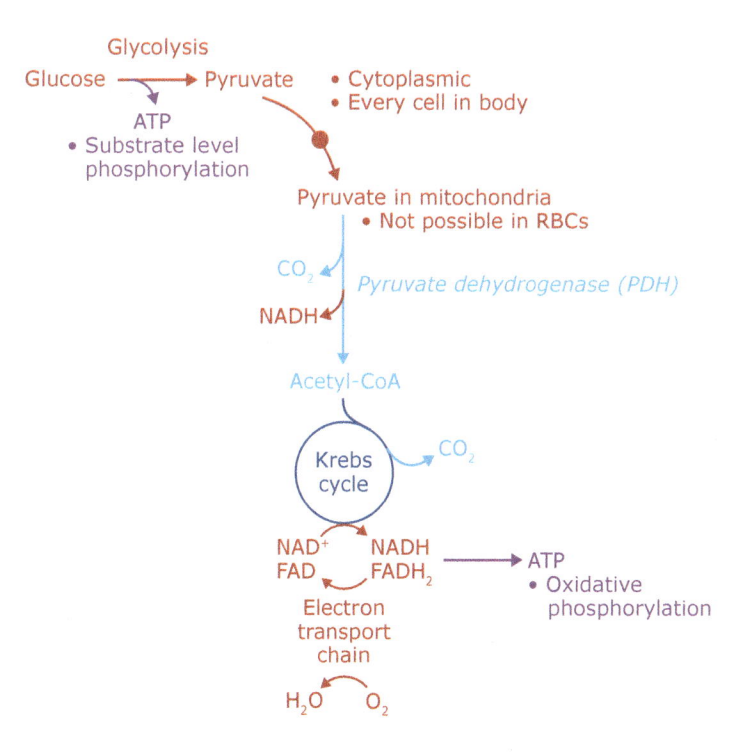

▲ Figure 3-3.1A ATP Generation in the Insulin World

- ↑ ATP in the Insulin World:
  - Liver makes energy stores:
    — Acetyl-CoA → Fatty acid synthesis
    — Glucose → Glycogen synthesis
  - Muscle also does glycogen and fat
  - Adipose stores fat made by liver:
    — Uses lipoprotein lipase (LPL)

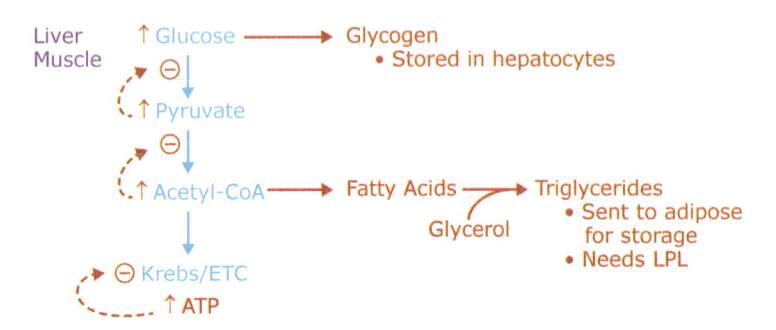

▲ **Figure 3-3.1B** High ATP in the Insulin World

3.2 Glucagon World of Biochemistry

- Postabsorptive phase:
  - Glucagon/epinephrine phosphorylate rate-limiting enzymes
- How do I make ATP?
  - Use fat and four pathways:
    — Mobilization from adipose by hormone sensitive lipase (HSL)
    — β-oxidation of fatty acids:
      - In mitochondria
      - Makes acetyl-CoA
    — Krebs Cycle
    — ETC
  - RBCs and CNS still use glucose to make ATP
- ↑ ATP in the Glucagon World:
  - Liver feeds extra-hepatic tissues:
    — Acetyl-CoA → Ketones
      - Ketones will be used by muscle, heart in particular
      - Ketones are also for renal cortex
    — Gluconeogenesis:
      - Converts amino acids, lactate, and glycerol to glucose
      - Glucose is released for RBCs and CNS
    — Glycogenolysis:
      - Short-term maintenance of blood glucose
      - Finite stores

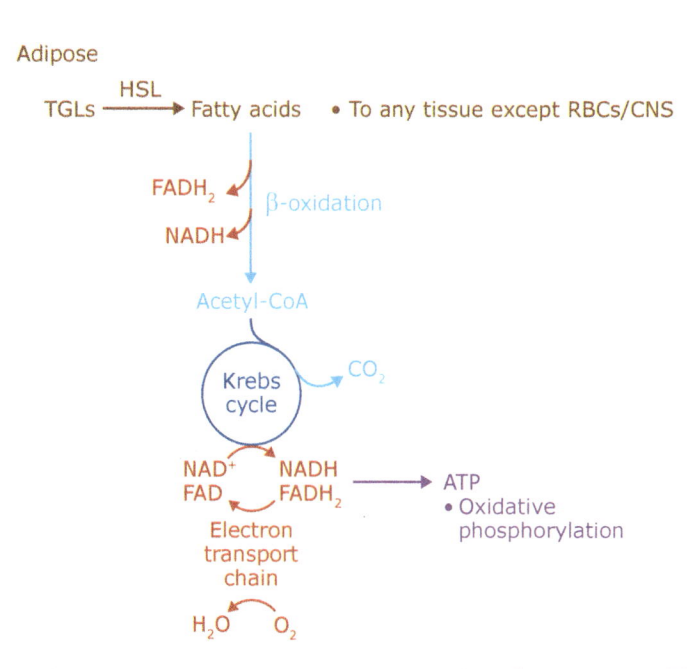

▲ Figure 3–3.2A ATP Generation in the Glucagon World

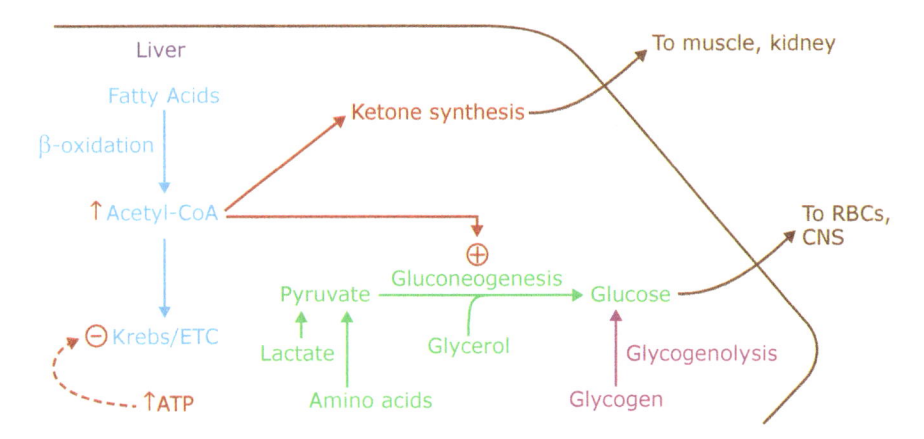

▲ Figure 3–3.2B High ATP in the Glucagon World

3.3 Protein Catabolism

- Occurs in the Insulin World:
  - Gives glycolysis, Krebs intermediates
  - Gives acetyl-CoA
- Occurs in the Glucagon World:
  - Gives substrates for gluconeogenesis
  - Gives acetyl-CoA for ketogenesis
- In either worlds, liver detoxifies ammonia through the urea cycle

Table 3-3.3 — Summary of Pathways Occurring in the Liver

Biochemistry World	How do I make ATP?	What Do I Do If ATP Is High?
Insulin World	Glycolysis PDH Krebs cycle ETC	• Glycogen synthesis • Fat synthesis
Glucagon World	β-oxidation Krebs cycle ETC	• Glycogenolysis • Gluconeogenesis • Ketogenesis

Metabolism: Making ATP

Unit 2

CHAPTER 4 — Krebs Cycle (Tricarboxylic Acid Cycle)

1 Overview

- Burns acetyl-CoA to CO_2 and produces 3 NADH, 1 $FADH_2$, and 1 GTP

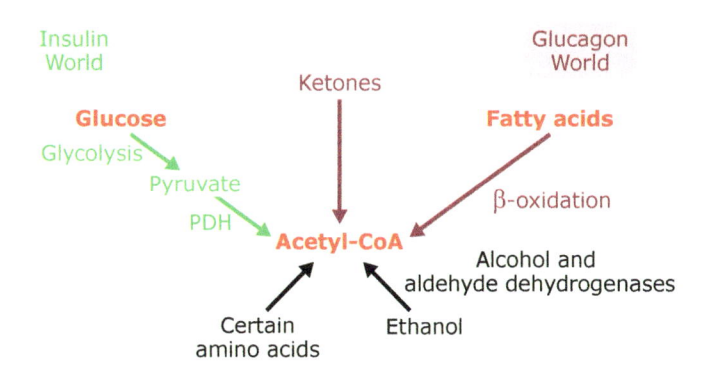

▲ **Figure 4–1.0A** Important Sources of Acetyl-CoA

- NADH and $FADH_2$ are then reoxidized (recycled to NAD, FAD) by the electron transport chain in presence of O_2 yielding a large amount of ATP (oxidative phosphorylation)
- The CO_2 produced is primarily trapped as bicarbonate thanks to carbonic anhydrases
  - Recall from *Physiology*:

$$PCO_2 \propto \frac{\text{Metabolic production}}{\text{Ventilation}}$$

  - Some CO_2 can bind the amino groups of Arg and Lys on Hb (carbamino groups)
- The intermediates of the Krebs cycle are not produced, not broken down by the cycle:
  - Amino acid catabolism is an important source
  - In presence of ↑ ATP, intermediates leave for other pathways
- Energy levels regulate the Krebs cycle, not insulin or glucagon

---

USMLE® Key Concepts

For Step 1, you must be able to:
- ▶ Describe Krebs cycle and its central relationship to general metabolism.
- ▶ Discuss sources and fate of Krebs cycle intermediates.
- ▶ Differentiate between niacin, thiamine, and riboflavin deficiencies.

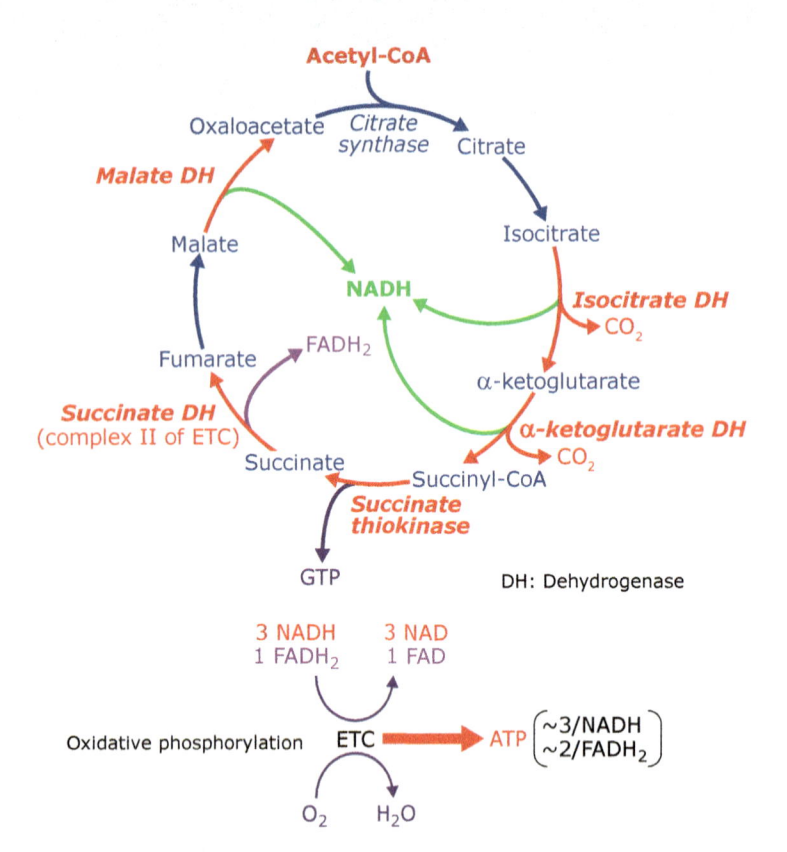

▲ Figure 4–1.0B Krebs Cycle/Electron Transport Chain

2 Key Enzymes

- Four dehydrogenases (DH):
  - Three produce NADH:
    - Isocitrate DH
    - α-ketoglutarate DH
    - Malate DH
  - One produces FADH$_2$:
    - Succinate DH
- One substrate-level phosphorylation:
  - Succinate thiokinase
  - Produces GTP

2.1 Isocitrate DH
- Major regulatory step in the cycle
- One C of acetyl-CoA released as CO_2
- Produces NADH

2.2 α-Ketoglutarate DH
- Enzyme complex similar to PDH
  - Requires:
    - Thiamine pyrophosphate (thiamine, vitamin B1)
    - Lipoic acid
    - CoASH (pantothenate, vitamin B5)
    - FAD (riboflavin, vitamin B2)
    - NAD (niacin, vitamin B3)
- Second C on acetyl-CoA released as CO_2
- Produces NADH

2.3 Succinate Thiokinase
- Succinyl-CoA is a high-energy substrate:
  - Like 1,3BPG and PEP from glycolysis
- Substrate-level phosphorylation:
  - Produces a GTP
  - GTP is equivalent to ATP
  - GTP could be used for translation (protein synthesis) or by G-proteins

2.4 Succinate DH
- The only step producing FADH$_2$
- Part of complex II (ETC)

2.5 Malate DH
- Produces third NADH
- Returns the oxaloacetate

Isocitrate
Ca^{2+} (muscle) ⊕ | ⊕ ADP
                    | ⊖ NADH
α-ketoglutarate

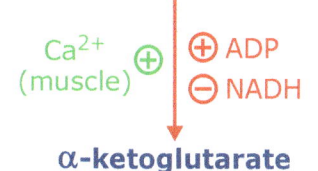

▲ Figure 4–2.1
Allosteric Regulation of Isocitrate Dehydrogenase

3 Krebs Cycle Intermediates

- Amino acids supply several intermediates of Krebs cycle

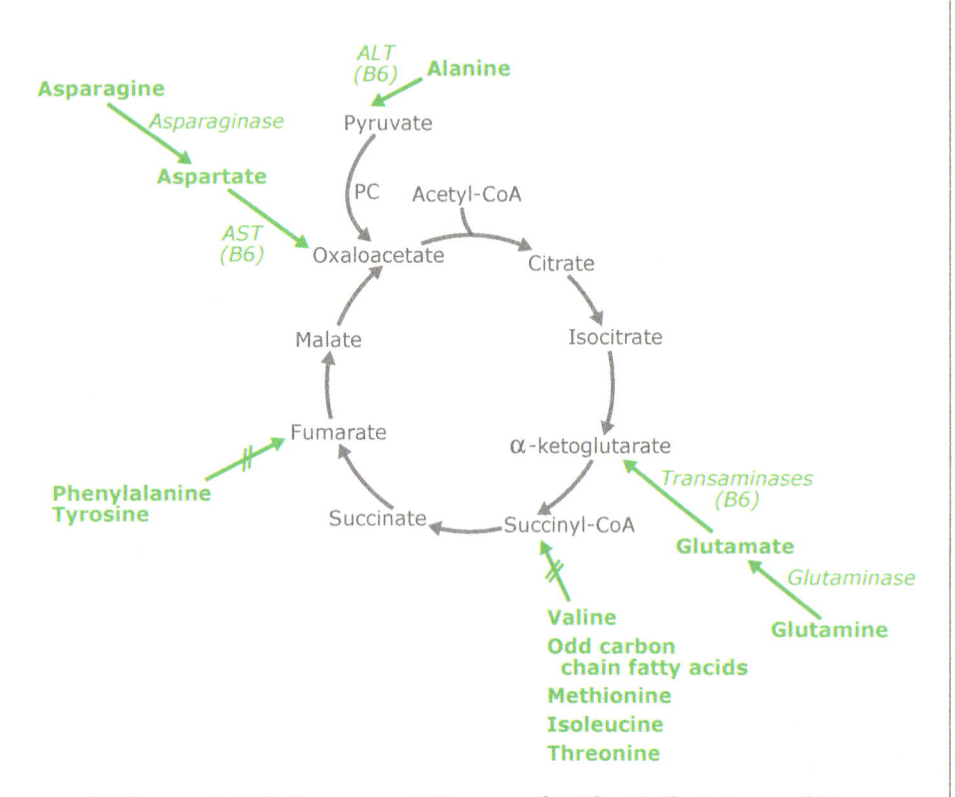

Figure 4–3.0 Important Sources of Krebs Cycle Intermediates

- Urea cycle can also supply fumarate
- Fatty acids cannot provide intermediates of Krebs cycle:
  - Oxidized to acetyl-CoA, which produces CO_2
  - Minor exception: 3C propionyl-CoA from odd C-chain fatty acid oxidation gives succinyl-CoA ("O" of VOMIT pathway)

Role of Key Intermediates Besides Krebs Cycle

- When ATP is high, Krebs cycle stops:
  - Intermediates may leave to participate in other pathways

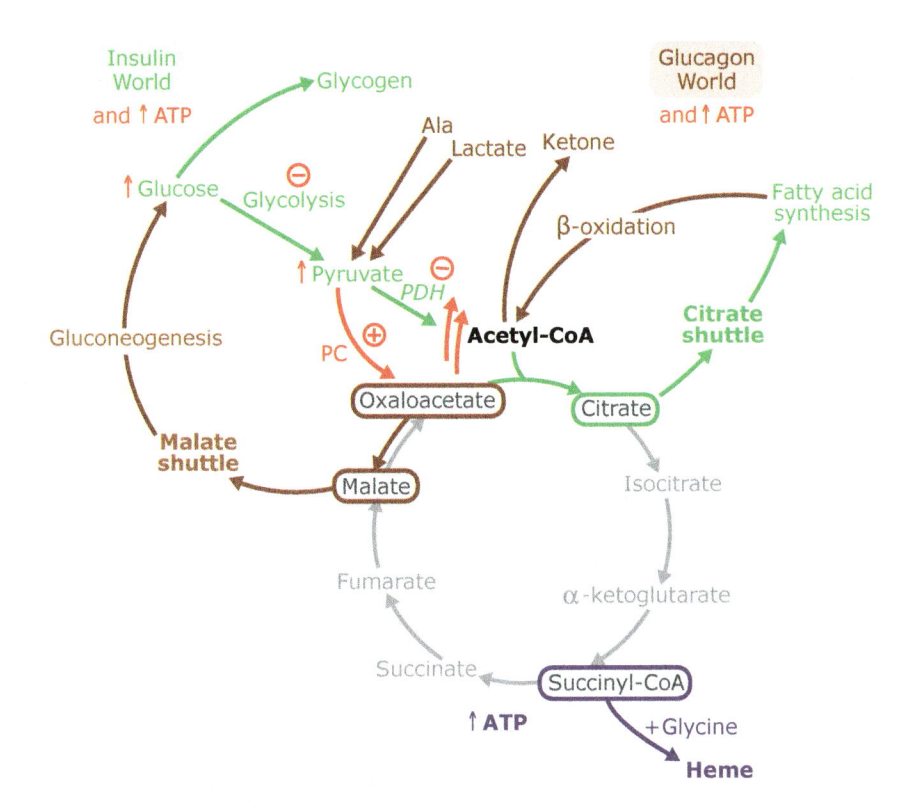

▲ Figure 4–4.0 Fate of Key Intermediates in Presence of ↑ATP

- Insulin + ↑ATP : Citrate → fatty acid synthesis
- Glucagon + ↑ATP : Malate → gluconeogenesis
- ↑ATP : Succinyl-CoA → heme synthesis

5 Clinical Significance of Krebs Cycle

- Critical for ATP production
- See pyruvate metabolism (Chapter 7) for pyruvate dehydrogenase and pyruvate carboxylase deficiencies:
  - Lactic acidemia and neurological symptoms
- Major roles for niacin, thiamine, and riboflavin

5.1 Niacin

- Needed for cofactors NAD and NADP
- Some synthesis from tryptophan:
  - Hartnup disease:
    —Autosomal recessive
    —SLC6A19 (chromosome 5) deficiency:
    - Solute carrier family 6 member 19
    - A Na$^+$/amino acid cotransporter
    - Present in kidney tubule and proximal intestine

    —Mild pellagra-like presentation
    —Rx: High-protein diet to overcome the transport deficiency
- Present in many foods, including liver, chicken, beef, fish, peanuts, beer, etc.
- Pellagra and the "4 Ds": Dietary niacin deficiency
  - Dementia
  - Dermatitis
  - Diarrhea
  - Death
- Niacin is used at pharmacologic doses to lower VLDL and raise HDL:
  - Blocks hormone-sensitive lipase, depriving hepatocytes from fatty acids
  - In turn, liver releases less fat to send out to storage
  - Excess niacin causes intense flushing and itching
    —Relieved by aspirin

5.2 Thiamine

- Present in bran (husk) of grains, pork, and legumes (peas, beans, lentils)
- Dietary deficiency results in beriberi:
  - Most common cause is chronic alcoholism
- TPP is an important cofactor for:
  - PDH
  - α-ketoglutarate DH
  - Branched chain ketoacid DH
  - Transketolase (only requires TPP; HMP shunt)
- Two clinical forms:
  - Dry beriberi: Neuromuscular
  - Wet beriberi: Cardiac failure
- Neurological findings include:
  - Wernicke encephalopathy:
    — Confusion
    — Ataxia
    — Ophthalmoplegia
  - Korsakoff syndrome:
    — Confabulation
    — Memory loss
    — Psychosis
- Neuropathological findings:
  - Multiple infarcts in mammillary bodies and medial dorsal thalamic nuclei
- Late cardiac complications:
  - Dilated cardiomyopathy
- Diagnosis:
  - RBC transketolase activity is decreased
- Treatment:
  - Supplementation
  - Required in managing hypoglycemia in a chronic alcoholic

5.3 Riboflavin

- Needed for cofactors FAD and FMN (complex I of ETC)
- Three important FAD reactions:
  - Succinate DH of Krebs cycle
  - Fatty acyl-CoA DH of β-oxidation
  - Mitochondrial glycerol-3 phosphate DH of glycerol phosphate shuttle
- Present in yeast extracts, milk, cheese, leafy vegetables, almonds, etc.
- Deficiency is dietary:
  - Stomatitis:
    - —Like pellagra but no widespread skin lesions
    - —Fissured, cracked lip (cheilosis)
    - —Painful glossitis (red tongue)
  - Sore throat:
    - —Edema of pharyngeal and oral mucosal membranes
  - Anemia:
    - —Normochromic, normocytic
    - —Mobilization of iron from ferritin stores requires an oxidoreductase that uses FMN
    - —Striking erythroid hypoplasia in marrow
    - —Absent or low reticulocytes in blood
- Treatment: Supplementation

5.4 Pantothenate

- Required for CoA production:
  - Critical for carbohydrate, lipid, and protein metabolism
- "Pan" tothen means "everywhere" in Greek:
  - Deficiency from diet is virtually impossible!
  - Energy production deficiency would affect multiple organ function

CHAPTER 5 — Electron Transport Chain

1 Overview

- Electrons from NADH and FADH$_2$ flow through a series of complexes:
  - Located in the inner mitochondrial membrane
- O$_2$ is the terminal acceptor of electrons
- The energy derived from the current created is used to pump protons out of the mitochondria:
  - H$^+$ create a chemical and electrical gradient
- H$^+$ rush back into the mitochondria through ATP synthase:
  - ATP is generated from ADP + Pi

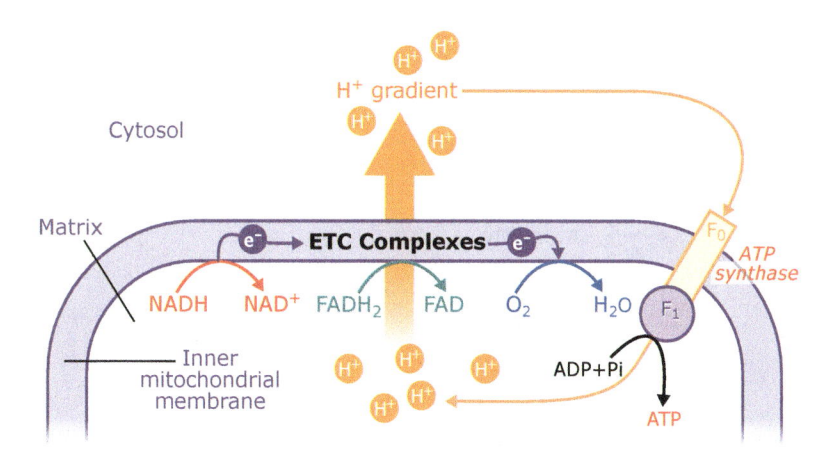

▲ Figure 5-1.0 Overview of Electron Transport Chain

USMLE® Key Concepts

For Step 1, you must be able to:

- Describe ETC and its regulation by energy.
- Differentiate inhibitors from uncouplers of ETC.
- Discuss hypoxia, mitochondrial disease, and free radical damage as they relate to ETC.

2 Important Sources of NADH and FADH$_2$

- Dehydrogenases can reduce NAD$^+$ and FAD to electron-rich NADH and FADH$_2$:
  - Must deliver electrons from within the mitochondria to ETC
  - Cytoplasmic NADH from glycolysis must be shuttled across the mitochondrial membrane
- Malate-aspartate shuttle:
  - Delivers electrons as NADH to ETC
  - Generates 3 ATP for each NADH shuttled
- Glycerol-3 phosphate shuttle:
  - Delivers electrons as FADH$_2$ to ETC
  - Generates 2 ATP for each NADH shuttled

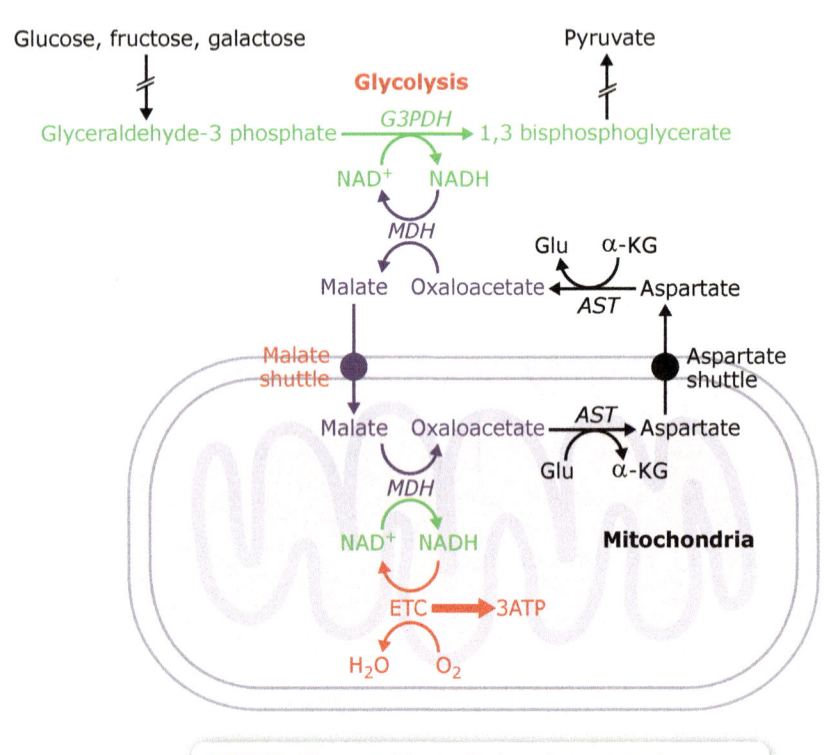

G3PDH: Glyceraldehyde-3 phosphate dehydrogenase
MDH: Malate dehydrogenase
AST: Aspartate transaminase

▲ Figure 5–2.0A Electron Shuttles: Malate Aspartate Shuttle

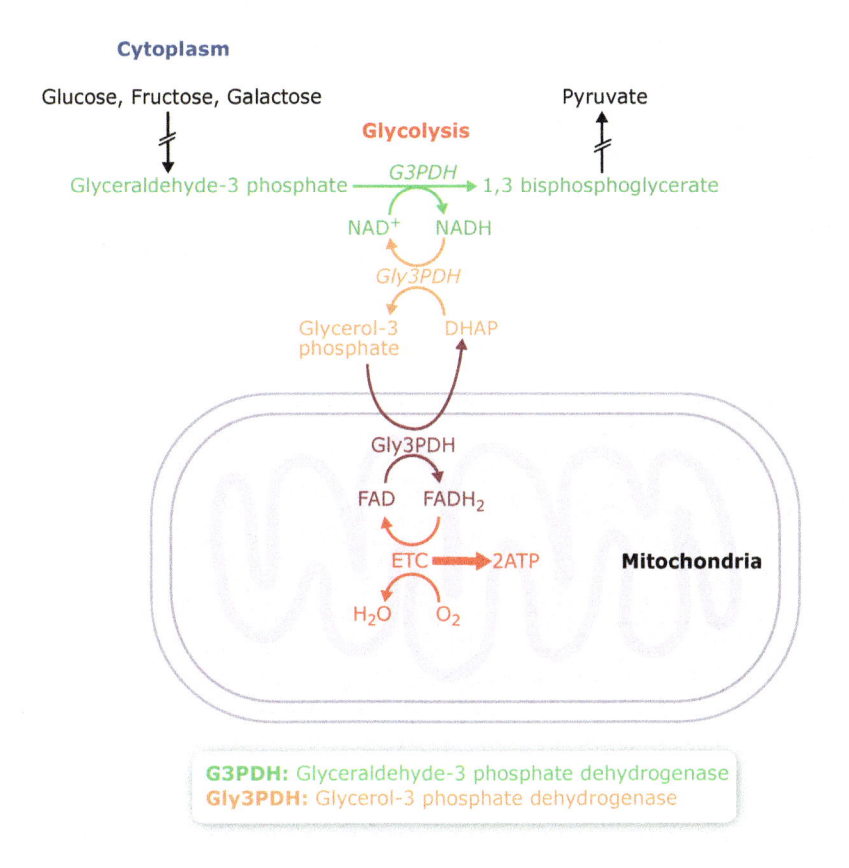

▲ Figure 5–2.0B Electron Shuttles: Glycerol-3 Phosphate Shuttle

G3PDH: Glyceraldehyde-3 phosphate dehydrogenase
Gly3PDH: Glycerol-3 phosphate dehydrogenase

Table 5-2.0 — Important Dehydrogenases (DH)

Enzyme	Pathway	Location	Cofactor
NADH			
Glyceraldehyde-3 phosphate DH	Glycolysis	Cytoplasm	NADH
Lactate DH	–	Cytoplasm	NADH
Glycerol-3P DH	Gluconeogenesis	Cytoplasm	NADH
Pyruvate DH	–	Mitochondria	NADH
Isocitrate DH	Krebs	Mitochondria	NADH
α-KG DH	Krebs	Mitochondria	NADH
Malate DH	Krebs	Mitochondria	NADH
Hydroxyacyl-CoA DH	β-oxidation	Mitochondria	NADH
FADH$_2$			
Fatty acyl-CoA DH	β-oxidation	Mitochondria	FADH$_2$
Succinate DH	Krebs	Mitochondria	FADH$_2$
Glycerol-3P DH	Electron shuttle	Mitochondria	FADH$_2$

3 Electron Transport Chain

- Succession of oxido-reduction steps to O_2:
    - Reduction: When e^- are accepted
    - Oxidation: When e^- are released to the next complex
- Components include:
    - FMN (flavin mononucleotide) and iron-sulfur centers of complex I
    - Coenzyme Q (ubiquinone), a lipid derived from cholesterol pathway
    - Heme-iron of cytochromes b/c1 (complex III), c, and a/a3 (complex IV)
- NADH delivers to complex I FMN
- $FADH_2$ delivers directly to CoQ

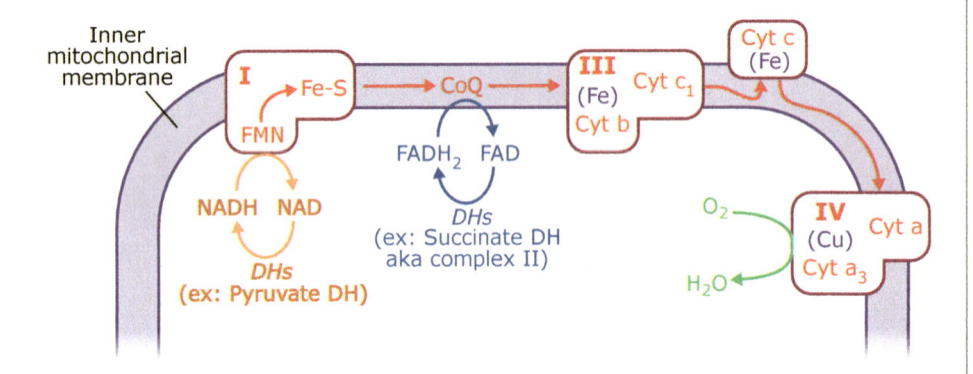

▲ Figure 5–3.0 Electron Transport Chain

- **NADH** gives electrons to complex I (NADH dehydrogenase):
    - FMN (from riboflavin) accepts electrons from NADH
    - FMN passes the electrons to iron-sulfur centers (FeS)
    - FeS centers pass electrons to CoQ
- **$FADH_2$** gives electrons directly to CoQ:
    - Succinate DH of Krebs cycle is a part of complex II of ETC
- **CoQ** is the only component of ETC that is not a protein:
    - It receives electrons from complex I and from $FADH_2$ reactions
- CoQ passes electrons to cytochromes:
    - Cytochromes are heme-containing proteins
    - Each heme contains iron:
        —Fe^{3+} accepts e^-, becomes reduced as Fe^{2+}
        —Fe^{2+} passes e^- on, becomes oxidized as Fe^{3+}
- Complex III contains cyt b and cyt c1
- Cytochrome c
- Complex IV (cytochrome oxidase) contains cyt a and cyt a3:
    - Copper moves the e^- in cytochrome oxidase to O_2
- O_2 is the final acceptor:
    - Cytochrome oxidase has a binding site for O_2
    - O_2 is reduced to H_2O

4 Proton Gradient and ATP Synthesis

- Complexes I, III, and IV can pump protons outside of the mitochondria
- Protons can only be pumped as electrons flow through the chain:
  - Electron transport and H+ gradient are "coupled"
- As positive charges from H+ leave for the intermembrane space they create a membrane potential and a pH gradient
- F_o, F_1 ATP synthase:
  - F_o is a H+ channel spanning the inner membrane
  - F_1 is a headpiece projecting in the mitochondria
  - As H+ flows through F_o, F_1 phosphorylates ADP and releases ATP
- ATP/ADP antiport:
  - ATP is transported out of mitochondria
  - ADP is brought in for recycling
- Coupling of ETC and ATP synthesis:
  - NADH, $FADH_2$ must be available to release electrons to ETC:
    —Metabolism must run
  - O_2 has to be delivered by RBC to accept e−
  - H+ gradient created must flow back through F_o, F_1 ATP synthase
  - ADP must be available to generate ATP while NADH and $FADH_2$ are reoxidized

5 Regulation

- Occurs through coupling: ADP ⊕, ATP ⊖
- ↑ ADP ⊕ H+ flow through F_o, F_1 ATP synthase
- ↓ H+ gradient ⊕ ETC complexes I, III, and IV
- ↑ NADH, $FADH_2$ oxidation to NAD+ and FAD:
  - ↑ O_2 consumption
  - ↑ Metabolic rate to regenerate NADH and $FADH_2$

6 Clinical Relevance

- Hypoxia
- Inhibitors of ETC
- Uncouplers of ETC
- Mitochondrial disorders
- Free radicals and oxidant stress

6.1 Hypoxia

- Hypoxic injury is the most common cellular injury
- Causes are fourfold:
  - Vascular
  - Cardiac
  - Pulmonary
  - Hematologic
- Lack of O_2 stops electron transfer from one complex to the next
- Without ETC, no H^+ gradient is generated
- Lack of H^+ through F_o shuts down ATP synthesis
- Substrate-level phosphorylations of anaerobic glycolysis become the sole source of ATP:
  - Provide a short adaptation/survival period during which reversible injury is observed
  - Treatment must reverse the cause of hypoxia prior to irreversible damage

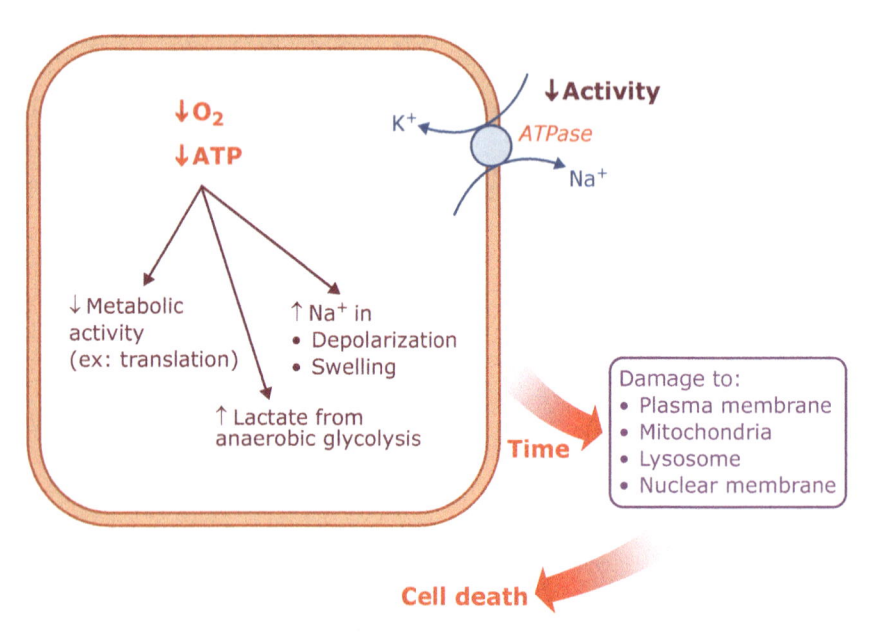

▲ Figure 5-6.1 Common Damage Mechanism From Hypoxia

6.2 Inhibitors of ETC

- Inhibition of ETC disrupts e⁻ flow through complexes:
  - NADH, FADH$_2$ build up and inhibit Krebs cycle and PDH
  - O$_2$ consumption decreases
  - H⁺ gradient is not made
  - ATP synthesis and metabolic rate drop

Table 5-6.2 — Site of Action of Selected Inhibitors of ETC

Site	Inhibitor	Comments
Complex I	Barbiturates	• Also GABA$_A$ agonists • Powerful CNS depression
	Rotenone	• Plant-derived insecticide, pesticide
	MPTP	• Neurotoxin produced during illicit opioid synthesis (MPPP, analog of meperidine) • Selectively taken up by dopamine transporter • Drug-induced parkinsonism
Complex II	Carboxin	• Agricultural fungicide • Oxathiin family (systemic)
Coenzyme Q	Atovaquone	• Antimalarial • Also used as backup drug against *P. jiroveci* • Ubiquinone analog
	Statins	• NOT INHIBITORS • ↓ Synthesis of CoQ • Basis for rhabdomyolysis
Complex III	Antimycin A	• Piscicide used in fish industry
Cytochrome C	—	• Release is associated with apoptosis • bcl-2 inhibits release • p53 stimulates release (through bax) • t(14;18) in follicular lymphoma

Complex IV	CO	• Burning of fossil fuels
		• Competes with O$_2$ binding to heme
		  — Hb (↓ saturation but ↑ affinity)
		  — Complex IV
		• Rx: Hyperbaric or 100% O$_2$ + ventilation

	CN⁻	• Naturally present in almonds • Byproduct of nitroprusside • Rx: Nitrites and thiosulfate or cobalamin
	Azide	• Preservative in sera and reagents
F$_o$	Oligomycins	• Macrolides blocking H⁺ channel of ATP synthase • Too toxic for therapeutic use
ATP-ADP translocase	Atractyloside	• Extremely toxic heteroglucoside from plants

Notes:
The neurotoxicity of methylmercury involves in part inhibition of complex II and decreased activity of free radical scavenging enzymes.
The cardiotoxicity of anthracyclines (daunorubicin, doxorubicin) involves in part interaction with CoQ and with complex III.

6.3 Uncouplers of ETC

- Uncoupling: ATP synthesis ↓ while metabolic rate ↑
- Uncouplers dissipate H^+ gradient:
  - Carry H^+ across inner mitochondrial membrane
  - H^+ bypass F_o which ↓ ATP synthase activity
  - ↓ ATP causes ↑ metabolic rate:
    - ↑ NADH, $FADH_2$ oxidation to NAD^+, FAD
    - ↑ O_2 consumption
    - Energy from ETC activity dissipated as heat
- Thermogenin:
  - Also known as uncoupling protein 1 (UCP1)
  - UCPs are a family of 5 proteins found throughout the body
  - Proton ionophore spanning inner mitochondrial membrane
  - UCP1 is found in brown adipose:
    - Brown adipose is found in infants: High mitochondria
- 2,4-dinitrophenol (2,4-DNP):
  - Pesticide used as a dieting aid
  - Resulted in many deaths
  - Still used illicitly in athletes to rapidly lose body fat
- Aspirin toxicity:
  - Only NSAID that is an uncoupler
  - 15–30 g: Moderate toxicity in adult
  - 30–50 g: Lethal
  - Much less in children (↓ Vd)

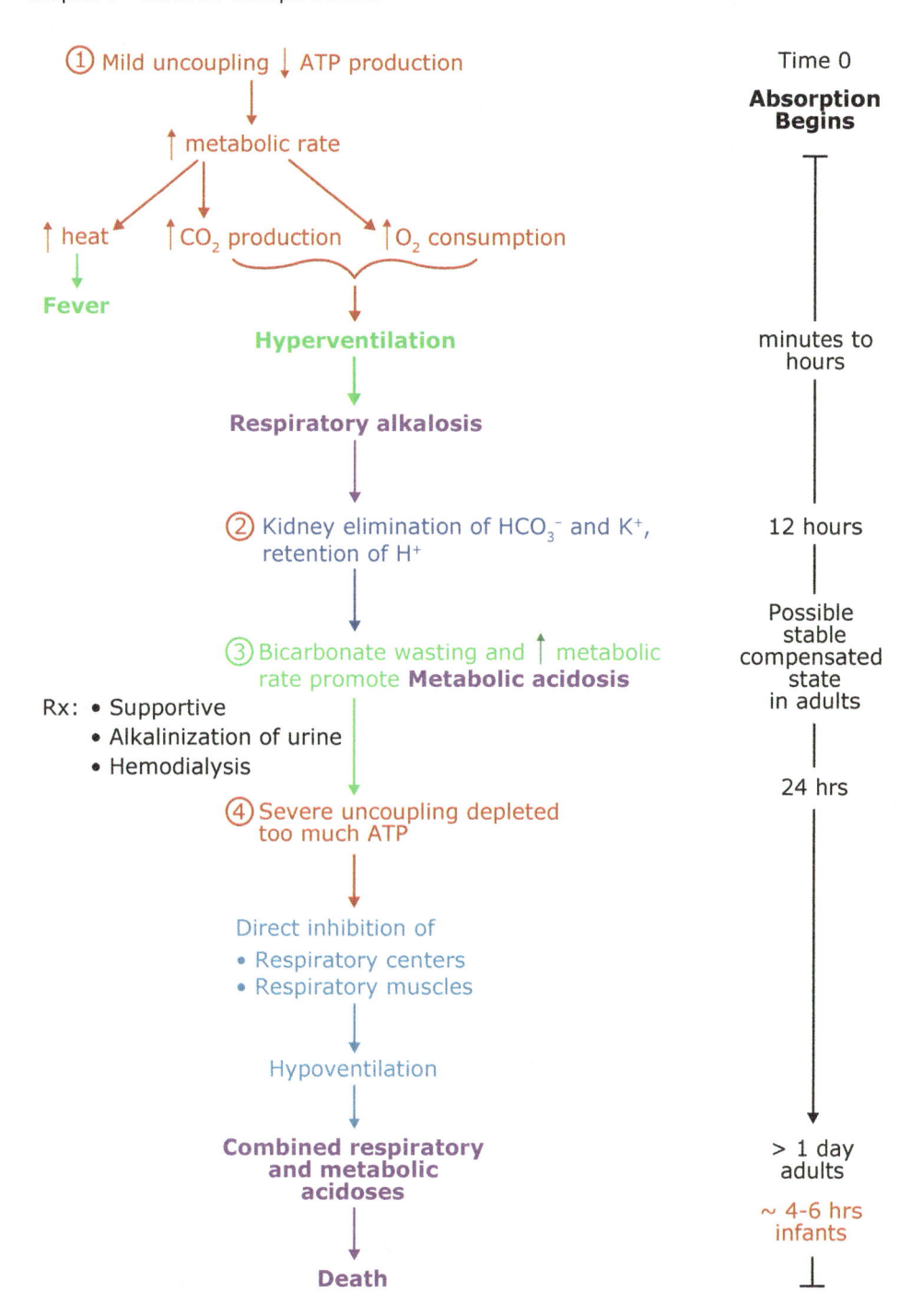

Chapter 5 • Electron Transport Chain — Biochemistry

① Mild uncoupling ↓ ATP production
↓
↑ metabolic rate
↓ ↓ ↓
↑ heat   ↑ CO_2 production   ↑ O_2 consumption
↓
Fever

↑ CO_2 production and ↑ O_2 consumption →
Hyperventilation
↓
Respiratory alkalosis
↓
② Kidney elimination of HCO_3^- and K^+, retention of H^+
↓
③ Bicarbonate wasting and ↑ metabolic rate promote **Metabolic acidosis**

Rx: • Supportive
• Alkalinization of urine
• Hemodialysis

↓
④ Severe uncoupling depleted too much ATP
↓
Direct inhibition of
• Respiratory centers
• Respiratory muscles
↓
Hypoventilation
↓
Combined respiratory and metabolic acidoses
↓
Death

Time 0
Absorption Begins

minutes to hours

12 hours

Possible stable compensated state in adults

24 hrs

> 1 day adults

~ 4-6 hrs infants

▲ **Figure 5-6.3** Chain of Events as Aspirin Toxicity Unfolds

6.4 Mitochondrial Disorders

- Mitochondrial DNA encodes several subunits of complexes of ETC
- Mitochondrial inheritance is maternal and dominant
- Neural and muscle tissues are primarily affected

Table 5-6.4 Selected Mitochondrial Diseases

Disease	Mutation	Symptoms
Leber hereditary optic neuropathy	Complex I	• Optic atrophy with sudden onset of visual loss in one eye followed by the other eye weeks later • Ganglion cell degeneration • Adult onset
MELAS	tRNA^{Leu}	• **M**itochondrial **e**ncephalomyopathy • **L**actic **a**cidosis • **S**troke-like episodes
MERRF	tRNA^{Lys}	• **M**yoclonic **e**pilepsy • **R**agged **r**ed **f**iber disease

6.5 Free Radical Generation, Damage, and Prevention

- Free radicals represent O_2 and N_2 toxicity to our cells:
  - Reactive oxygen species (ROS):
    - Superoxide: $O_2^{\bullet-}$ (ETC)
    - Hydrogen peroxide: H_2O_2 (reacts with Me^{2+}: Fenton reaction)
    - Hydroxyl radical: $^{\bullet}OH$ (most reactive ROS)
  - Reactive nitrogen-oxygen species (RNOS):
    - Nitric oxide: NO (NO synthase)
    - Peroxynitrite: $ONOO^-$ (formed from NO and H_2O_2)
- Sources of free radicals:
  - ETC (CoQ)
  - Oxidases (xanthine oxidase and reperfusion injury)
  - Peroxidases
  - CYP450 (acetaminophen and CCl_4 hepatotoxicity)
  - Ionizing radiation
- Free radicals trigger chain reactions:
  - Membrane damage through lipid peroxidation increases cellular permeability and calcium entry
  - Proteins and DNA structure are altered by the radicals:
    - Oxidation of cysteines, strand breaks in nucleic acids

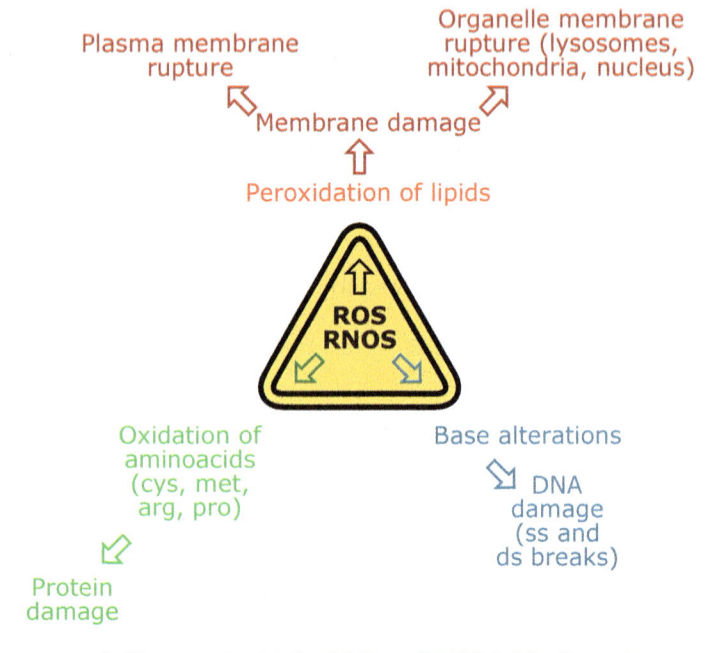

▲ **Figure 5–6.5A** ROS and RNOS-Mediated Cellular Alterations

6.5.1 Free Radicals and Inflammation

- **Respiratory burst:** Most important mechanism of digestion in a phagolysosome
- **NADPH oxidase** and **myeloperoxidase:**
  - Produce $O_2^{\bullet-}$ and $HOCl^{\bullet}$
  - NADPH oxidase deficiency = Chronic granulomatous disease
    - X-linked recessive
    - Lack of $O_2^{\bullet-}$ results in a negative NBT test (does not turn blue) or abnormal dihydrorhodamine flow cytometry
    - ↑ Catalase ⊕ infections
    - Antibiotic prophylaxis (co-trimoxazole, azole antifungals)
  - Myeloperoxidase deficiency:
    - Autosomal recessive
    - Lack of bleach ($HOCl^{\bullet}$) but presence of $O_2^{\bullet-}$ yields a positive NBT test
    - ↑ Candida infections

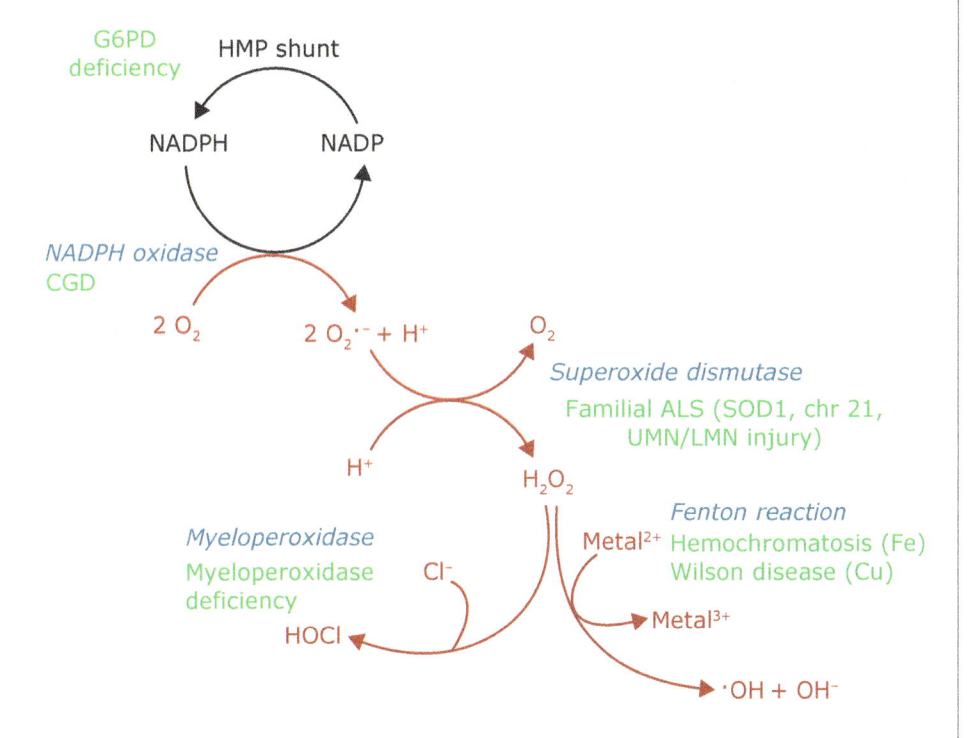

▲ **Figure 5-6.5B** ROS Generation and Disease Association

6.5.2 Defenses Against Free Radical Damage

- Superoxide dismutases (SOD) produce H_2O_2 from two molecules of $O_2^{•-}$

Table 5-6.5 Three SOD Enzymes and Their Locations

SOD	Location	Cofactor	Disease Association
1	Cytosol	Copper and zinc	Familial amyotrophic lateral sclerosis
2	Mitochondria	Manganese	Possible roles in neuromuscular diseases and cancer
3	Extracellular	Copper and zinc	

- Catalase converts peroxide into O_2 and H_2O
- Glutathione peroxidase and reductase:
  - Glutathione is a tripeptide:
    - Glu – Cys – Gly
    - Two forms: Reduced GSH and oxidized GS-SG
  - Requires selenium (peroxidase) and NADPH (reductase):
    - Se is a cofactor for the thyroid-hormone deiodinases
    - Se is used in topical antifungal preparation (to treat *Malassezia* dermatomycoses)

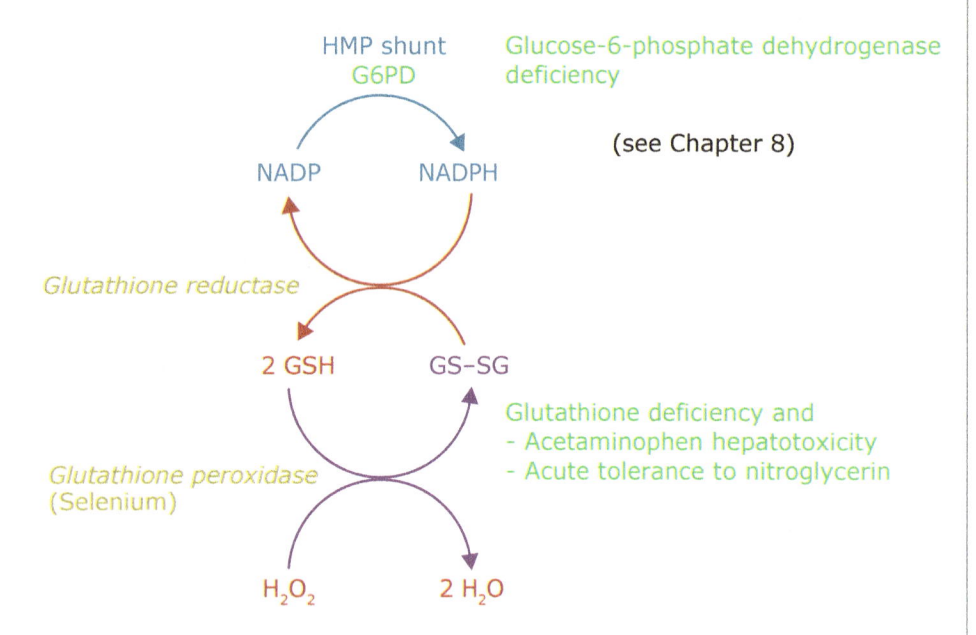

▲ **Figure 5–6.5C** Role of Glutathione in Detoxification of H_2O_2 and Associated Diseases

- Antioxidant vitamins:
  1. Vitamin E:
     — Lipid soluble
     — α-tocopherol, most potent
     — γ-tocopherol, most abundant
     — Found in oil (corn, soy, sunflower, etc.)
     — Protects against membrane peroxidation

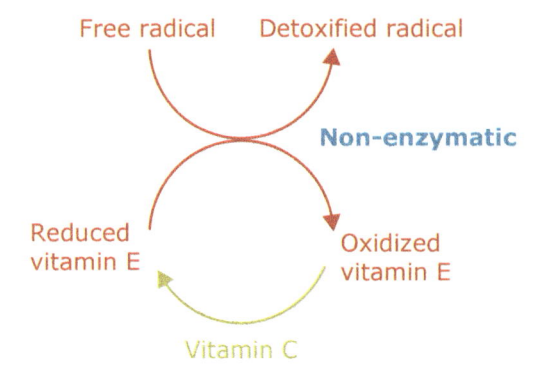

     ▲ Figure 5–6.5D Role of Antioxidant Vitamins

     — Deficiency can result from fat malabsorption:
       • Pancreatic insufficiency: Cystic fibrosis, chronic pancreatitis
       • Abetalipoproteinemia: Deficiency in ApoB-48 and B-100
     — Vitamin E deficiency presentation is secondary to oxidant stress on cell membrane lipids:
       • Anemia: Hemolytic with acanthocytosis
       • Retinopathy: Vitamin E is present in rod cell outer segment
       • Neurologic and muscular disease: Can mimic B12 deficiency
       • Impaired immune response
     — Vitamin E and clotting:
       • Vitamin E quinone is a potent inhibitor of vitamin K-dependent γ-carboxylase
       • Daily vitamin E supplementation enhances warfarin effects and can cause bleeding
  2. Vitamin C:
     — Helps recycle vitamin E
     — Water soluble: See Chapter 17 on collagen synthesis for deficiency
  3. Carotenoids:
     — Organic plant pigments
     — β-carotene is a precursor of vitamin A
     — Other carotenoids include lutein and zeaxanthin:
       • Lutein and zeaxanthin protect macula neurons from UV light

Insulin World

Unit 3

CHAPTER 6: Carbohydrate Digestion and Glycolysis

1 Overview

- Three sugars enter glycolysis:
  - Glucose
  - Fructose
  - Galactose
- Cytoplasmic pathway
- Produces ATP through substrate-level phosphorylation:
  - All cells can carry out glycolysis
  - Only source of ATP in hypoxic conditions
  - Only source of ATP in RBCs
- Comprises two sections:
  - First half consumes ATP
  - Second half produces ATP
- Six key enzymes:
  - Four kinases:
    - Hexokinase
    - Phosphofructokinase
    - Phosphoglycerate kinase
    - Pyruvate kinase
  - Two dehydrogenases:
    - Glyceraldehyde-3 phosphate dehydrogenase
    - Lactate dehydrogenase

USMLE® Key Concepts

For Step 1, you must be able to:

- Describe carbohydrate digestion.
- Know key glycolytic enzymes and their regulation.
- Integrate enzyme deficiencies of carbohydrate metabolism.

Chapter 6 • Carbohydrate Digestion and Glycolysis

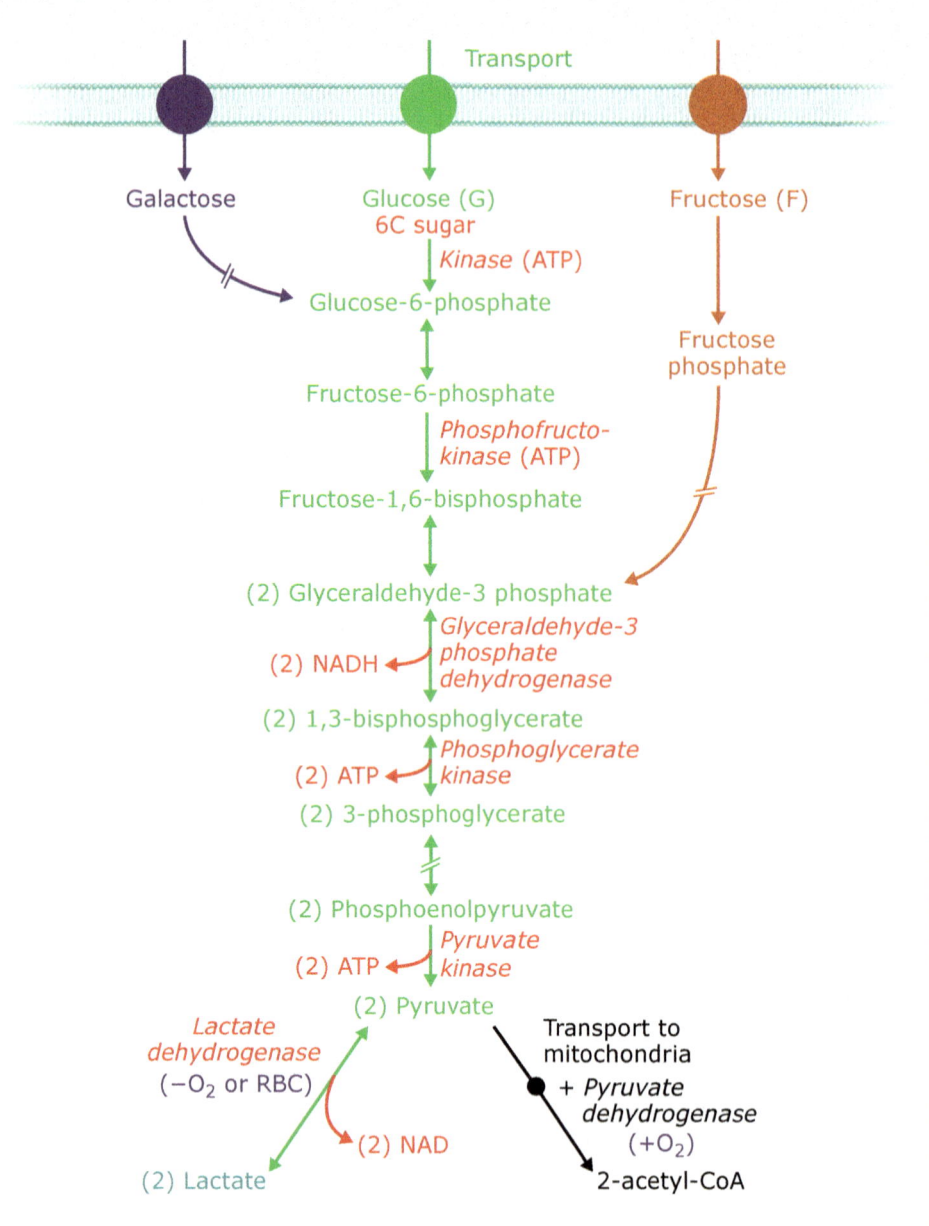

▲ **Figure 6-1.0** Overview of Glycolysis

2 Dietary Carbohydrates and Digestion

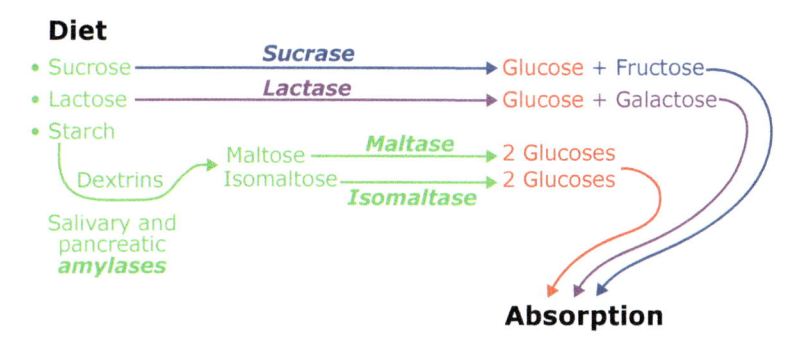

▲ Figure 6–2.0 Digestion of Major Dietary Carbohydrates

2.1 Types of Dietary Carbohydrates

- Starches:
  - Equivalent of glycogen for plants
  - Amylose:
    — Long chains of glucoses
    — α-1,4 linkage
  - Amylopectin:
    — α-1,4 linkage (linear)
    — α-1,6 linkage (branch)
- Sucrose:
  - Table sugar, fruits
  - Made of fructose and glucose
- Lactose:
  - Dairy products
  - Made of galactose and glucose
- Fibers:
  - Nondigestible carbohydrates
  - Consists of soluble and insoluble fibers:
    — Soluble fibers:
      - Pectins, mucilages, and gums
      - Can be digested by bacteria and absorbed by gut
    — Insoluble fibers:
      - Cellulose and lignin
      - Bulk of feces
- Average carbohydrate dietary requirements (2,000 kcal/day diet):
  - 45%–65% of total calories
  - Contribute 4 kcal/g
  - Absorbable sugars: 225–325 g/day
  - Fiber requirements: 20–35 g/day

2.2 Clinical Relevance

- Lactase deficiency:
  - Lactose intolerance is common:
    - Ranges from a few percent in Northern Europeans to 90% in Africans and Asians
    - Most become intolerant after weaning
    - Congenital lactase deficiency is very rare
  - Bloating, flatulence, diarrhea within 30 minutes to 2 hours of ingestion

- Obesity:
  - Dietary fibers promote early and prolonged satiety signals:
    - Bulking effects
  - Dietary fibers ↓ calorie intake:
    - Insoluble fibers are NOT absorbed
    - Less blood glucose = Less insulin demand
  - Rapid absorption of sugars leads to greater fat production

3 Absorption and Cellular Transport

- Two forms of transport:
  - Sodium-dependent:
    —Secondary active
  - Glucose transporters:
    —Facilitated diffusion

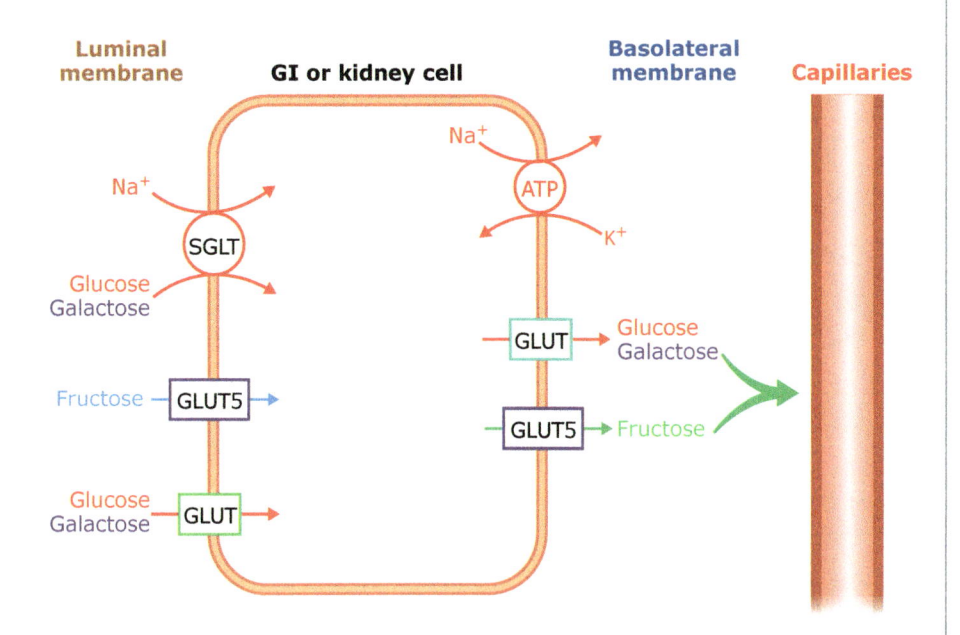

▲ Figure 6–3.0 Transport of Dietary Sugars Across Cell Membranes

3.1 Sodium-Dependent Glucose Uptake
- SGLT1:
  - Enterocytes of small intestine
  - Straight part of renal proximal tubule
- SGLT2:
  - Renal proximal convoluted tubule
  - Responsible for > 90% glucose reabsorption
- Allow transport of glucose and galactose:
  - Depend on Na$^+$/K$^+$ ATPase
  - Can concentrate Glc and Gal in cell

3.2 GLUT Family

- Uniporters for dietary sugars
- Sugars move down a concentration gradient
  - Can be bidirectional
- 12 different GLUTs in humans:
  - GLUT1-4: Glucose and galactose
  - GLUT5: Fructose
  - Other GLUTs are primarily intracellular (organelle transport)

GLUT1
- RBC
- Blood-brain barrier
- Blood-placental barrier

GLUT2
- Low affinity
- Liver
- β-cells of pancreas
- Kidney and GI (basolateral side)

GLUT uniporters

GLUT3
- Neurons

GLUT4
- Adipocytes
- Heart and skeletal muscle
- Insulin up-regulated

GLUT5
- Fructose
- Widely distributed

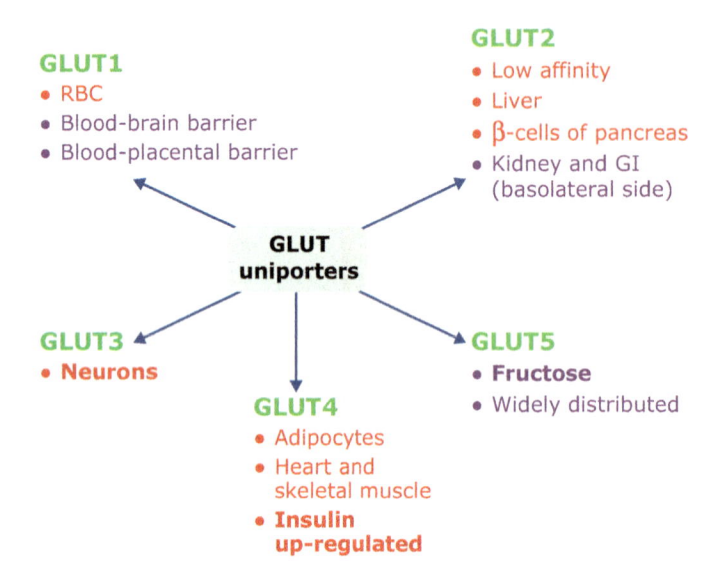

▲ **Figure 6-3.2** GLUT Distribution in Humans

3.3 Clinical Relevance

- SGLT2 and type 2 diabetes:
  - Blocked by "-gliflozins"
    - Canagliflozin, dapagliflozin
    - Type 2 diabetes
    - Decrease glycemia
    - Cause glucosuria:
      - ↑ Risk of UTIs
- GLUT1 deficiency:
  - De Vivo disease:
    - Low glucose in CSF/brain
    - Autosomal dominant
    - Refractory infantile seizures
    - Microcephaly
    - Mental and motor dysfunction
    - Rx: Ketogenic diet
      - Ketones are alternative fuel for brain cells
- GLUT2 deficiency:
  - Fanconi-Bickel syndrome:
    - Glycogen storage disease type XI
    - Hepatic GLUT2 is bidirectional
      - Used in glycogenolysis and gluconeogenesis
    - Fasting hypoglycemia
    - Hepatomegaly
    - Nephropathy
- GLUT4 and diabetes:
  - Lack or resistance to insulin ↓ GLUT4 in membrane
    - Adipocytes:
      - Glucose required for TGLs synthesis and storage
      - Hyperlipidemia, hyperglycemia
    - Striated muscle:
      - Decreased uptake
      - Hyperglycemia
- GLUT4 and exercise:
  - In striated muscle, AMP-dependent kinase ↑ GLUT4
    - Upregulation is not only insulin dependent
    - ATP utilization increases AMP
    - AMP upregulates GLUT4
    - Normalizes glycemia

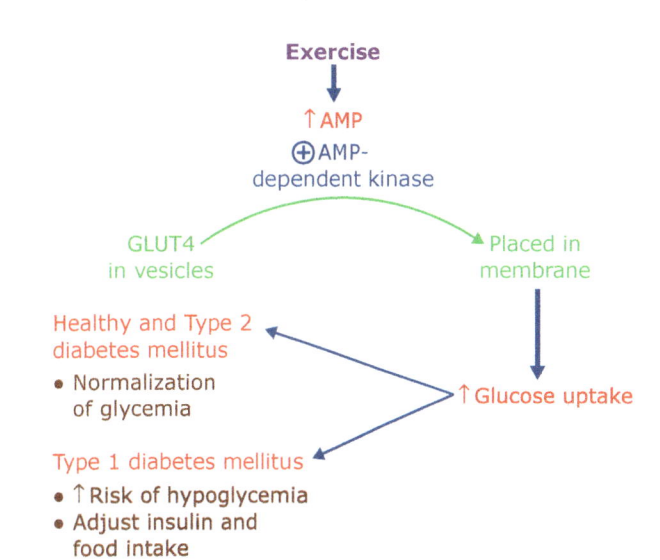

▲ Figure 6–3.3 Effect of Exercise on Glucose Uptake

4 Glycolysis

4.1 Trapping Sugars in Cells

- Phosphorylation effectively traps dietary sugars in cells
- Hexokinases phosphorylate carbon 6
- Phosphotransferases phosphorylate carbon 1
- Require ATP and Mg^{2+}:
  - All enzymes using or making ATP require Mg^{2+} as a catalyst
- Are irreversible
- Are locally inhibited by their product
- Glucokinase:
  - Subtype of hexokinase
  - Lower affinity for glucose (↑ Km)
  - β cells of pancreas and liver
  - Glucokinase regulatory protein (GKRP) regulates availability of glucokinase
- Galactokinase and fructokinase:
  - Phosphotransferases
  - High specificity for galactose and fructose
- Phosphatases are required to free intracellular sugars:
  - Critical for liver gluconeogenesis and glycogenolysis

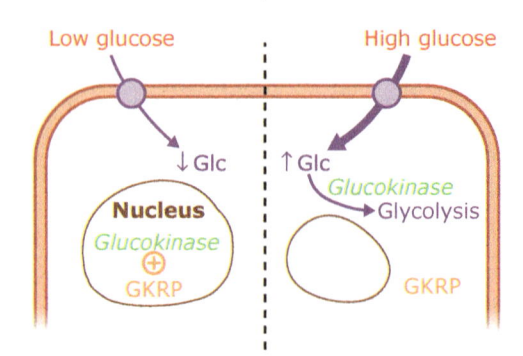

▲ Figure 6–4.1A Glucokinase Regulation by GKRP

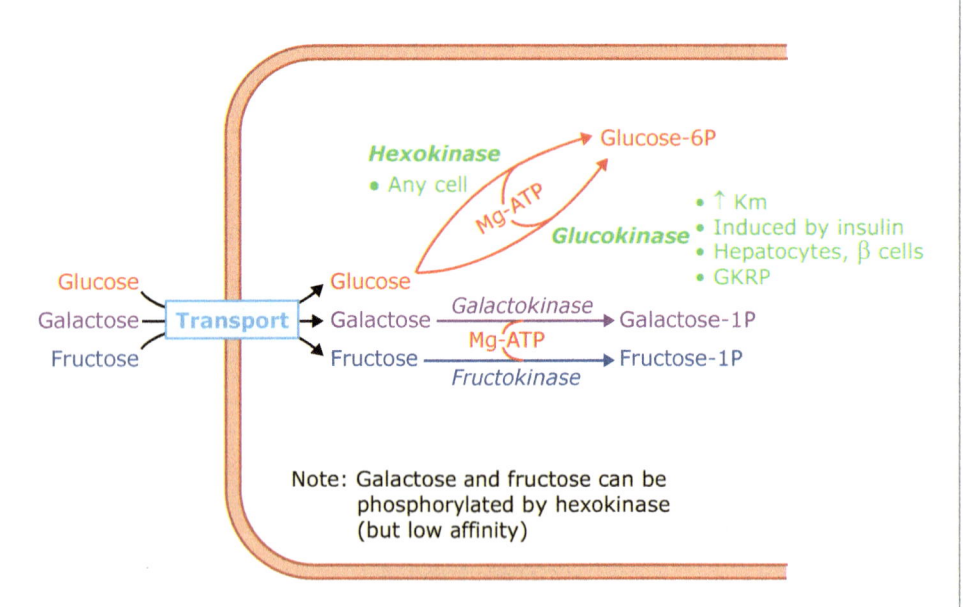

▲ Figure 6–4.1B Phosphorylation Traps Dietary Sugars in Cells

4.2 Conversion of Glucose-6-Phosphate to Fructose-1,6-bisphosphate

- Glucose-6P is isomerized to fructose-6-phosphate
- Fructose-6P is phosphorylated to fructose-1,6bisP:
  - Phosphofructokinase-1 (PFK-1) is rate-limiting
  - Irreversible
  - Requires ATP (and Mg^{2+})
- Fructose-2,6bisP is an allosteric activator of PFK-1:
  - Produced by PFK-2
- Local PFK-1 regulation:
  - ATP, citrate ⊖
  - AMP ⊕

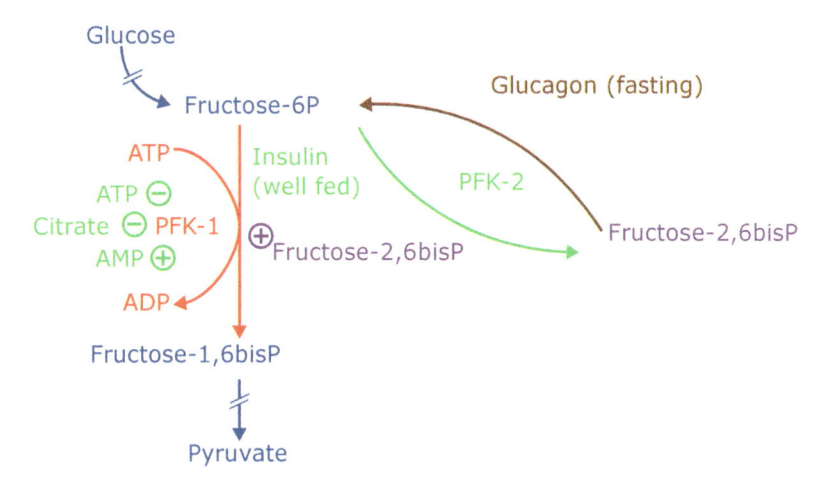

▲ Figure 6-4.2 Phosphofructokinase-1 (PFK-1)

- PFK-2 is bifunctional:
  - Has both a kinase domain and a phosphatase domain
  - Glucagon phosphorylates PFK-2 and activates the phosphatase domain:
    —Glucagon ↓ fructose-2,6bisP production
    —Lack of fructose-2,6bisP ⊖ PFK-1
  - Insulin dephosphorylates PFK-2 and activates the kinase domain:
    —Insulin ↑ fructose-2,6bisP production
    —Fructose-2,6bisP ⊕ PFK-1

4.3 Conversion of Fructose-1,6bisP to Triosephosphate

- Fructose-1,6bisP is cleaved to two 3C sugars:
  - Dihydroxyacetone phosphate (DHAP)
  - Glyceraldehyde-3 phosphate (GAP)
  - Done by aldolase
  - DHAP and GAP can be isomerized into one another
- One glucose can give rise to two GAPs

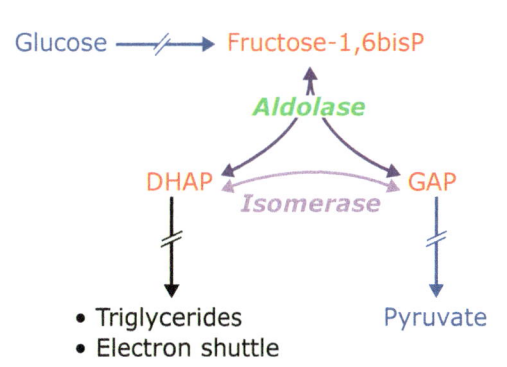

▲ Figure 6-4.3 Conversion of Fructose-1,6bisP to DHAP and GAP

Chapter 6 • Carbohydrate Digestion and Glycolysis

4.4 Glyceraldehyde-3P Dehydrogenase

- Oxidizes GAP to 1,3-bisphosphoglycerate (1,3BPG):
  - 1,3BPG is a high-energy-level substrate
- Uses NAD^+:
  - Produces NADH
  - NADH can enter mitochondrial ETC
- First potential for energy in glycolysis:
  - Requires mitochondria and O_2
  - Can provide ~3 ATP/NADH
- Site of glycolysis stall in hypoxia:
  - Requires lactate dehydrogenase (LDH)
  - LDH replenishes NAD^+ for glycolysis to continue

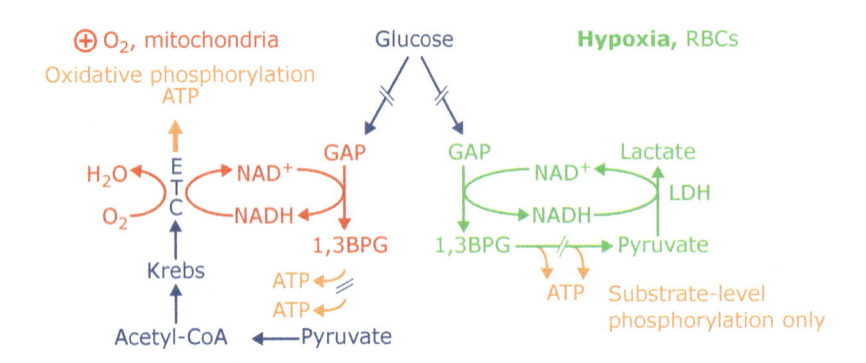

▲ Figure 6–4.4 Glyceraldehyde-3 Phosphate Dehydrogenase and LDH

4.5 Phosphoglycerate Kinase

- First substrate-level phosphorylation:
  - Provides ATP without the need for O_2 or mitochondria
- Reversible
- Produces 3-phosphoglycerate (3-PG)

▲ Figure 6–4.5 Phosphoglycerate Kinase (PGK)

4.6 Pyruvate Kinase

- Second substrate-level phosphorylation
- Irreversible
- 3-phosphoglycerate is converted to 2-phosphoglycerate by a mutase
- 2-phosphoglycerate is dehydrated to phosphoenolpyruvate (PEP) by enolase
- PEP is converted to pyruvate by pyruvate kinase:
  - ATP is produced
  - Last step of aerobic glycolysis
  - Controlled step

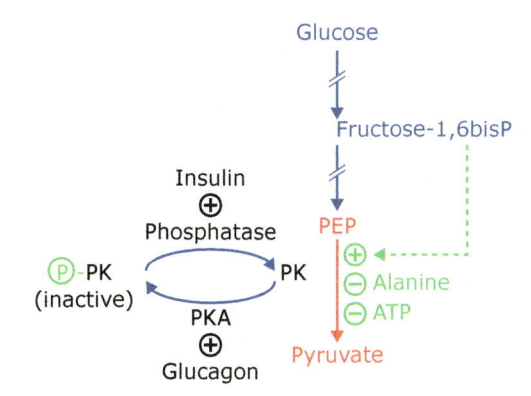

▲ Figure 6-4.6 Control of Pyruvate Kinase (PK)

4.7 Glycolysis in RBCs

- RBCs do anaerobic glycolysis:
  - SLPs are sole source of ATP
  - Glucose is converted to lactate
- RBCs have BPG mutase:
  - 2,3BPG decreases HbA's affinity for O_2

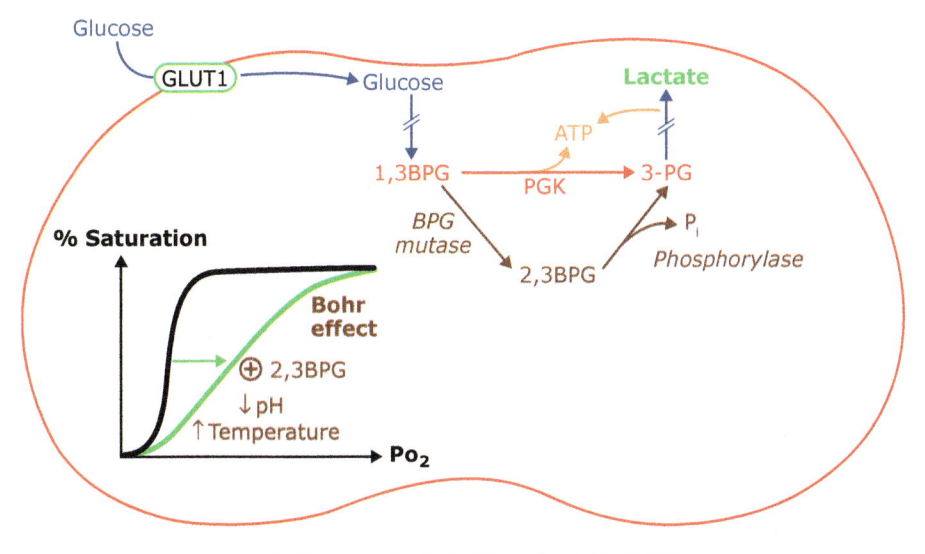

▲ Figure 6-4.7 Glycolysis in RBCs

4.8 Clinical Relevance of Glycolysis

4.8.1. Arsenic Poisoning

- Arsenite, AsO_3^{2-}:
  - Trivalent arsenic
  - Binds -SH groups
    — Lipoic acid makes CoASH
    — CoASH is required for several dehydrogenases:
      - PDH
      - α-ketoglutarate DH

- Arsenate, AsO_4^{3-}:
  - Pentavalent arsenic
  - Substitutes for phosphate during ATP synthesis

- Both compounds decrease ATP synthesis:
  - Whether oxidative (PDH, Krebs cycle)
  - Or non-oxidative (GAPDH, glycolysis)

- Contaminated groundwater is the greatest exposure risk:
  - Neurologic and cardiovascular toxicities
  - Dermatologic (melanosis, keratosis)
  - Carcinogen: Bladder cancer from drinking contaminated H_2O
  - Skin, lung, GI, liver, hematopoietic, and lymphatic cancers as well

- Acute exposure is treated with chelators (dimercaprol, succimer)
- Prevention is by decontamination of groundwater

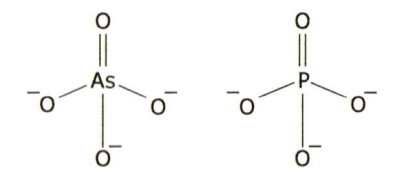

Arsenate inhibits glyceraldehyde-3-phosphate dehydrogenase

▲ Figure 6–4.8A Similarities Between Arsenate and Phosphate

4.8.2 Pyruvate Kinase Deficiency

- Hemolytic anemia:
  - Second most common cause after glucose-6P dehydrogenase deficiency
- Autosomal recessive in most cases
- Lack of ATP causes chronic hemolysis:
  - Jaundice, icterus (↑ bilirubin)
  - Gallstones
  - Splenomegaly
  - ↑ Erythropoiesis, reticulocytosis
  - Echinocytes (membrane damage)
- Rx: Blood transfusions or splenectomy

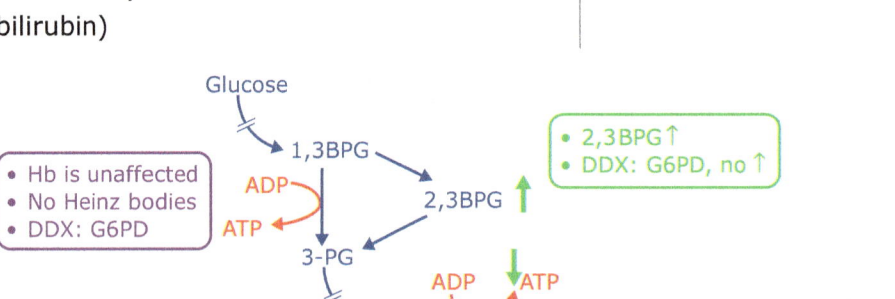

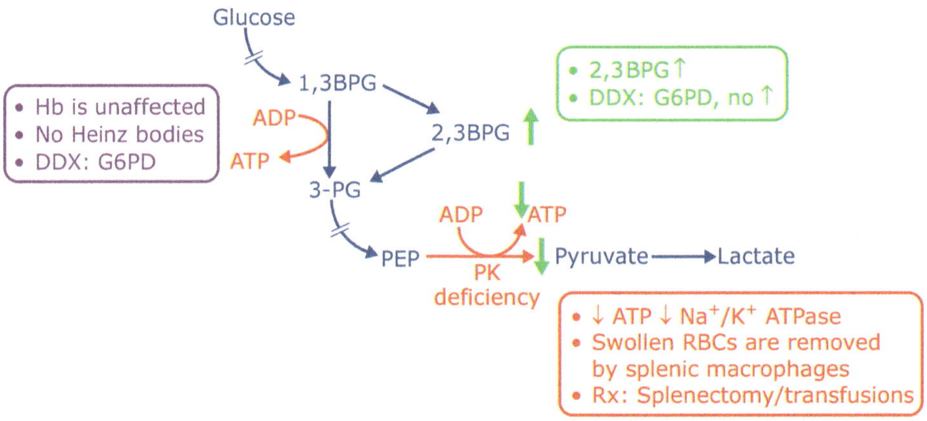

- Hb is unaffected
- No Heinz bodies
- DDX: G6PD

- 2,3BPG ↑
- DDX: G6PD, no ↑

- ↓ ATP ↓ Na^+/K^+ ATPase
- Swollen RBCs are removed by splenic macrophages
- Rx: Splenectomy/transfusions

▲ Figure 6–4.8B RBC Pyruvate Kinase Deficiency

5 Fructose and Galactose

5.1 Metabolism

- Both fructose and galactose require a kinase to be phosphorylated:
  - Hexokinase can phosphorylate fructose and galactose, but slowly
  - Fructokinase and galactokinase (see Topic 4.1)
- Both enter glycolysis:
  - Fructose as a DHAP or GAP
  - Galactose as glucose-6P
- Fructose is a ketose sugar:
  - Cannot be reduced
- Galactose is an aldose sugar:
  - Can be reduced to galactitol
  - Aldose reductase

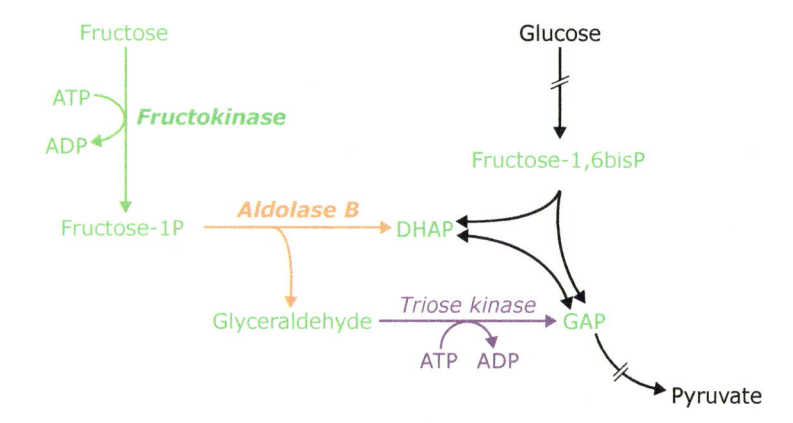

▲ Figure 6–5.1A Fructose Metabolism

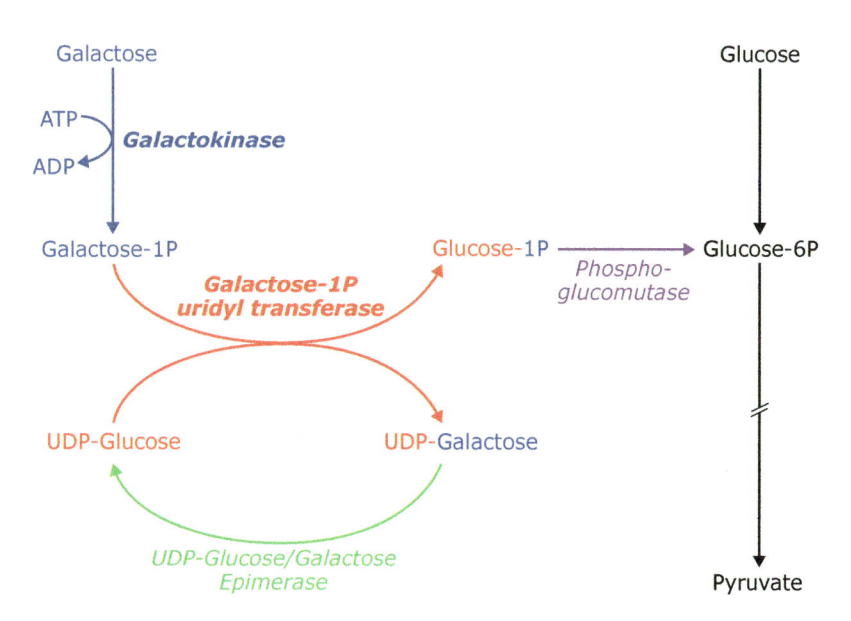

▲ Figure 6–5.1B Galactose Metabolism

5.2 Clinical Relevance: Enzyme Deficiencies

- Kinase deficiencies are benign:
  - Cataracts in galactokinase deficiency
- Aldolase B and galactose-1P uridyltransferase deficiencies:
  - Severe
  - Multi-organ damage
  - Galactosemia has cataracts and neurologic failure
- Galactosemia presents at birth
- Fructosemia presents after introduction of solid foods in diet

Table 6-5.2 Comparison Between Genetic Deficiencies in Fructose and Galactose Metabolism

Fructose Metabolism	Galactose Metabolism
Fructokinase deficiency	**Galactokinase deficiency:**
— Essential fructosuria	— Galactosemia type 2
— Autosomal recessive	— Autosomal recessive
— Benign	— Benign
— No cataracts	— Cataracts from galactitol in infant (wks old)
— Excess fructose is cleared by the kidney	— Rx: Lactose- and galactose-free diet
Aldolase B deficiency	**Gal-1P uridyltransferase deficiency**
— Hereditary fructose intolerance	— Galactosemia type 1
— Accumulation of fructose-1P	— Accumulation of gal-1P
• Osmotic damage	• Osmotic damage
• ↓ ATP production	• ↓ ATP production
— Symptoms start with the introduction of fruits in the diet	— Symptoms start shortly after birth
• Hepatomegaly	• Hepatomegaly
• Jaundice	• Jaundice
• Hypoglycemia	• Hypoglycemia
• Hyperuricemia	• Hyperuricemia
• Renal failure	• Renal failure
	• Cataracts
	• Vomiting
	• Seizures
	• Encephalopathy
— Autosomal recessive	— Autosomal recessive
— Rx: Fructose-free diet	— Rx: Lactose- and galactose-free diet
	Galactose epimerase deficiency:
	— Galactosemia type 3
	— Identical to type 1
	— Diagnosed through blood testing

Polyol (Sorbitol) Pathway

- Glucose is a source of fructose
- Involves two enzymes:
  - Aldose reductase
  - Sorbitol dehydrogenase
- Occurs in many tissues:
  - Critical in seminal vesicles
  - Spermatozoa use fructose as fuel

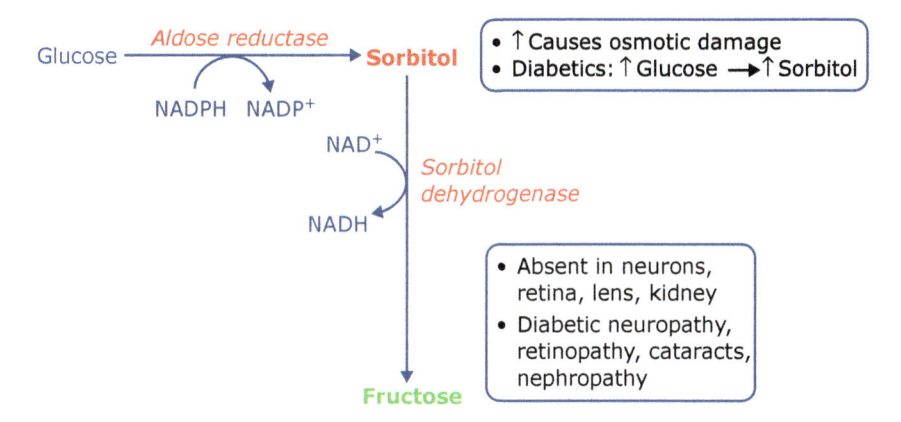

Glucose → (Aldose reductase; NADPH → NADP$^+$) → **Sorbitol** → (Sorbitol dehydrogenase; NAD$^+$ → NADH) → **Fructose**

- ↑ Causes osmotic damage
- Diabetics: ↑ Glucose → ↑ Sorbitol

- Absent in neurons, retina, lens, kidney
- Diabetic neuropathy, retinopathy, cataracts, nephropathy

▲ **Figure 6–6.0** Polyol Pathway and Clinical Relevance

CHAPTER 7 Pyruvate Metabolism

1 Overview

- Important crossroad in metabolism
- Two key enzymes: Pyruvate dehydrogenase and pyruvate carboxylase
- Sources of pyruvate:
  - Glycolysis endpoint
  - Lactate (LDH)
  - Alanine (ALT)
- Fates of pyruvate:
  - Acetyl-CoA through pyruvate dehydrogenase complex (PDH):
    —Acetyl-CoA enters Krebs cycle if ATP is needed
    —Acetyl-CoA can be converted to fatty acids when insulin is present and ATP is high
  - Oxaloacetate through pyruvate carboxylase (PC):
    —Oxaloacetate enters Krebs cycle if ATP is needed
    —Oxaloacetate combines the excess acetyl-CoA to leave mitochondria as a citrate and go to fatty acid synthesis
    —Oxaloacetate leaves mitochondria as a malate and goes to gluconeogenesis if ATP and glucagon are present
  - Lactate (LDH)
  - Alanine (ALT)

> **USMLE® Key Concepts**
>
> For Step 1, you must be able to:
> - Recognize the sources and fates of pyruvate.
> - Discuss the role of hormones and ATP in pyruvate metabolism.
> - Know pyruvate metabolism enzyme or vitamin deficiencies.

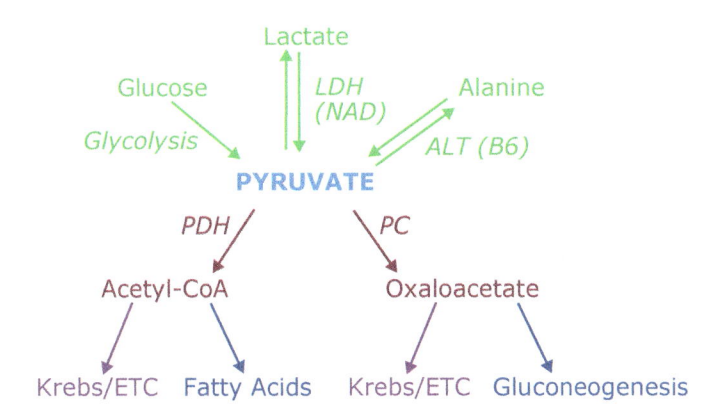

▲ Figure 7–1.0 Pyruvate Metabolism

2 Pyruvate Dehydrogenase: Biochemistry

- Links glycolysis to Krebs cycle
- PDH is irreversible
- PDH is mitochondrial
  - Cytosolic pyruvate is actively transported by pyruvate translocase
- PDH is a complex of three enzymes: E_1, E_2, and E_3
- E1 is the rate-limiting step and uses thiamine pyrophosphate (TPP)
- Insulin and glucagon control PDH:
  - Dephosphorylation by insulin activates the enzyme
  - Phosphorylation by glucagon inactivates the enzyme
  - The complex comes with its own PDH phosphatase and PDH kinase
  - The addition or removal of phosphates occurs on serine residues
- Levels of energy locally control PDH:
  - ADP, NAD, and CoA activate PDH (low energy)
  - ATP, NADH, and acetyl-CoA inhibit PDH (high energy)
- PDH complex requires five cofactors:
  - Thiamine pyrophosphate (E_1)
  - Lipoate and coenzyme A (E_2)
  - FAD and NAD (E_3)
  - Similar requirements for α-ketoglutarate dehydrogenase and branched chain keto acid dehydrogenase (deficient in maple syrup urine disease)

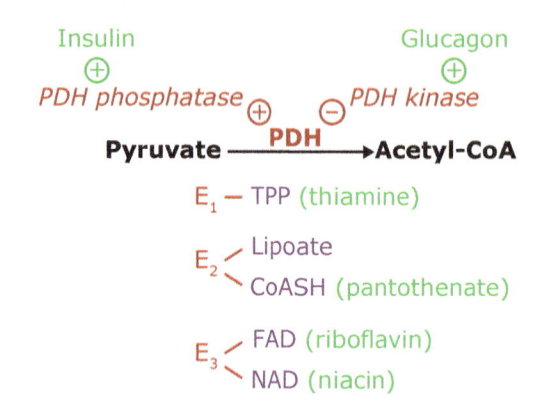

```
           Insulin                    Glucagon
              ⊕                          ⊕
      PDH phosphatase ⊕      ⊖   PDH kinase
                         PDH
         Pyruvate ─────────→ Acetyl-CoA

              E₁ — TPP (thiamine)

              E₂ ⟨ Lipoate
                   CoASH (pantothenate)

              E₃ ⟨ FAD (riboflavin)
                   NAD (niacin)
```

▲ Figure 7–2.0 Pyruvate Dehydrogenase

3 Pyruvate Dehydrogenase: Clinical Relevance

3.1 PDH Deficiency
- X-linked E_1 deficiency
- Neurodegenerative pathology
  - Seizures, intellectual disability, microcephaly, blindness, etc.
- Systemic lactic acidosis
- Treatment:
  - Alternative source of acetyl-CoA: Ketones
  - Decreased lactate production: Low carbohydrates
  - Supportive management of metabolic acidosis

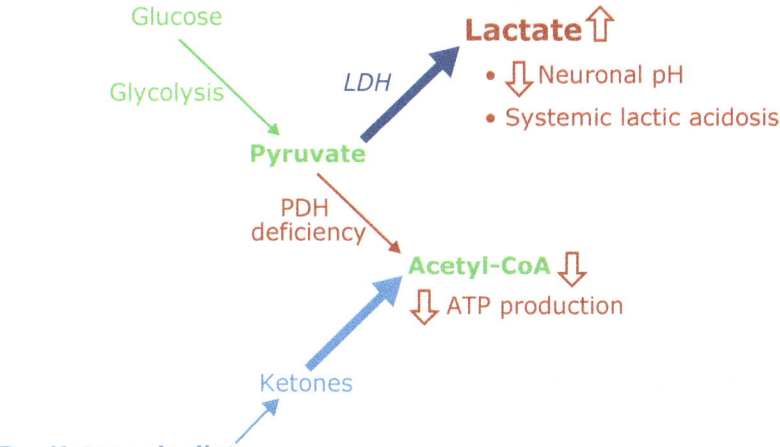

▲ Figure 7–3.1 PDH Deficiency

3.2 Vitamin Deficiencies
- Thiamine and niacin deficiencies decrease acetyl-CoA production from pyruvate
- Neurons, muscle, and cells with high ATP requirements are mostly targeted
- See beriberi and pellagra in Chapter 4

3.3 Primary Biliary Cirrhosis
- E_2 is the primary target of antimitochondrial antibodies

4. Pyruvate Carboxylase

- Links pyruvate to fatty acid synthesis and gluconeogenesis
- Irreversible
- Requires three cofactors (as do all carboxylases):
    1. ATP
    2. Biotin
    3. CO_2
- Is not clearly controlled by insulin and glucagon
- See Chapter 11 on gluconeogenesis or Chapter 8 on fatty acid synthesis

5 Pyruvate Carboxylase: Clinical Relevance

5.1 Pyruvate Carboxylase Deficiency
- Autosomal recessive
- Fasting hypoglycemia (↓ gluconeogenesis)
- Lactic acidosis (↑ LDH)
- Defects in myelin (↓ fatty acid synthesis)

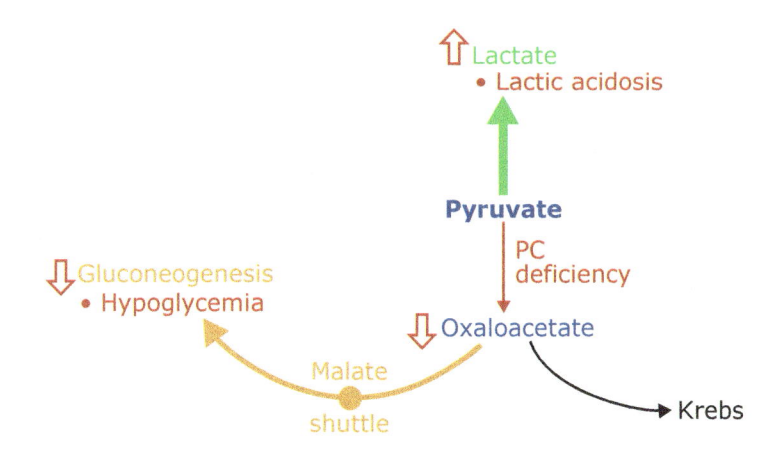

▲ Figure 7–5.1 Pyruvate Carboxylase Deficiency

5.2 Biotin Deficiency
- Required for all carboxylases (pyruvate, propionyl-CoA, and acetyl-CoA carboxylases on Step 1)
- Involved in fatty acid synthesis, gluconeogenesis
- Rare deficiency:
  - Avidin from egg whites prevents biotin absorption
  - Anticonvulsants and antibiotics
  - Rashes/seborrheic dermatitis
  - Alopecia
  - Paresthesia
  - Anemia
  - CNS symptoms (hallucinations, depression)

CHAPTER 8: Glycogen Synthesis and Fatty Acid Synthesis

1 Overview

- Insulin world and ↑ ATP from burning glucose:
  - Excess dietary glucose converted to glycogen
  - Excess acetyl-CoA converted to fatty acids

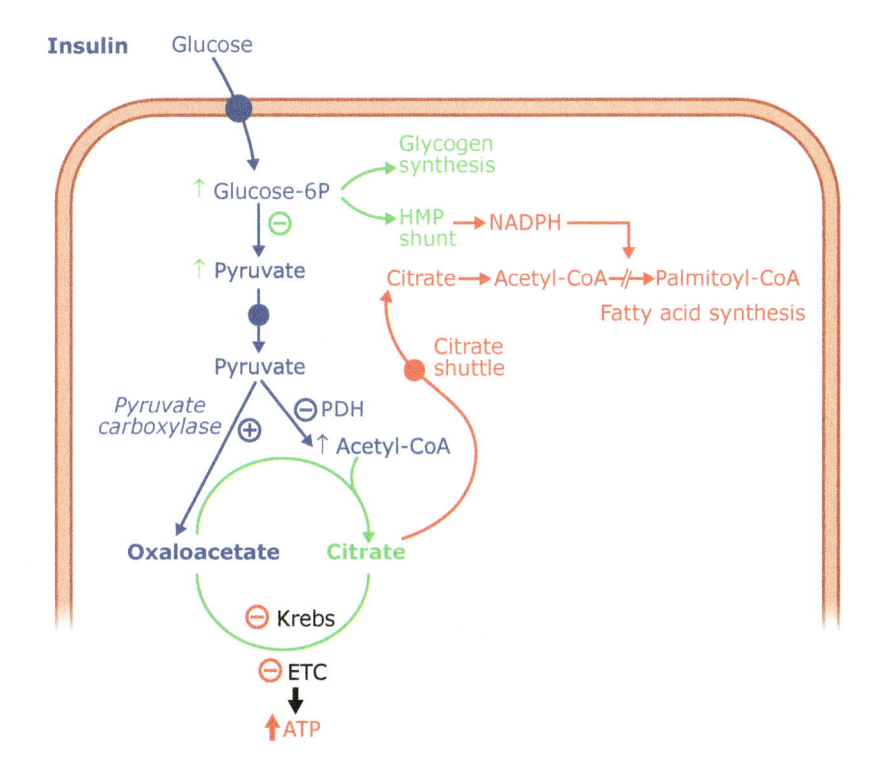

▲ Figure 8–1.0 Glycogen and Fatty Acid Synthesis

USMLE® Key Concepts

For Step 1, you must be able to:
- ▶ Understand the regulation of glycogen and fatty acid synthesis.
- ▶ Understand the roles of the HMP shunt.
- ▶ Identify important clinical correlations.

- ↑ ATP ⊖ glycolysis, PDH, Krebs, and ETC:
  - ↑ Acetyl-CoA ⊖ PDH, ⊕ PC:
    - Pyruvate is converted to oxaloacetate
    - OA combines with acetyl-CoA to form citrate
    - Citrate leaves through citrate shuttle
    - Cytoplasmic citrate initiates fatty acid synthesis
  - ⊖ Glycolysis PFK-1 causes ↑ G6P:
    - G6P enters glycogen synthesis
    - G6P enters HMP shunt
    - HMP shunt provides NADPH for fatty acid synthesis

2 Glycogen Synthesis

- Major storage form of glucose in animals, humans, and fungi:
  - Analog of plant starch
  - Branched polymer of glucose
  - Core protein: Glycogenin
- Requires energy as UTP:
  - UDP-glucose is precursor
- Cytoplasmic process
- Most cells make glycogen
- Liver and muscle are primary storage sites:
  - Fate of liver glycogen:
    — Maintenance of blood glucose on fasting
    — Used by extrahepatic tissues
  - Fate of muscle glycogen:
    — Used as a local source of energy by muscle
    — No participation in maintenance of fasting blood glucose levels

2.1 Glycogen Synthase and Branching Enzyme

- Glycogen synthase:
  - Rate-limiting
  - Makes α-1,4 bonds between glucoses
  - Uses UDP-glucoses
  - UDP is not incorporated in glycogen
- Branching enzyme:
  - A glycosyltransferase
  - Two-step process
    — Break α-1,4
    — Transfer as α-1,6

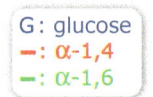

G : glucose
— : α-1,4
— : α-1,6

① Glycogen synthase made linear glycogen > 11 residues

12 11 10 9 8 7 6 5 4 3 2 1
G—G—G—G—G—G—G—G—G—G—G—G

② Branching enzyme cleaves α-1,4, transfers to α-1,6:

6 5 4 3 2 1
G—G—G—G—G—G
|
G—G—G—G—G—G
12 11 10 9 8 7

▲ Figure 8–2.1A Branching Enzyme

- Cycles of glycogen synthase and branching enzyme result in highly branched glycogen granule

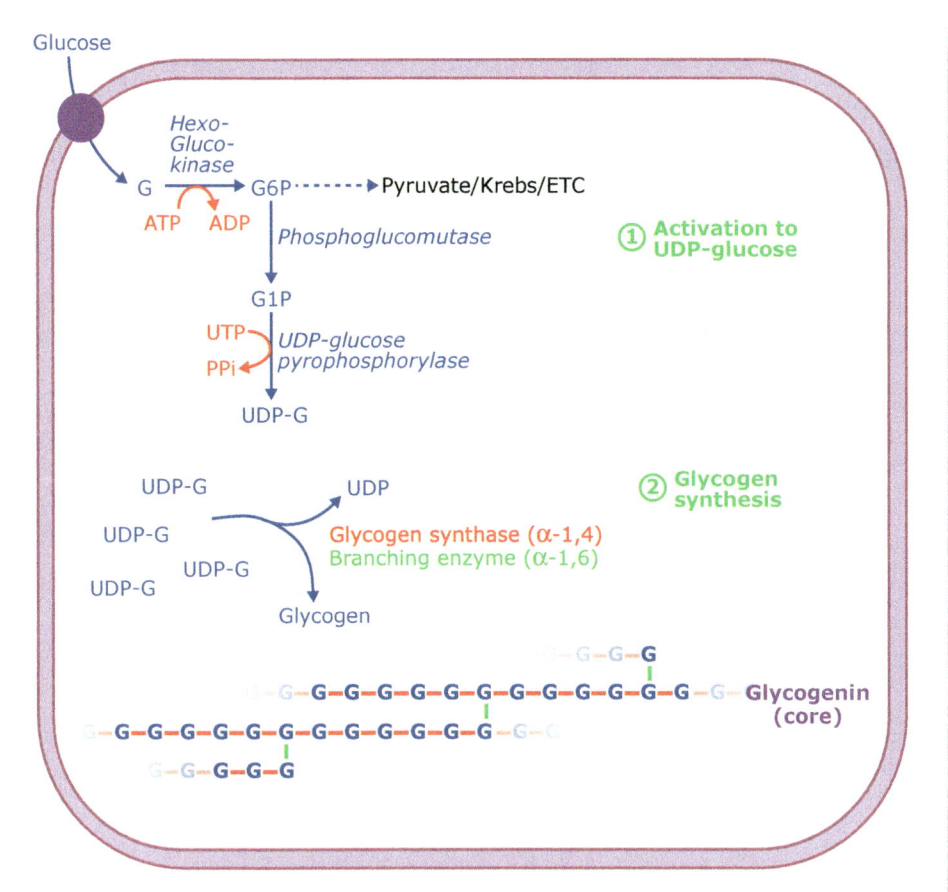

▲ Figure 8-2.1B Glycogen Synthesis

2.2 Control of Glycogen Synthase

- Insulin dephosphorylates and activates the enzyme:
  - Dephosphorylation by protein phosphatase 1
- Glucagon phosphorylates and inactivates the enzyme
  - Phosphorylation by protein kinase A
- Local regulation:
  - Feed forward activation by glucose-6P
    — ↑ G6P occurs in presence of ↑ ATP

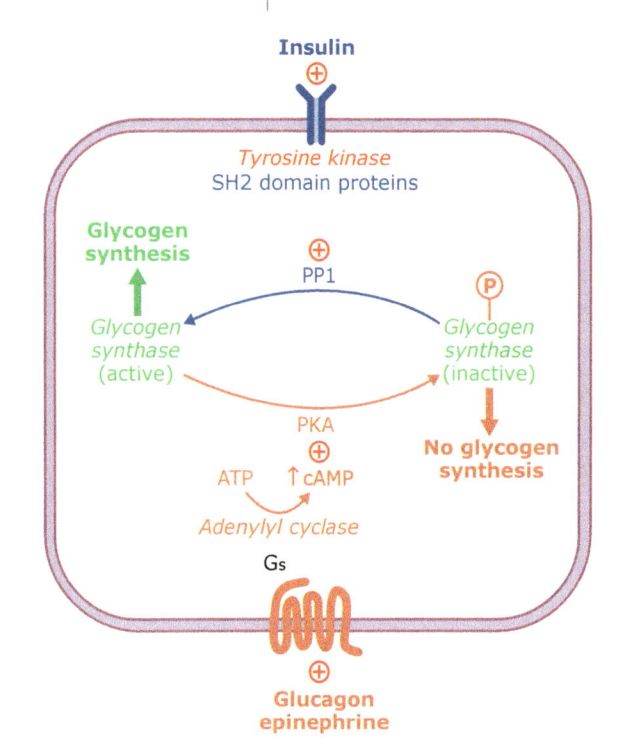

▶ Figure 8-2.2 Hormonal Control of Glycogen Synthase

2.3 Clinical Relevance

2.3.1 Glycogen Synthase Deficiency
- Also known as glycogen storage disease type 0:
  - Although no storage issue, many similar clinical characteristics
- Two genes:
  - *GYS1* in muscle
  - *GYS2* in liver

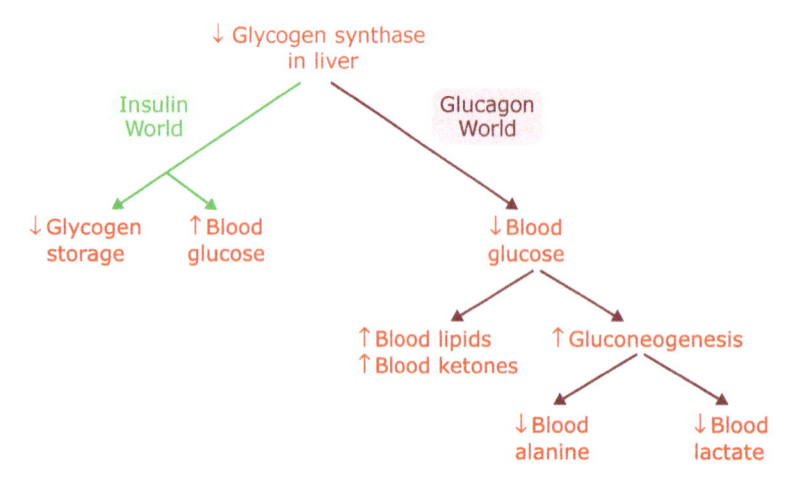

▲ Figure 8–2.3 Effects of *GYS2* Mutations

2.3.2 Branching Enzyme Deficiency
- Also known as Andersen disease or glycogen storage disease type IV
- Affects liver and muscle, including heart, CNS
  - Long linear glycogen builds up in liver
    - Hepatomegaly
    - Hepatic damage
    - Cirrhosis
    - Rarely hypoglycemia
  - Dilated cardiomyopathy
  - Neuromuscular variants exist
- Autosomal recessive
- Dx in first few months of life
- Poor prognosis, supportive Rx

3. Fatty Acid Synthesis

- Three major steps:
  - Citrate shuttle
  - Acetyl-CoA carboxylase
  - Fatty acid synthase

3.1 Citrate Shuttle

- Mitochondrial acetyl-CoA from glucose builds up due to ↑ ATP
- Activation of pyruvate carboxylase converts pyruvate to oxaloacetate
- Oxaloacetate combines with acetyl-CoA to make citrate
- Citrate leaves mitochondria
- Citrate lyase releases acetyl-CoA and oxaloacetate in cytoplasm
- Oxaloacetate is recycled to pyruvate by malic enzyme:
  - Produces NADPH for fatty acid synthase

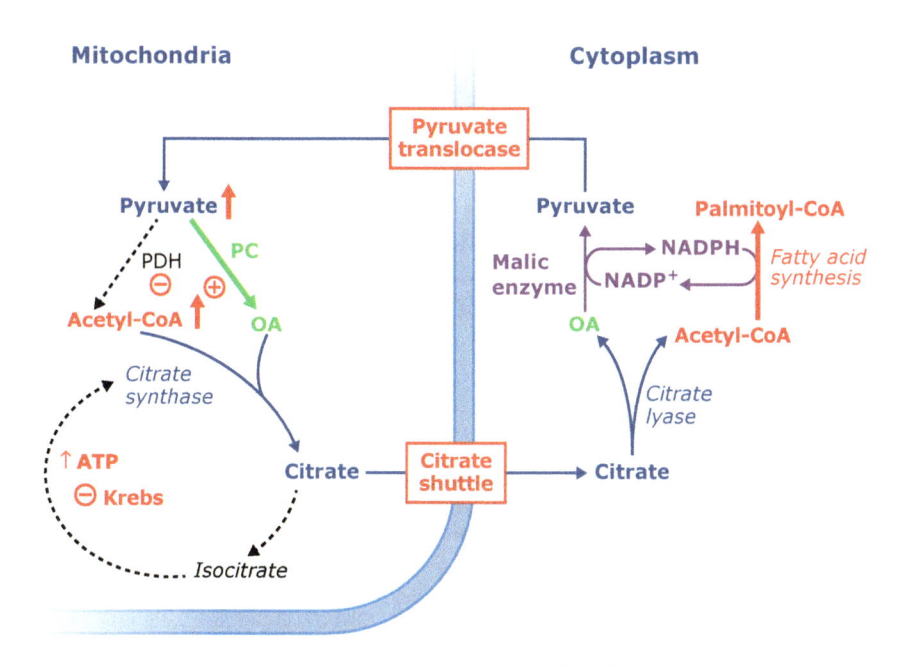

▲ Figure 8–3.1 Citrate Shuttle

3.2 Acetyl-CoA Carboxylase

- Rate-limiting step:
  - Insulin dephosphorylates to activate acetyl-CoA carboxylase:
    —Dephosphorylation is by protein phosphatase 2, not PP1
- Glucagon phosphorylates to inhibit acetyl-CoA carboxylase:
  —Phosphorylation is by AMP-activated kinase, not PKA
  - Citrate activates acetyl-CoA carboxylase
- Requires ATP, biotin, CO_2 (ABC enzyme)
- Makes malonyl-CoA

3.3 Fatty Acid Synthase Complex

- Multi-enzyme complex:
  - Cytosolic
  - Contains phosphopantetheine
    - Derived from pantothenic acid (vitamin B5)
    - Part of acyl carrier protein (ACP)
  - Contains a critical cysteine residue
  - Only uses the 2C of acetyl-CoA to build a 16C palmitoyl-CoA
    - 7 cycles
    - CO_2 used by acetyl-CoA carboxylase is not incorporated in fatty acid
  - Requires 2 NADPH per cycle
    - Provided by HMP shunt and malic enzyme
  - Insulin induces complex

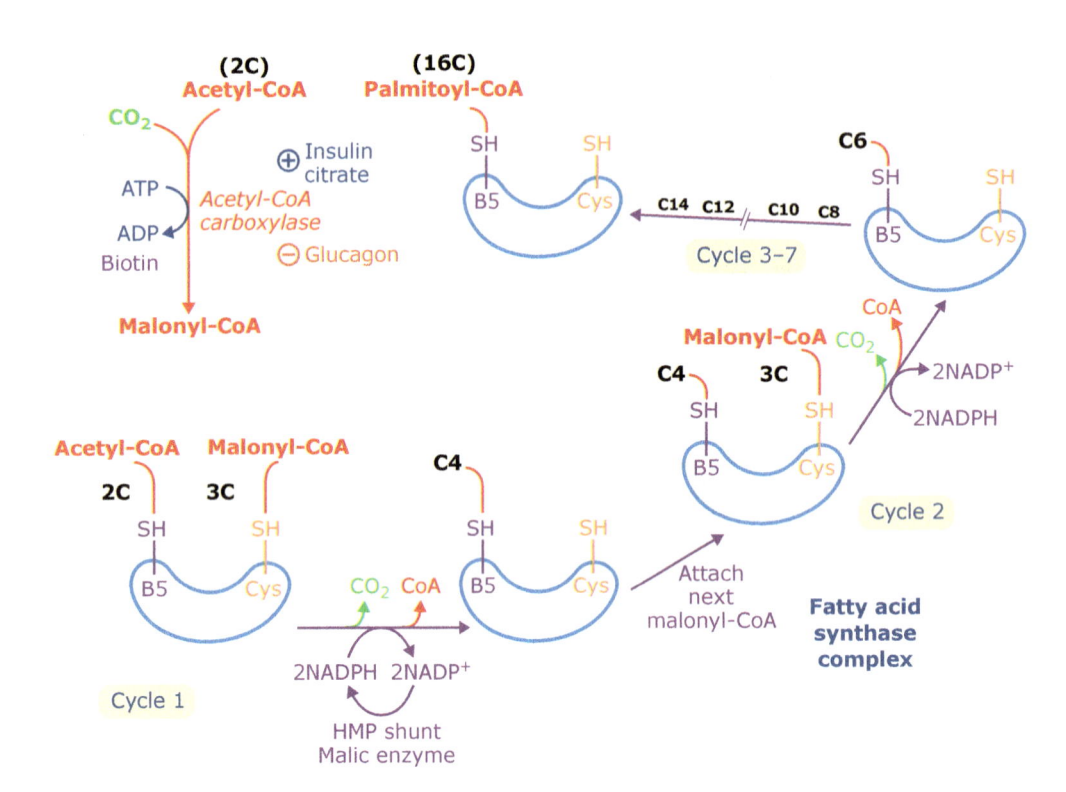

▲ Figure 8-3.3 Fatty Acid Synthesis

3.4 Elongation and Desaturation of Fatty Acids

- Occurs in endoplasmic reticulum
- Elongation:
  - Malonyl-CoA provides 2C fragments
  - NADPH is required
- Desaturation:
  - Requires O_2, NADH and cytochrome b_5
  - Cannot put a double bond past position 9

Chapter 8 • Glycogen Synthesis and Fatty Acid Synthesis

3.5 Clinical Relevance

- **Insulin controls many steps in carbohydrate and lipid metabolism:**
  - Upregulates GLUT4
  - Induces glucokinase
  - Activates PFK-2/PFK-1
  - Activates pyruvate kinase
  - Activates pyruvate dehydrogenase
    - → ↑ ATP and acetyl-CoA
  - Activates acetyl-CoA carboxylase
  - Induces fatty acid synthase
    - → Promotes conversion of excess dietary glucose to fat
  - Induces lipoprotein lipase
    - → ↑ Storage of fat
    - → WEIGHT GAIN
- Food that rapidly increases glucose and ATP levels results in greater fat storage:
  — Basis of "glycemic index" and "insulin index"
- Visceral (central) obesity:
  — Key feature of metabolic syndrome
  — Correlated to CV risk and strokes
  — Correlated to type 2 diabetes

4 Hexose-Monophosphate Shunt

- **Produces NADPH and ribose 5-phosphate**
- G6P leaves glycolysis into shunt
- Shunt returns to glycolysis as F6P or GAP

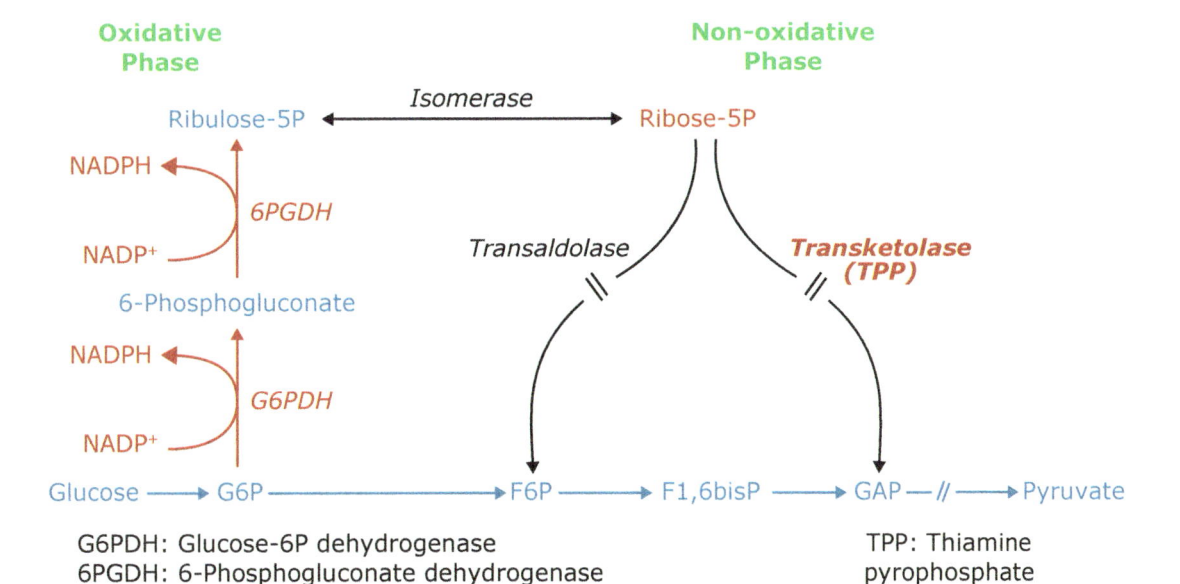

Oxidative Phase — **Non-oxidative Phase**

Ribulose-5P ←Isomerase→ Ribose-5P

6PGDH: NADP⁺ → NADPH
6-Phosphogluconate

G6PDH: NADP⁺ → NADPH

Transaldolase / **Transketolase (TPP)**

Glucose → G6P → F6P → F1,6bisP → GAP —//→ Pyruvate

G6PDH: Glucose-6P dehydrogenase
6PGDH: 6-Phosphogluconate dehydrogenase
TPP: Thiamine pyrophosphate

▲ Figure 8–4.0 Hexose-Monophosphate Shunt

4.1 Clinical Relevance

4.1.1 Thiamine Deficiency
- ↓ PDH and α-KGDH activity
- ↓ Transketolase activity:
    — Used as diagnostic test
- Most common cause is chronic alcoholism
- Can be dietary
- Affects ATP production
- Must be supplemented prior to correction of hypoglycemia in chronic alcoholics

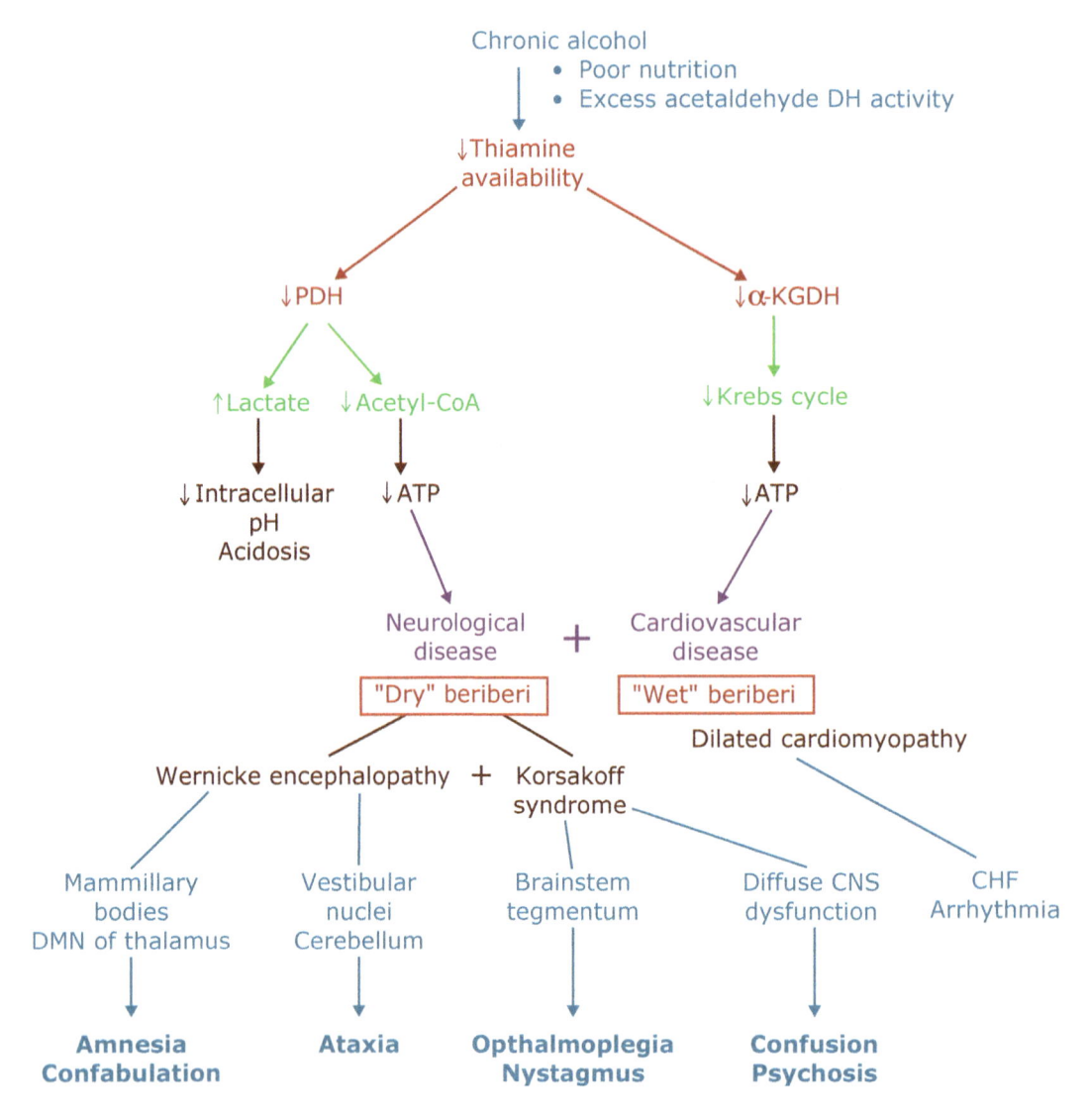

▲ Figure 8–4.1A Thiamine Deficiency

4.1.2 Glucose-6-Phosphate Dehydrogenase Deficiency

- X-linked recessive
- Also known as favism
- Epidemiology:
  - Mediterranean populations
  - African descent
- Hemolytic anemia:
  - Triggers:
    - No. 1: Infections
    - Drugs and chemicals:
      - Antimalarials (quinine group)
      - Sulfonamides
      - Isoniazid, dapsone, aspirin
      - Napthalene, methylene blue
    - Fava beans:
      - Vicine and convicine alkaloids
  - Rarely chronic hemolysis (severe deficiency, < 10%)
    - Mimics CGD
- Mechanisms of hemolysis:
  - NADPH is required for glutathione reductase in RBCs
- Rx: Avoid triggers
- 6PGDH deficiency is identical in presentation, but is autosomal recessive

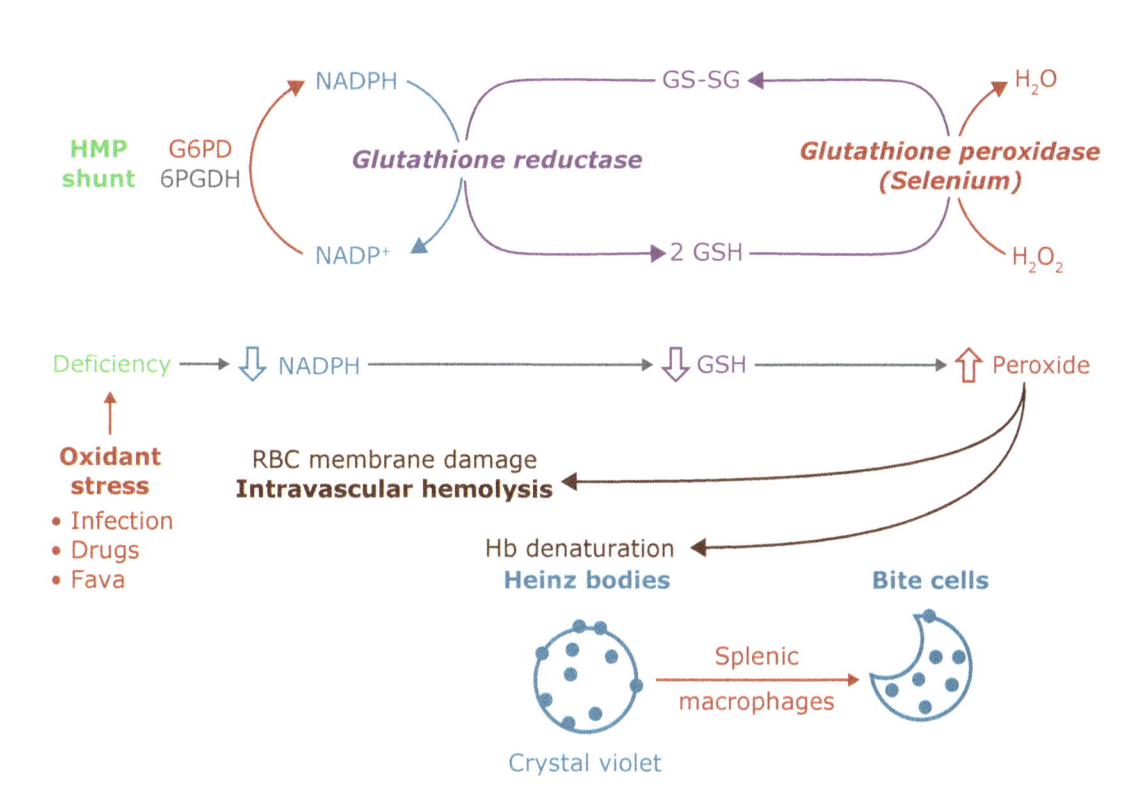

▲ Figure 8-4.1B G6PD Deficiency in RBCs

CHAPTER 9: Lipid Digestion and Lipoprotein Metabolism

1 Overview

- Diverse group of water insoluble chemicals
- Two sources:
  - Diet (exogenous)
  - Endogenous synthesis
- Major dietary lipids:
  - **Triglycerides (TGLs):**
    - Storage form of energy
    - Source of acetyl-CoA during fasting
    - Contribute 9 kcal/g
    - Represent 20%–35% of total caloric intake
  - **Cholesterol:**
    - Important precursor:
      - Membrane fluidity
      - Steroid hormones
      - Vitamin D
      - Bile salts
      - Myelin
    - Less than 200–300 mg/day from diet:
      - Liver makes 80% of needed daily cholesterol
  - **Lipid soluble vitamins: A, D, E, and K**
  - **Essential fatty acids:**
    - Linoleic acid (ω-6):
      - Source of arachidonic acid
    - Linolenic acid (ω-3)
- Endogenously produced lipids:
  - Triglycerides
  - Cholesterol
  - Phospholipids
  - Sphingolipids
  - Prostaglandins
  - Leukotrienes
- **Lipoproteins:**
  - Major form of transport
  - LDL is the main form of distribution of cholesterol
  - VLDL and chylomicrons transport triglycerides
  - HDL removes cholesterol from fatty streaks

USMLE® Key Concepts

For Step 1, you must be able to:

- Describe exogenous and endogenous lipoprotein metabolism.
- Differentiate the variety of apoproteins and their roles.
- Describe cholesterol synthesis and its control.
- Understand the roles of LDL and HDL with respect to atherosclerosis.
- Describe genetic and acquired hyperlipidemias.

2 Lipid Digestion

2.1 Role of Pancreatic Enzyme and Intestinal Cholecystokinin

- Pancreas plays critical role:
  - Stimulated by intestinal cholecystokinin
  - Secretes lipase and colipase as well as proteases and amylase
  - Secretes bicarbonate to neutralize gastric acid
- Triglycerides:
  - Hydrolyzed by lipases to free fatty acids and 2-monoacylglycerol
- Cholesterol esters:
  - Hydrolyzed by esterases to free cholesterol
- Membrane phospholipids:
  - Hydrolyzed by phospholipase A_2 to lysophospholipids
- Emulsification by bile salts required for absorption

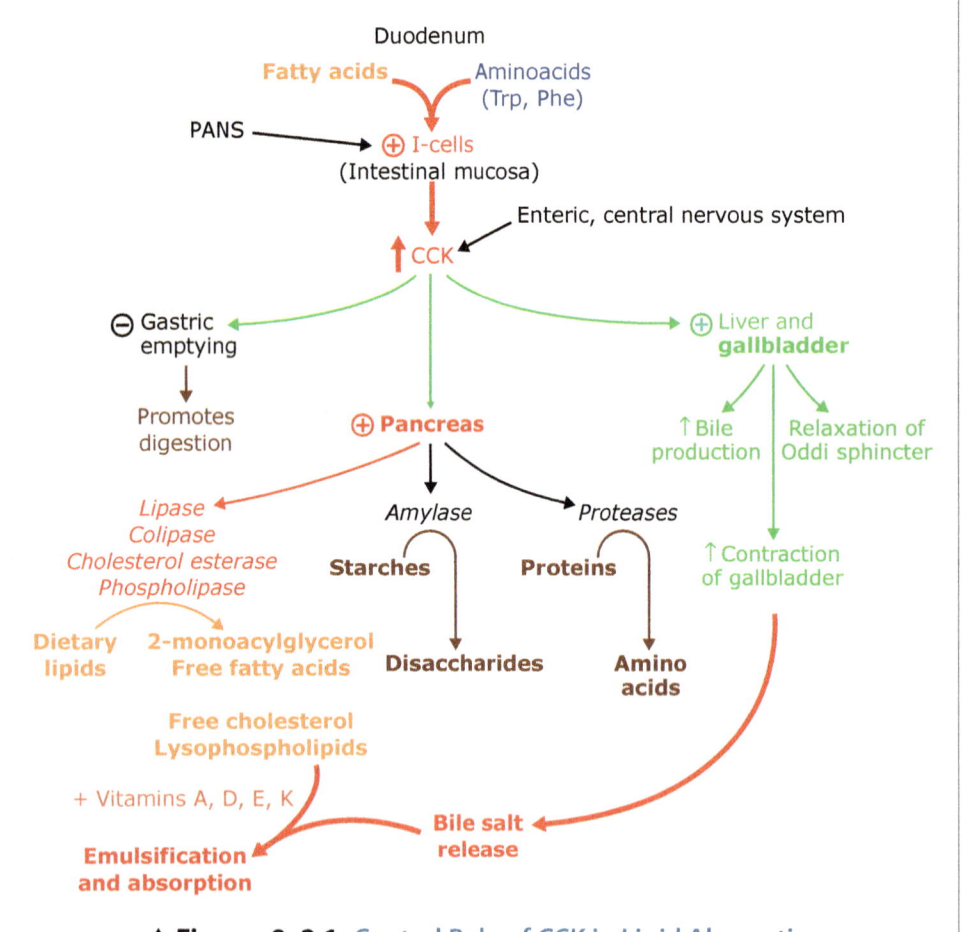

▲ Figure 9–2.1 Central Role of CCK in Lipid Absorption

2.2 Clinical Relevance: Fat Malabsorption
- Steatorrhea
- Deficiency of fat-soluble vitamins
- Deficiency of essential fatty acids
- Causes include:
  - Pancreatic insufficiency:
    — Chronic alcoholism (adults)
    — Cystic fibrosis (children)
  - Gallbladder disease
    — Cirrhosis:
      - ↓ Synthesis
    — Obstruction:
      - Stones
      - Strictures
  - Cholestyramine and other bile-sequestering resins:
    — Side effect from cholesterol-lowering resins
  - Small bowel disease

3 Lipoprotein Metabolism

3.1 Chylomicrons
- Exogenous lipids are packaged as chylomicrons:
  - Enterocytes activate free fatty acids to fatty acyl-CoA
    — Thiokinase
- Fatty acyl-CoAs bind to 2-monoacylglycerol and form triglycerides
- Fatty acyl-CoA esterifies cholesterol in cholesterol esters
- ApoB-48
    — Expressed in enterocytes
    — Allows secretion in lymph/blood

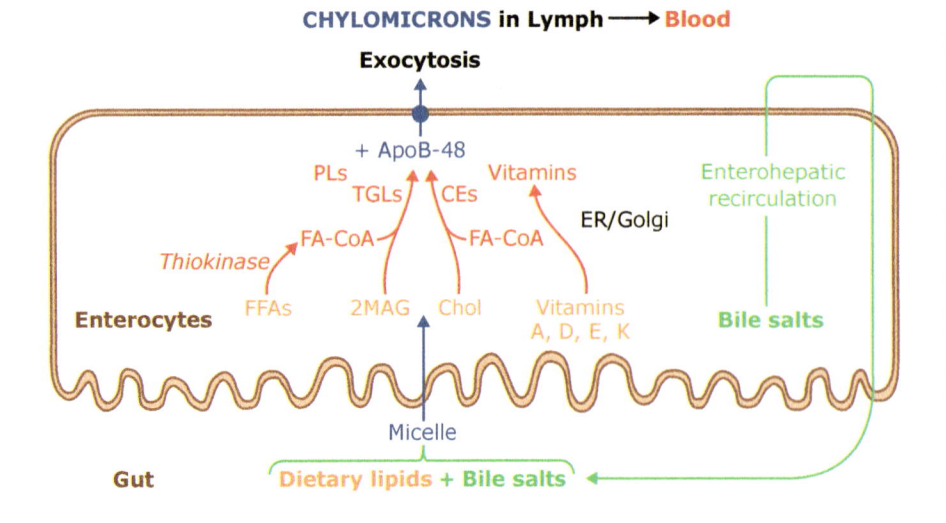

▲ Figure 9-3.1 Synthesis of Chylomicrons

- Chylomicrons are the least dense of all lipoproteins:
  - Greatest TGLs content
  - Least protein
  - Clinical relevance:
    — Density gradient and zonal ultracentrifugation
    — Separates lipoproteins based on density:
      - Lighter at top, heavier at bottom
    — In order of increasing density:
      Chylomicrons - VLDL - IDL - LDL - HDL

3.2 VLDL

- Endogenous lipids are packaged as VLDL:
  - Produced by the liver
  - Excess dietary glucose is converted to fatty acids and cholesterol
- Fatty acids are converted to TGLs, cholesterol to CES
- ApoB-100 allows secretion in blood

3.2.1 Sources of Hepatic Glycerol-3P

- TGLs are made of glycerol and three fatty acids
- Two hepatic sources:
  - Glycerol from blood lipases activity:
    — Glycerol kinase makes it glycerol-3P
    — Glycerol kinase is not found in adipocytes
  - DHAP from glycolysis:
    — Glycerol-3P dehydrogenase converts DHAP to glycerol-3P

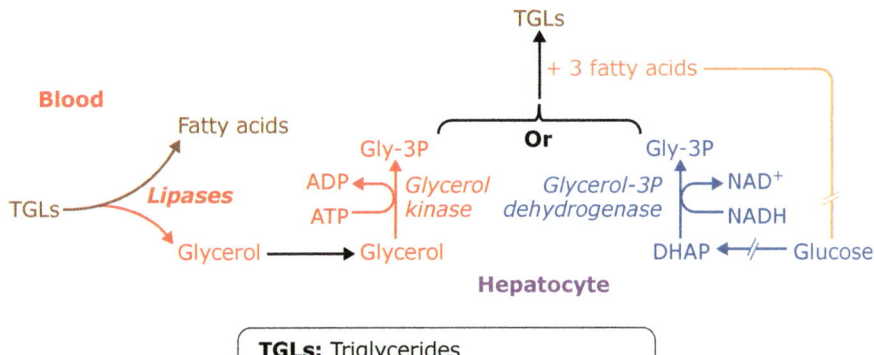

TGLs: Triglycerides
Gly-3P: Glycerol-3 phosphate
DHAP: Dihydroxyacetone phosphate

▲ Figure 9–3.2A Synthesis of Hepatic Triglycerides

3.2.2 Triglycerides and Cholesterol Esters

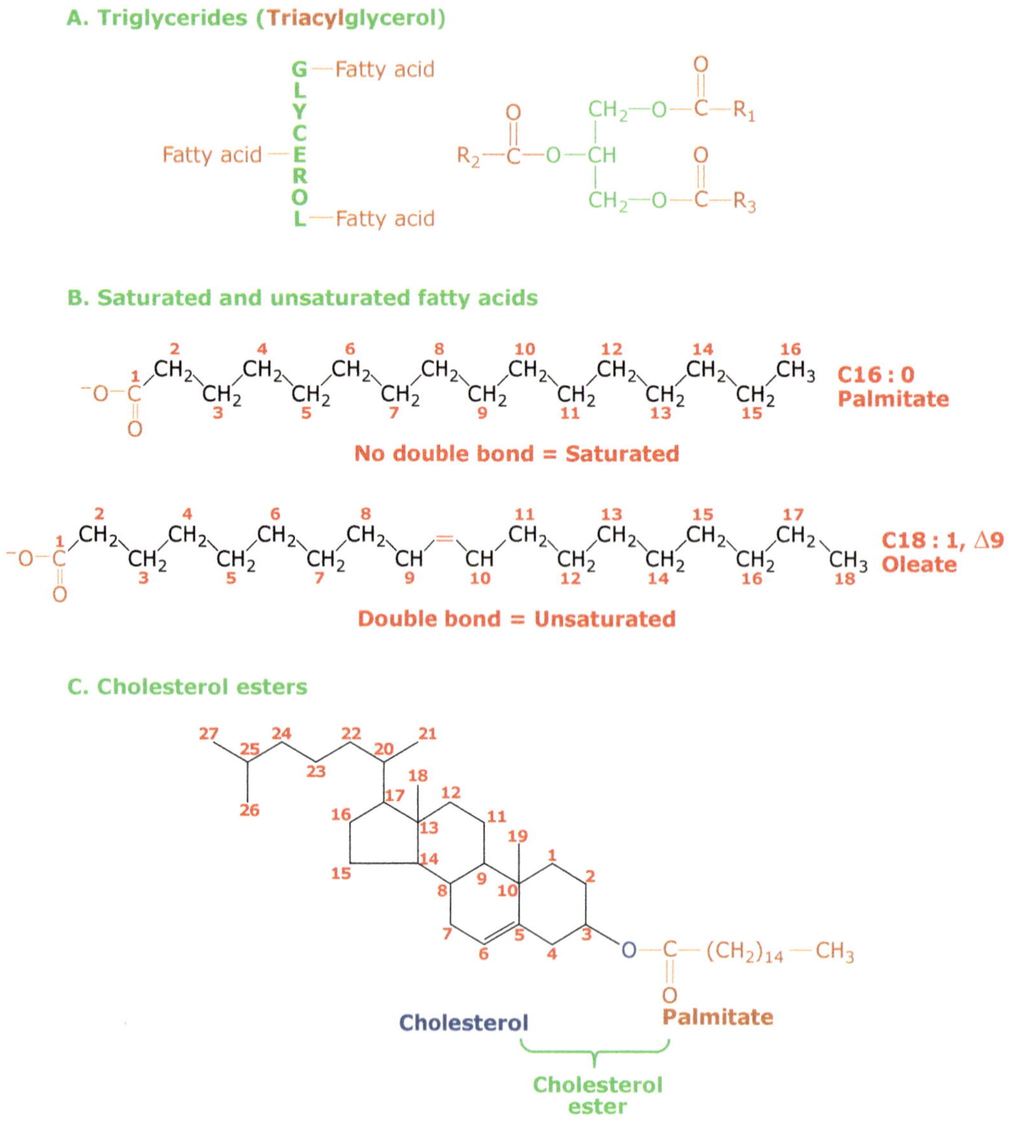
A. Triglycerides (Triacylglycerol)
G—Fatty acid
GLYCEROL
Fatty acid—E
L—Fatty acid
$CH_2—O—C(=O)—R_1$
$R_2—C(=O)—O—CH$
$CH_2—O—C(=O)—R_3$
B. Saturated and unsaturated fatty acids
C16 : 0
Palmitate
No double bond = Saturated
C18 : 1, Δ9
Oleate
Double bond = Unsaturated
C. Cholesterol esters
$O—C—(CH_2)_{14}—CH_3$
Cholesterol
Palmitate
Cholesterol ester

▲**Figure 9–3.2B** Structure of Triglycerides, Fatty Acids, and Cholesterol Esters

4 Storage of Dietary and Endogenous Triglycerides

- Blood chylomicrons and VLDLs receive ApoC-II and ApoE from HDL
- ApoC-II activates lipoprotein lipase (LPL):
  - Located in adipose and muscle capillaries
  - ApoC-II is a cofactor of LPL
  - LPL is also induced by insulin
- LPL releases free fatty acids and glycerol:
  - Glycerol can be recycled by hepatic glycerol kinase
  - Free fatty acids must become TGLs for storage
- TGLs synthesis in adipocytes:
  - The only source of glycerol-3P in adipocytes is DHAP
  - To spare DHAP from glycolysis, ↑ ATP is required
  - Depends on adequate GLUT4-mediated glucose uptake
  - Clinical relevance:
    —Diabetes and hyperlipidemia:
    - ↓ Insulin or insulin response ↓ GLUT4
    - Less glucose in adipocytes means less ATP
    - Less ATP results in less DHAP sparing
    - Less fat storage = ↑ blood lipids

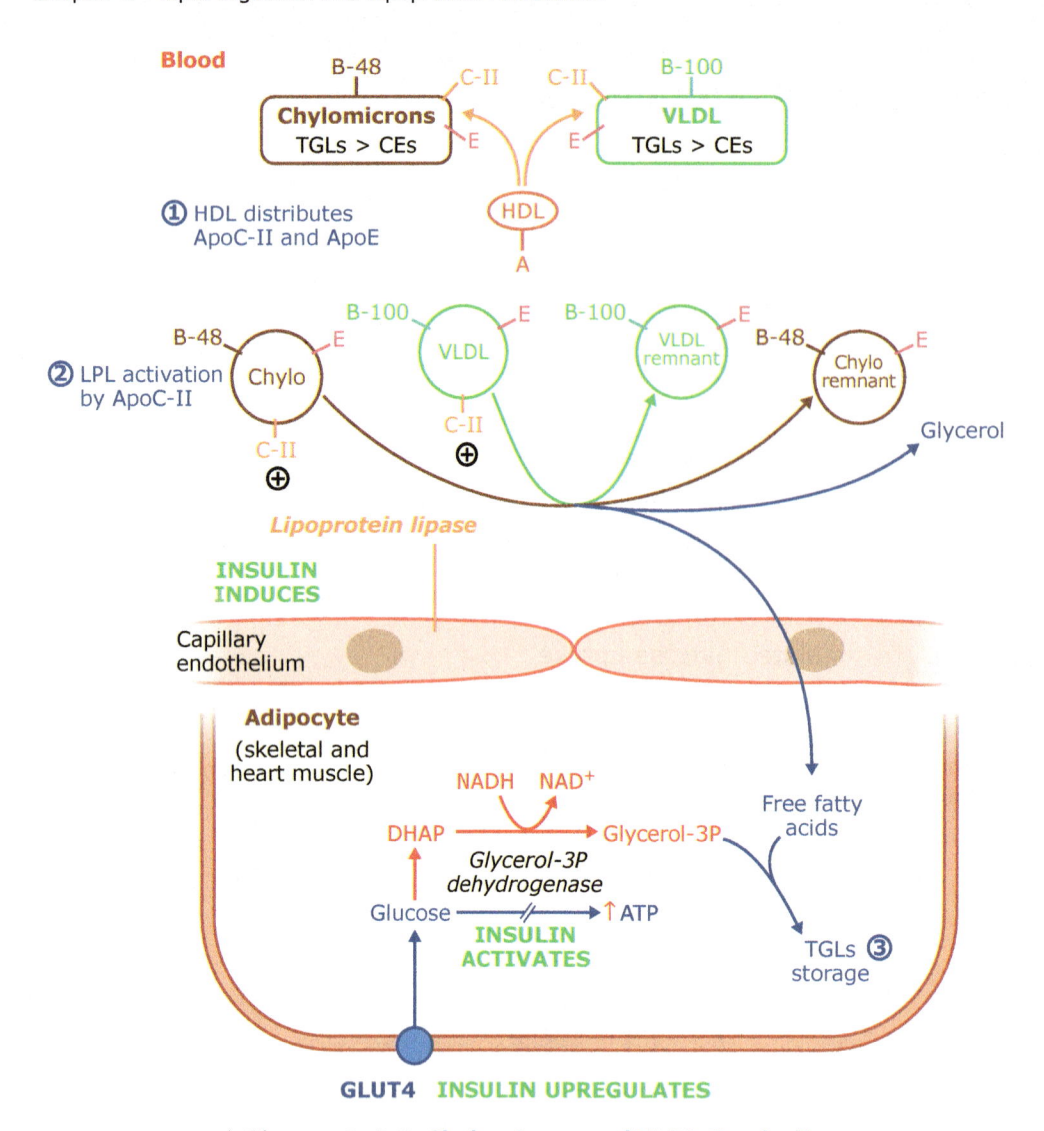

Chapter 9 • Lipid Digestion and Lipoprotein Metabolism

Figure 9-4.0 Chylomicron and VLDL Catabolism

5 Hepatic Uptake of VLDL and Chylomicron Remnants

- VLDL remnants and chylomicron remnants have ApoE:
- ApoE receptors mediate endocytosis of remnants:
  - Contain primarily cholesterol esters (CEs)
  - Hepatic lipases release the remaining fatty acids
- All dietary cholesterol enters liver
- About 50% of VLDL remnants can become IDL and LDL

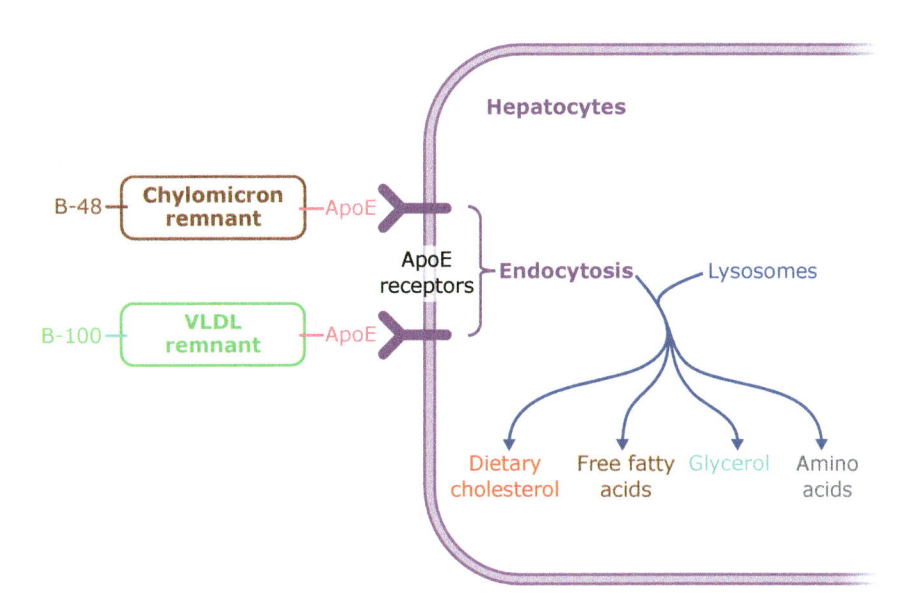

▲ Figure 9–5.0 Liver Uptake of Chylomicron and VLDL Remnants

6 IDL and LDL Production

- 50% of VLDL remnants do not enter liver through ApoE receptors
- Hepatic lipases remove the remainder of TGLs in VLDL remnants:
  - Form IDL
- Cholesterol ester transfer protein (CETP) enriches IDL in CEs:
  - Forms LDL
- LDL can be taken up by tissues expressing LDL receptors:
  - LDL receptors bind to ApoB-100
  - 60% of LDL is taken up by the liver
  - 40% of LDL is taken up by extrahepatic tissue
    —Adrenal cortex
    —Gonads
    —Any cell
- Unused LDL can become oxidized LDL:
  - Sheds free cholesterol
  - Forms fatty streaks

7 HDL Production and Role

- HDL is produced by liver, intestine, as well as free ApoA-1
- ApoA-1 stimulates lecithin cholesterol acyltransferase (LCAT):
  - LCAT scavenges free cholesterol from fatty streaks
  - LCAT esterifies cholesterol to CEs
  - HDL becomes CE rich
- CETP transfers these CEs to IDLs and forms LDL
- HDL also shuttles apoproteins:
  - ApoC-II
  - ApoE
  - Distribution to chylomicrons and VLDL
- HDL uptake through SR-B1 receptors:
  - Distributes cholesterol
  - SR-B1 only found in liver and steroidogenic tissues
- Benefit of HDL:
  - Pick up cholesterol from fatty streaks
  - Return cholesterol to liver
  - "Reverse cholesterol transport"

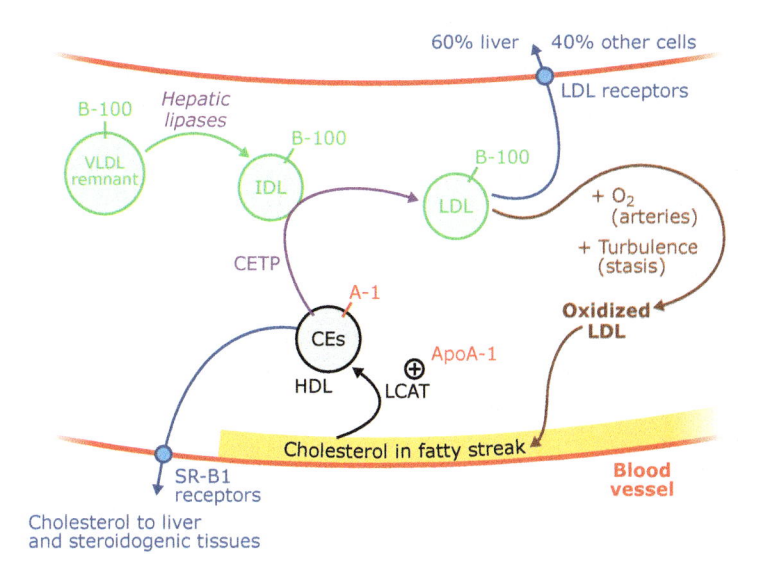

▲ **Figure 9–7.0** Relationship Between IDL, LDL, and HDL

Table 9-7.0	Lipoproteins and Roles
Lipoprotein and Associated Apoproteins	**Role**
Chylomicrons	Transport dietary lipids
ApoB-48	Secretion into lymph/blood
ApoC-II	Cofactor of LPL: – Puts TGLs in storage – Makes chylomicron remnants
ApoE	Liver uptake of remnants
VLDL	Transport endogenous lipids
ApoB-100	Secretion into blood
ApoC-II	Cofactor of LPL: – Puts TGLs in storage – Makes VLDL remnants
ApoE	Liver uptake of remnants
IDL	• Return endogenous lipids to liver • Precursor of LDL
ApoB-100	
ApoC-II	
ApoE	
LDL	Cholesterol delivery to tissues
ApoB-100	Endocytosis by LDL receptors
HDL	• Reverse cholesterol transport • Shuttles ApoC-II, ApoE • Delivers cholesterol to steroidogenic tissues.
ApoA-1	Activates LCAT

8 De Novo Synthesis of Cholesterol

8.1 Synthesis

- Acetyl-CoA provides all the carbons of cholesterol
- Synthesis is cytoplasmic:
  - Requires ATP and NADPH
- Conversion of acetyl-CoA to mevalonate is the rate-limiting step:
  - Catalyzed by HMG CoA-reductase
    - —↓ Intracellular sterols ↑ transcription and vice versa
    - —↑ Sterol and bile salts ↑ proteolysis
    - —Glucagon phosphorylates and inhibits
    - —Insulin dephosphorylates and activates
    - —Inhibited by statins
- Mevalonate is then converted to isoprenes
  - Requires ATP
  - Isoprenes are used to make CoQ and dolichol phosphate
- Several isoprenes are condensed into squalene
- Squalene is converted to cholesterol
  - Multiple steps
  - An intermediate is lanosterol
- Fate of cholesterol varies with cell types

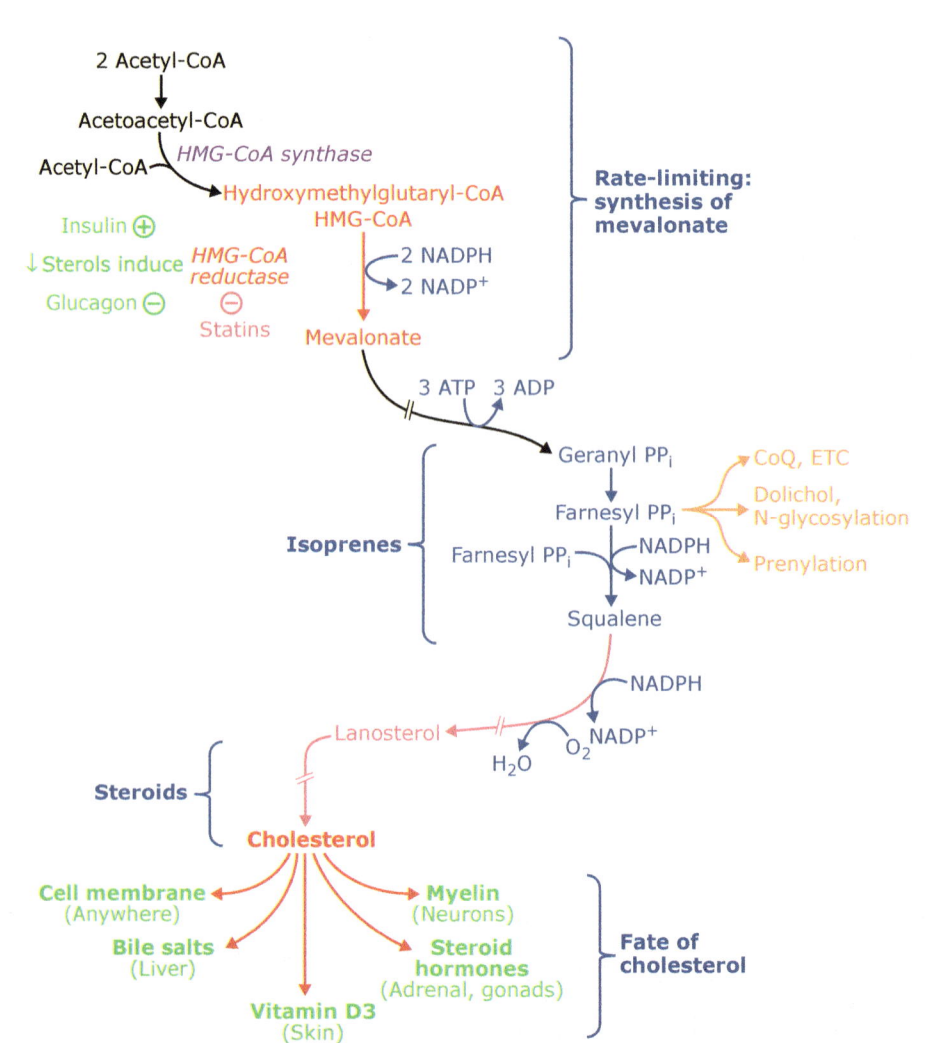

▶ Figure 9–8.1
Cholesterol Synthesis

8.2 Clinical Relevance

- **Smith-Lemli-Optiz syndrome:**
  - 7-dehydrocholesterol reductase deficiency
  - Autosomal recessive mutations in *DHCR7* gene, chromosome 11
  - Last step converting 7-dehydrocholesterol to cholesterol
  - Symptoms are correlated to:
    - —Low level of cholesterol
    - —Accumulation of 7-dehydrocholesterol
    - —Microcephaly, cleft lip/palate, polydactyly and syndactyly, and ambiguous genitalia
    - —Agenesis of corpus callosum and cerebellar hypoplasia
    - —Cardiac, renal, pulmonary, liver, and eye abnormalities
  - Rx is supportive:
    - —High cholesterol in diet
    - —Statins to ↓ levels of 7-DHC

- **Statins:**
  - Main class of cholesterol-lowering medication
  - Benefits:
    - —Reduces risks of heart attacks and stroke
  - ⊖ HMG CoA-reductase and ↓ mevalonate synthesis
  - Side effect of myalgia:
    - —↓ CoQ synthesis
    - —↓ ETC, ↓ ATP in skeletal muscle
    - —Cells swell, burst, myositis
    - —If too many, rhabdomyolysis and ATN/ARF
    - —Directly proportional to dosage and potency:
      - Atorvastatin and rosuvastatin are most potent
  - Rare hepatotoxicity
  - High risk of drug interactions

8.3 Bile Acids Synthesis

- Also referred to as bile salts:
  - Bile pigments are breakdown products of bilirubin
    — Heme degradation
- Needed for dietary lipid absorption
- Two types:
  - Chenodeoxycholic acid
  - Cholic acid
- Conjugation of bile salts:
  - With taurine
  - With glycine
  - Makes them good detergents
  - Can emulsify lipids
- Enterohepatic recirculation
- Clinical relevance: Bile sequestering resins
  - Cholestyramine, colestipol, colesevelam
  - Trap bile salts in gut
  - Prevent recirculation
  - Force hepatocytes to consume more cholesterol to make more bile salts
  - Lower intracellular cholesterol upregulates LDL receptors
    — ↓ Blood LDL
  - Side effects:
    — Steatorrhea
    — Vitamin K deficiency

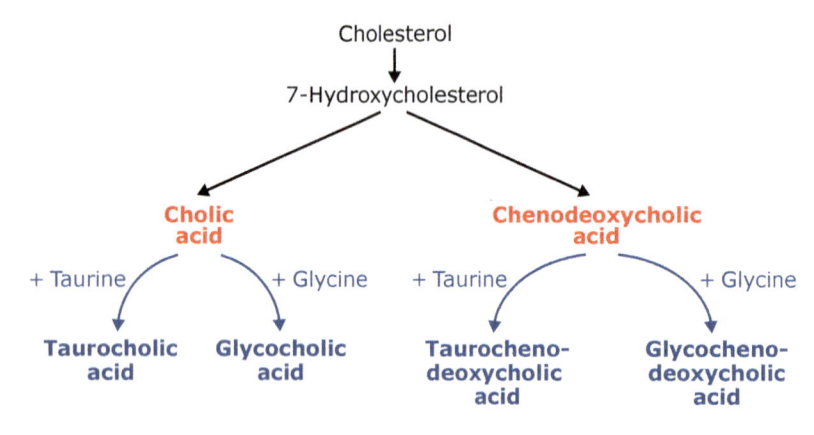

```
                    Cholesterol
                        ↓
                7-Hydroxycholesterol
                   ↙           ↘
              Cholic         Chenodeoxycholic
               acid                acid
           ↙        ↘          ↙           ↘
      +Taurine   +Glycine   +Taurine     +Glycine
         ↓          ↓          ↓            ↓
     Taurocholic Glycocholic Taurocheno-  Glycocheno-
        acid       acid     deoxycholic  deoxycholic
                                acid         acid
```

▲ **Figure 9-8.3** Bile Salts

9 Hyperlipidemias

- Acquired or genetic disorders of blood lipids/lipoproteins:
  - Primary hyperlipidemias are genetic
  - Secondary hyperlipidemias are acquired:
    —Diabetes
    —Obesity
- Two broad clinical consequences:
  - ↑ TGLs: ↑ Pancreatitis
  - ↑ Cholesterol: ↑ Cardiovascular/cerebrovascular risk
- Fredrickson classification of primary hyperlipidemia:
  - Based on electrophoresis or ultracentrifugation lipoprotein pattern
  - 5 types (I through V)

Table 9-3.1B — Fredrickson Classification of Familial Hyperlipidemias

Type		Name	Lipoproteins	Mechanism
I	I_a	Familial hyperchylomicronemia	Chylomicrons	↓ LPL
	I_b	Familial ApoC-II deficiency		↓ ApoC-II
II	II_a	Familial hypercholesterolemia	LDL	↓ LDL receptor
	II_b	Familial combined hyperlipidemia	LDL and VLDL	↓ LDL receptor and ↑ ApoB
III		Familial dysbetalipoproteinemia	IDL	↓ ApoE-2
IV		Familial hypertriglyceridemia	VLDL	↑ Production ↓ elimination
V		Familial mixed hyperlipidemia	VLDL and chylomicrons	↑ Production ↓ LPL

9.1 Familial Hypercholesterolemia

- Autosomal dominant
  - 1/500 (heterozygous)
- LDL receptor gene mutation:
  - Chromosome 19
  - >1,000 mutations known:
    —No expression (class I)
    —Stuck in ER/Golgi (class II)
    —Problem binding LDL (class III)
    —Defective endocytosis (class IV)
    —Lack of recycling (class V)
- ↑ Blood LDL ↑ chances of oxidation:
  - Early atherosclerosis

- Laboratory findings:
  - Heterozygous: Two- to three-fold ↑ in total cholesterol
  - Homozygous: Five- to six-fold ↑ in total cholesterol
- Physical signs:
  - Xanthelasma
  - Corneal arcus
  - Tendon xanthoma:
    — Pathognomonic
  - Ischemic disease:
    — Angina/MI
    — PVD
    — TIAs/strokes
- Treatment with lipid-lowering medication
  - HMG CoA-reductase inhibitors
    — +/− Bile sequestering resins
    — Ezetimibe:
      - ↓ Dietary cholesterol transport
    — Niacin, fibrates
  - Mipomersen:
    — Homozygous familial hypercholesterolemia only
    — Antisense RNA against ApoB-100 mRNA

9.2 Familial Hyperchylomicronemia
- Rare autosomal recessive disorder
- ↑ Chylomicrons = ↑ TGLs
  - Eruptive skin xanthomas
  - Acute pancreatitis
- Serum appearance:
  - Turbid with creamy supranate
  - Serum is clear in familial hypercholesterolemia
  - Rx: Diet

9.3 Diabetes as a Cause of Acquired Hyperlipidemia
- Similar to type V hyperlipidemia:
  - Mixed hyperlipidemia
- ↓ Insulin or insulin resistance:
  - ↓ Catabolism of VLDL and chylomicrons
  - ↓ LPL activity and ↑ HSL activity
  - ↑ Blood VLDL increases conversion to LDL
- Treatment:
  - Statins
  - Fibrates:
    — ⊕ PPARα
    — ↑ LPL expression

10 Abetalipoproteinemia

- Autosomal recessive
- Mutation in microsomal triglyceride transfer protein (MTP):
  - Required to manufacture chylomicrons and VLDL
  - Catalyzes binding of ApoB-48 and ApoB-100 to lipids
- Blood findings:
  - ↓ VLDL
  - ↓ Chylomicrons
- Symptoms/signs are secondary to decrease absorption of dietary fats:
  - Vitamins A, D, E, and K deficiencies:
    —Retinitis pigmentosa (↓ vitamin A)
    —Acanthocytosis (↓ vitamin E)
    —Degeneration of spinocerebellar tracts and dorsal columns (↓ Vitamin E)
    —Scoliosis (↓ vitamin D)
  - Steatorrhea
  - ↓ Linoleic and linolenic acids
  - Hypocholesterolemia
- Rx aims at supplementing essential lipids and vitamin E in particular

Glucagon World

Unit 4

CHAPTER 10 — Lipid Catabolism and Ketone Bodies

1 Overview

- **Glucagon world** pathways:
  - **Mobilization** of fat occurs upon fasting
  - **β-oxidation** of fatty acids supplies acetyl-CoA to generate ATP
  - In presence of ↑ ATP:
    — Excess hepatic acetyl-CoA is converted to **ketone bodies**
    — Ketones are a primary fuel for renal cortex and muscle
    — Ketones can become significant as CNS fuel during prolonged starvation
- β-oxidation and ketone body production occur at the same time as hepatic gluconeogenesis and glycogenolysis

USMLE® Key Concepts

For Step 1, you must be able to:
- Describe β-oxidation of fatty acids.
- Describe the consequences of defects in β-oxidation.
- Understand the role of liver-produced ketones as fuel for extrahepatic tissues.

2 Mobilization of Lipids

- **Hormone-sensitive lipase (HSL):**
  - ↓ Insulin, ↑ epinephrine, ↑ ACTH activate
  - Activation through cAMP and PKA
- Releases free fatty acids (FFAs) and glycerol
  - FFAs enter β-oxidation or ketogenesis (in liver)
  - Glycerol enters gluconeogenesis

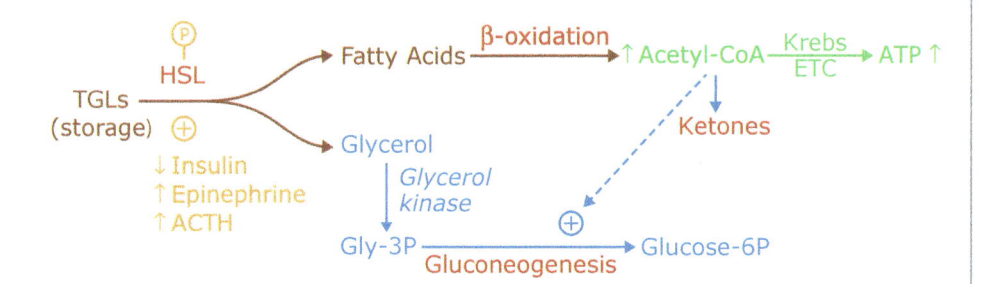

▲ Figure 10–2.0 Mobilization of Intracellular Lipids by HSL

3 β-Oxidation of Fatty Acids

- Occurs in mitochondria of all tissues except:
  - RBCs (no mitochondria)
  - CNS (fatty acids-albumin complex too large to cross the blood-brain barrier)
- Three-step process:
  - Activation to fatty acyl-CoA
  - Transport through carnitine shuttle
  - Oxidation to acetyl-CoA
- Levels of energy are primary control:
  - ↑ ATP inhibits
  - ↑ AMP activates
- Other modes of oxidation include:
  - ω-oxidation
  - α-oxidation
  - Peroxisomal oxidation

3.1 Activation of FFAs

- Carries in blood on albumin
- Released, enter cytosol
- Fatty acyl-CoA synthetase
  - Requires ATP
  - Generate a fatty acyl-CoA

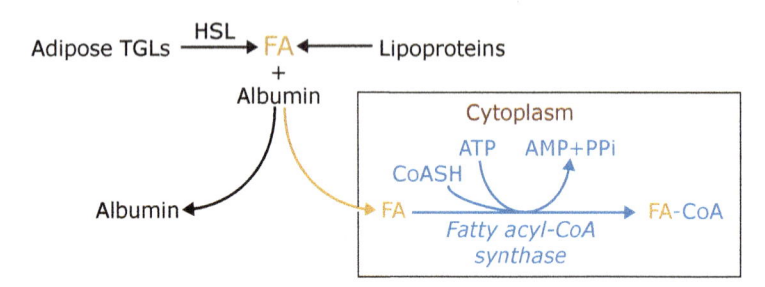

▲ Figure 10–3.1 Activation of Fatty Acids

3.2 Carnitine Shuttle

- Consists of 2 carnitine acyltransferases (CAT):
  - CAT I:
    - Outer mitochondrial membrane
    - Grabs the activated fatty acid
    - Rate-limiting:
      - Malonyl-CoA ⊖ CAT I
  - CAT II:
    - Mitochondrial matrix
    - Releases fatty acid as a fatty acyl-CoA
    - Regenerates free carnitine transporter
- CATs are also known as carnitine palmitoyltransferases (CPT)
- Relevance of malonyl-CoA ⊖ of CAT I
  - Malonyl-CoA is produced by acetyl-CoA carboxylase in fatty acid synthesis
  - Insulin ↑ malonyl-CoA
  - Glucagon ↓ malonyl-CoA
  - Indirect hormonal control of β-oxidation
  - Fatty acids cannot be made and broken at the same time

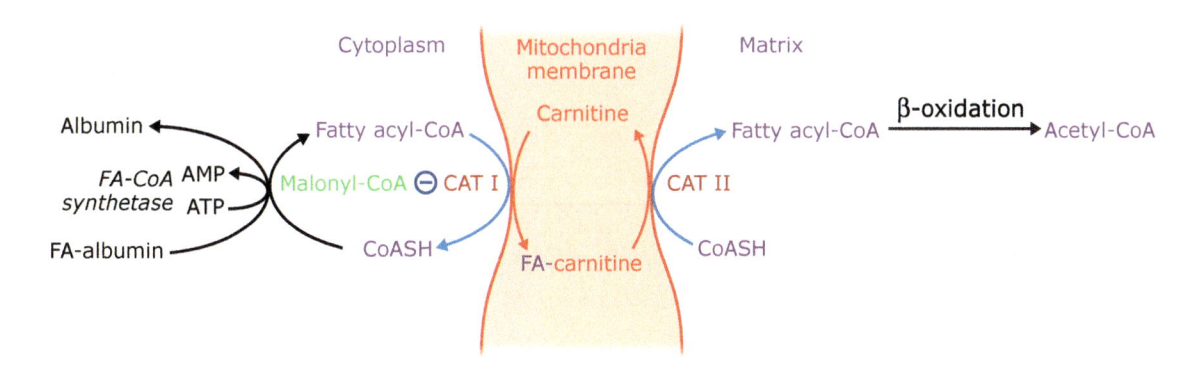

▲ Figure 10–3.2A Carnitine Shuttle

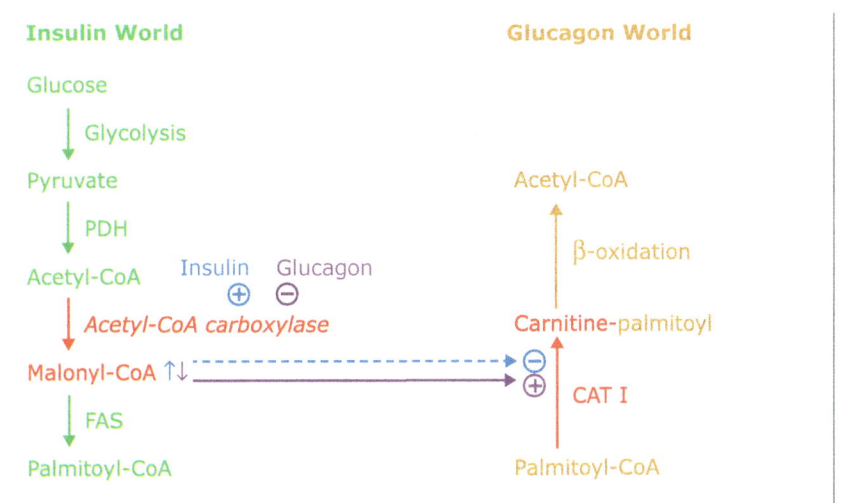

▲ Figure 10–3.2B Insulin and Glucagon Control of Lipid Metabolism

3.3 β-Oxidation of Even C-Chain Saturated Fatty Acids

- Four-step cycles inside mitochondria
- Produces FADH$_2$, NADH, and 1 acetyl-CoA per cycle
- Occurs in mitochondria
- The longer the fatty acid, the greater the amount of ATP generated
- Oxidation of 16C-long palmitate:
  - 7 NADH, 7 FADH$_2$, 8 acetyl-CoA
  - Approximately 129 ATPs (−2 for activation, 3/NADH, 2/FADH$_2$, 1/GTP)

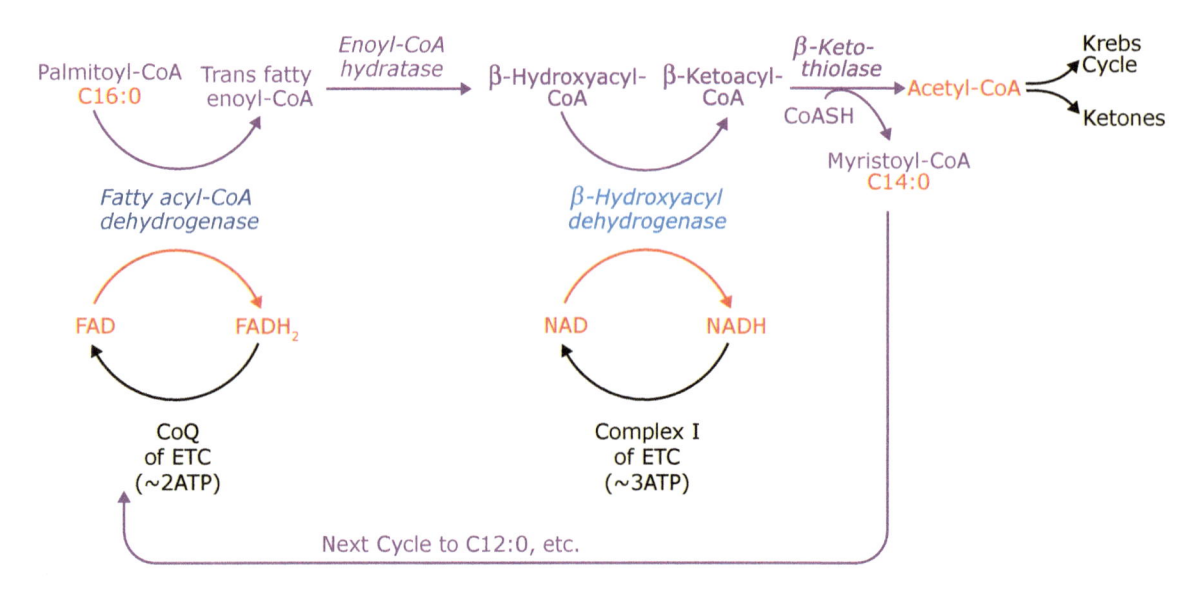

▲ Figure 10-3.3 β-Oxidation of Palmitoyl-CoA (C16:0)

3.4 Oxidation of Odd C-Chain Fatty Acids

- Produces acetyl-CoA and propionyl-CoA:
  - β-oxidation until production of C3 fragment propionyl-CoA
- Propionyl-CoA carboxylase and methylmalonyl-CoA mutase:
  - Convert propionyl-CoA to methylmalonyl-CoA and succinyl-CoA
- Succinyl-CoA can enter gluconeogenesis:
  - Exception to the rule that fatty acids cannot make glucose
- Propionyl-CoA carboxylase requires ATP, biotin, and CO_2
- Methylmalonyl-CoA mutase requires vitamin B12:
  - Methylmalonic aciduria is diagnostic of B12 deficiency

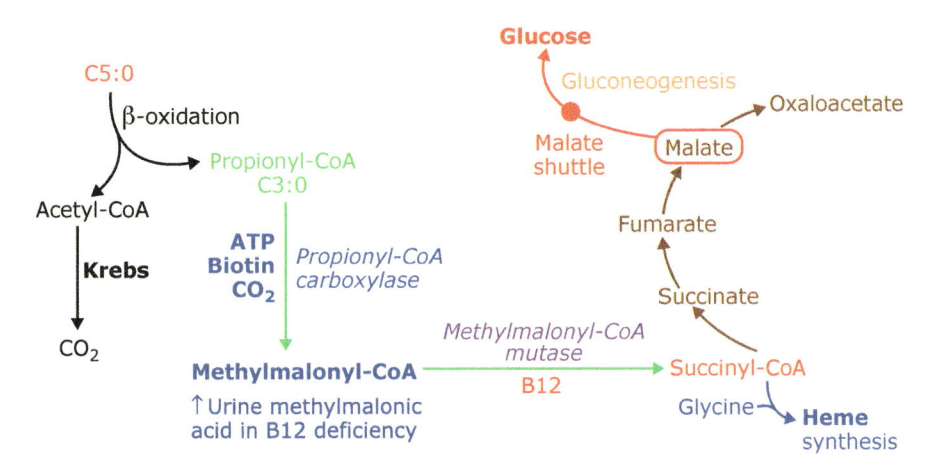

▲ Figure 10–3.4 Terminal Oxidation of Odd C-Chain Fatty Acids

3.5 Oxidation of Unsaturated Fatty Acids

- Requires extra enzymes to handle double bonds
- Yields less ATP than saturated fatty acids

3.6 ω-Oxidation of Fatty Acids

- The ω-carbon is the terminal –CH3 carbon of the fatty acid:
  - C16 of palmitate, for example
- ω-carbon is oxidized to a –COOH in the ER:
  - Forms a dicarboxylic acid
- Allows β-oxidation in mitochondria to proceed from the other end

3.7 α-Oxidation of Fatty Acids

- Specialized oxidation for branched chain fatty acids
- Common in CNS

3.8 Peroxisomal Oxidation of Fatty Acids

- Occurs in peroxisomes
- Uses O_2 and forms H_2O_2
- Starts oxidation of very-long-chain fatty acids (> 22C)
  - Once short enough, sent to mitochondria for β-oxidation

4 Clinical Relevance of Oxidation of Fatty Acids

- Several defects exist in catabolism of fatty acids
- These include:
  - Carnitine deficiency
  - Medium-chain acyl-CoA dehydrogenase (MCAD) deficiency
  - Peroxisomal disorders:
    - Adrenoleukodystrophy
    - Zellweger syndrome

4.1 Carnitine Deficiency

Several forms

- Systemic carnitine deficiency
- Autosomal recessive
  - Symptoms within a few hours of life:
    - Seizures
    - Arrhythmia
    - SIDS
    - Hypoketotic hypoglycemia
    - Similar to MCAD deficiency

- Carnitine palmitoyltransferase II deficiency:
  - Autosomal dominant
  - Myopathic only:
    - Affects skeletal muscle
    - Hereditary myoglobinuria
  - Severe form can be lethal early
  - Milder form presents later in life
  - Muscle weakness, cramping on prolonged exercise
    - ↓ ATP from lack of β-oxidation in type I muscle fibers
  - Rhabdomyolysis and ATN/ARF possible

Table 10-4.1 **Myopathic Carnitine Deficiency vs. McArdle Disease**

	Carnitine Deficiency	McArdle Disease
Enzyme	CPTII	Muscle glycogen phosphorylase
Muscle Type	Type I (slow twitch)	Type II (fast twitch)
Presentation	Weakness and cramping with prolonged exercise	Weakness and cramping at onset of exercise
Laboratory finding	↑ Blood acyl carnitine	↓ Blood lactate
Biopsy	↑ Muscle triglycerides	↑ Muscle glycogen
Rx	• Avoid fasting • Restrict lipid intake	• Avoid fasting • Sucrose prior to exercise

4.2 MCAD Deficiency

- Autosomal recessive
- MCAD is responsible for oxidation of C6–C12 fatty acids
- Affects liver ATP production
  - First fasting is associated with:
    - Profound hypoglycemia
    - Absence of ketones
    - Ketones would be ↑ in von Gierke disease
  - Greater ω-oxidation:
    - Dicarboxylic acidemia:
      - Urine adipic (6C) and suberic (8C) acids
  - ↑ Medium-chain acylcarnitine in blood
- Symptoms:
  - Hepatomegaly:
    - ↑ Medium-chain fatty acids
  - Vomiting, lethargy
  - Seizures, coma
  - SIDS
  - Precipitated by overnight fast, or infection with vomiting
- Rx:
  - Frequent feedings
  - Diet with slow-release carbohydrates (starches)

4.3 Peroxisomal Disorders

4.3.1 Adrenoleukodystrophy

- X-linked recessive
- *ABCD1* gene defect:
  - Peroxisome membrane transporter
- Accumulation of very-long-chain fatty acids:
  - Affects CNS, adrenal cortex, and Leydig cells
- Progressive demyelination leads to death
- Adrenal insufficiency (Addison) and sexual dysfunction
- Supportive Rx and poor prognosis

4.3.2 Zellweger Syndrome

- Cerebrohepatorenal syndrome
- A type of leukodystrophy
- Autosomal recessive:
  - PEX mutations:
    - *PEX* genes are involved in the genesis of peroxisomes
  - Impaired CNS development with hypomyelination
  - Hepatomegaly
  - Renal cysts
- Elevated very-long-chain fatty acids in plasma
- Rx is supportive

5 Ketogenesis and Ketogenolysis

- Ketogenesis takes place in the liver:
  - Glucagon world, ↑ ATP from the β-oxidation of fatty acids
  - Acetyl-CoA builds up and is used to make ketones
- Ketogenolysis occurs in extrahepatic tissues:
  - Muscles, kidney use ketones as a source of acetyl-CoA
  - Brain uses ketones in extreme starvation (> 4–5 days)

5.1 Ketogenesis in Hepatocytes

- Occurs in mitochondria
- Acetyl-CoA from β-oxidation is condensed to form:
  - Acetoacetate
  - β-hydroxybutyrate
  - Normal ratio in blood is 1:1
- Acetone is a by-product
  - Spontaneous decarboxylation of acetoacetate
  - Volatile
  - Imparts "fruity" smell to breath in diabetics

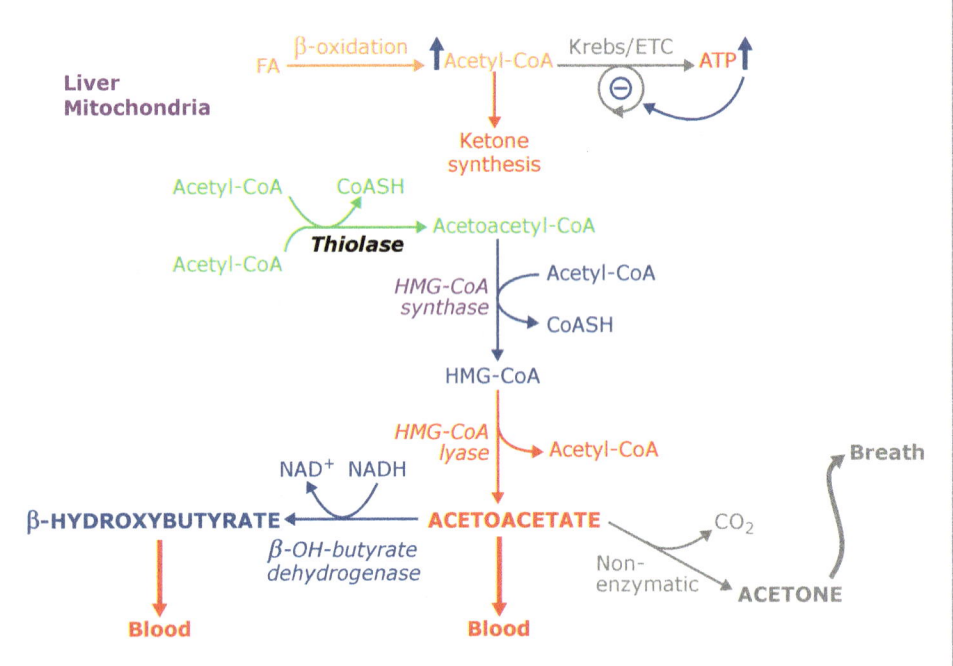

▲ Figure 10–5.1 Ketogenesis

5.2 Ketogenolysis

- **Extrahepatic mitochondria only:**
  - Muscle
  - Kidney
  - GI
  - Brain
- **Acetoacetate and β-hydroxybutyrate are transported into cells:**
  - Oxidation to acetyl-CoA
  - Mitochondrial matrix
  - Used in Krebs cycle
- **Succinyl-CoA:acetoacetate CoA transferase:**
  - Thiotransferase, also known as thiophorase
  - Critical in activation of ketone bodies
  - Absent in liver
  - No GTP formed
- Two cell types do not use ketones:
  - RBCs (no mitochondria)
  - Hepatocytes (no thiophorase)

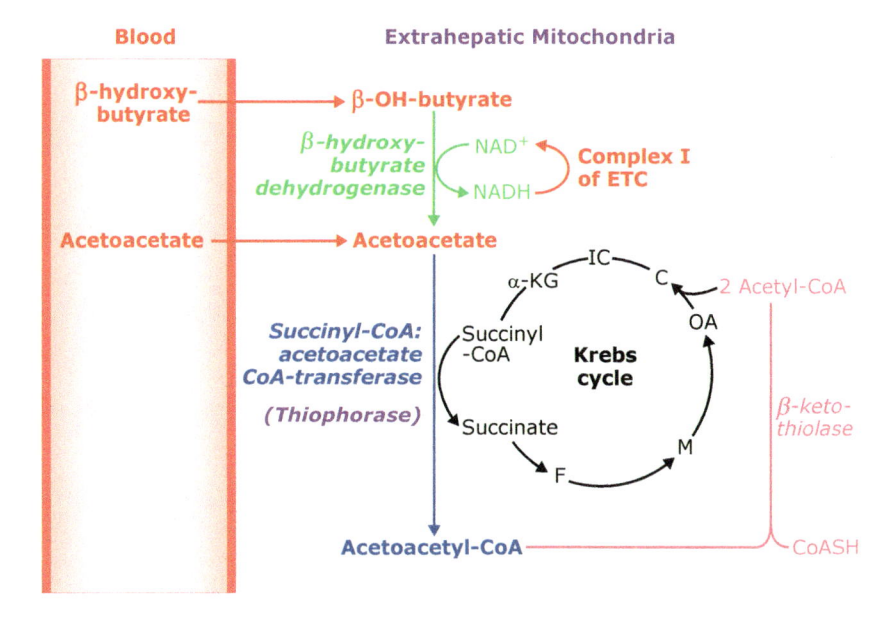

▲ **Figure 10–5.2A** Ketogenolysis

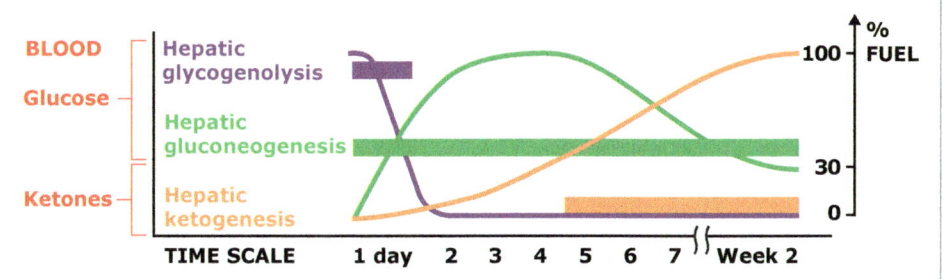

- In prolonged starvation, ketones will represent two thirds of fuel used by CNS
- Glucose from gluconeogenesis will represent one third, sparing muscle proteins

▲ **Figure 10–5.2B** Pattern of Fuel Used by Brain During Fasting

5.3 Clinical Relevance

5.3.1 Ketoacidosis

- Two common types:
  - Type 1 diabetes
  - Alcoholism
- Type 1 diabetes:
  - Lack of insulin world
  - Formation exceeds use
  - Accompanied by severe hyperglycemia:
    —Glucosuria and osmotic diseases
    —Hypokalemic state masked by mild hyperkalemia:
    - Acidosis causes intracellular K^+ shift outside
    - Secondary hyperaldosteronism due to osmotic diuresis wastes K^+
  - Metabolic acidosis with increased serum anion gap
  - Presentation:
    —Fruity breath odor
    —Vomiting
    —Dehydration (tachycardia, ↓ BP)
    —Confusion
    —Kussmaul breathing (deep, gasping)
    —Coma
  - Rx:
    —IV glucose + insulin
    —Fluid
    —K^+, HCO_3^-
- Alcoholism:
  - Alcohol ↓ gluconeogenesis:
    —Hypoglycemia ↑ mobilization of fatty acids
    —↑ Hepatic conversion to ketones
    —Dehydration exacerbates ketoacidosis
- Ketotic hypoglycemia of childhood:
  - Enzyme deficiencies:
    —Maple syrup urine disease
    —von Gierke disease
    —Galactosemia
    —Hereditary fructose intolerance

5.3.2 Ketogenic Diets

- High-fat diets:
    - Fat:carbohydrate ratio 3:1
- Used to ↓ epileptic seizures in children
- Ketones can be used by brain to make acetyl-CoA:
    - ↑ ATP, stabilizes membrane potential
    - Precursor of acetylcholine
- Used in PDH deficiency:
    - Ketones become source of acetyl-CoA
- Medium-chain TGLs induce ketosis most efficiently

CHAPTER 11: Gluconeogenesis and Glycogenolysis

1 Overview

- Maintenance of blood glucose during fasting:
  - Performed by liver glycogenolysis and gluconeogenesis
  - Required for RBCs and neurons
- Energy required to maintain blood glucose:
  - Hepatocytes exclusively burn fat to provide ATP for gluconeogenesis
- Glycogen is a finite store:
  - Main source of fasting glucose for 8–12 hours
  - Exhausted within a day or so
- Gluconeogenesis represents a net synthesis of glucose:
  - Within 4 hours of a meal, gluconeogenesis supplies increasing percentage of fasting blood glucose
  - By 30 hours of fasting, gluconeogenesis becomes the sole source of blood glucose
- Hormonal changes during fasting:
  - Insulin decreases
  - Glucagon, epinephrine, and cortisol increase
  - These hormonal changes promote gluconeogenesis and glycogenolysis
  - They also promote mobilization of fat and lipolysis, as well as ketone body synthesis

USMLE® Key Concepts

For Step 1, you must be able to:

- Describe gluconeogenesis.
- Contrast glycogenolysis in liver vs. muscle.
- Discuss glycogen storage diseases.

Chapter 11 • Gluconeogenesis and Glycogenolysis

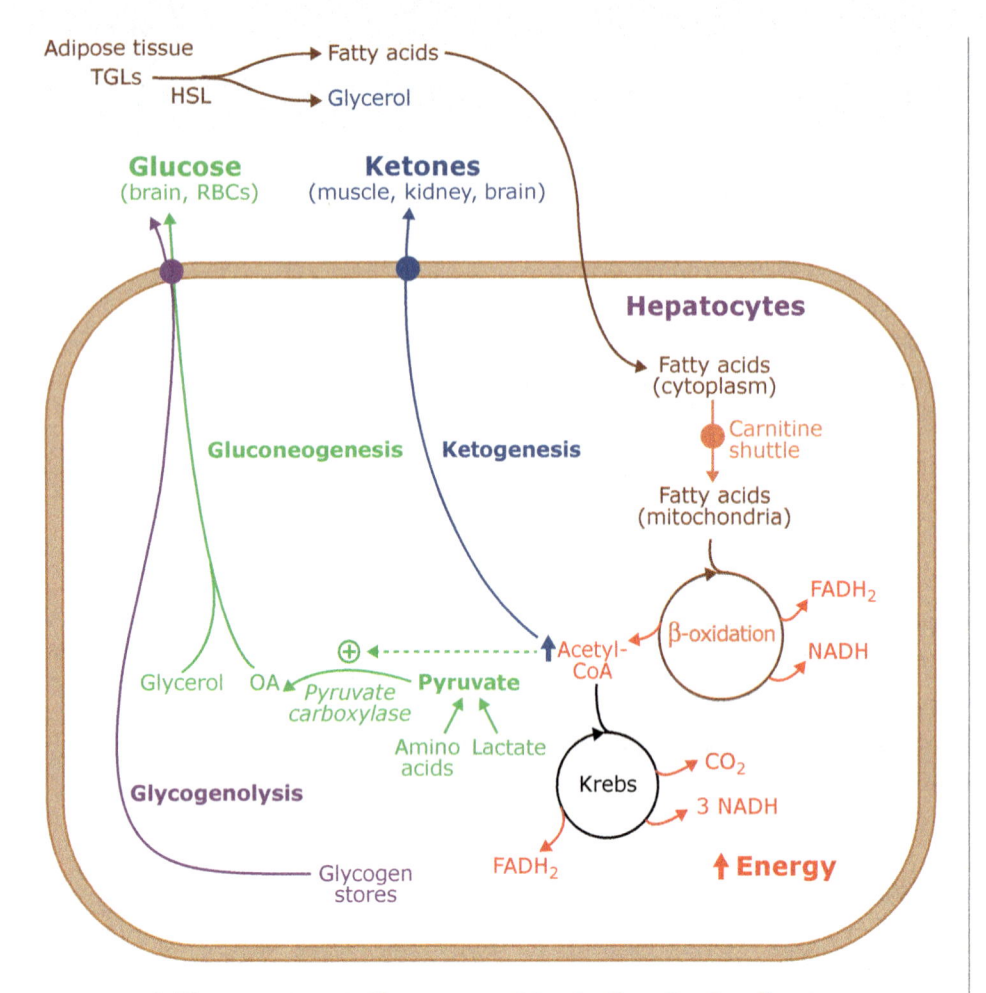

▲ **Figure 11-1.0** Hepatocyte Metabolism During Fasting

2 Glycogenolysis

2.1 Glycogen Phosphorylase and Debranching Enzyme

- **Glycogen phosphorylase:**
  - Rate limiting
  - Breaks α-1,4 bonds between glucoses
  - Releases glucose-1P
  - Stops 4 glucose units short of a branching point
- **Debranching enzyme:**
  - Has two enzymatic activities:
    — Glucosyltransferase
    — α-1,6 glucosidase
  - Glucosyltransferase removes 3 glucose residues:
    — Transfers them to the end of another chain
    — Attaches through α-1,4 linkage
  - **α-1,6 glucosidase cleaves the single branch residue:**
    — Releases a free glucose
- Cycles of phosphorylase/debranching continue until glycogen is exhausted

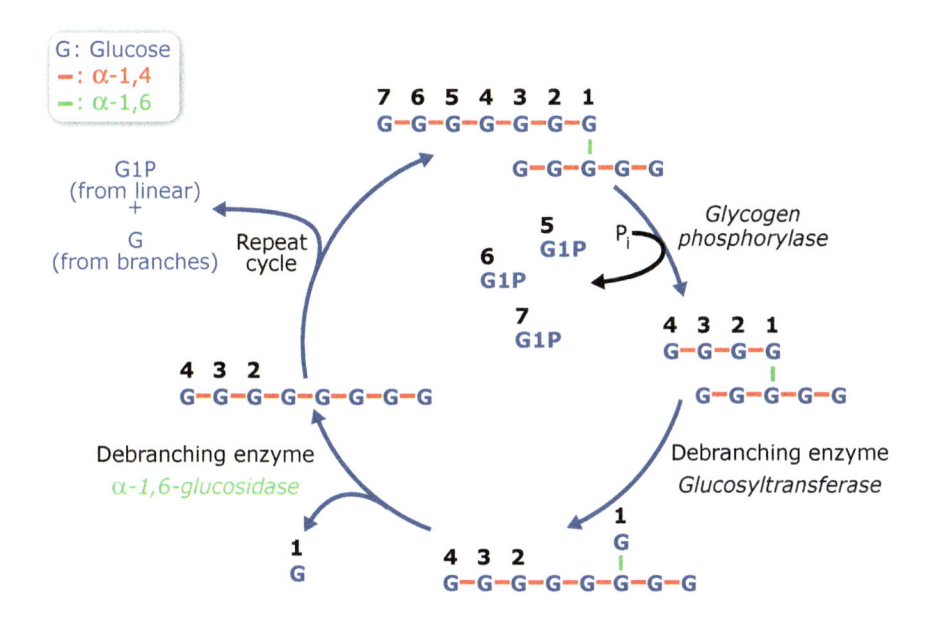

▲ **Figure 11–2.1** Actions of Glycogen Phosphorylase and Debranching Enzyme

2.2 Fate of Glucose Released in Glycogenolysis

- Hepatic glycogenolysis:
  - Liver releases all glucose units in blood:
    — For extrahepatic use only
  - Liver has glucose-6-phosphatase:
    — Untraps sugar
- Muscle glycogenolysis:
  - Muscle uses glucose for itself
  - Muscle does not have glucose-6-phosphatase

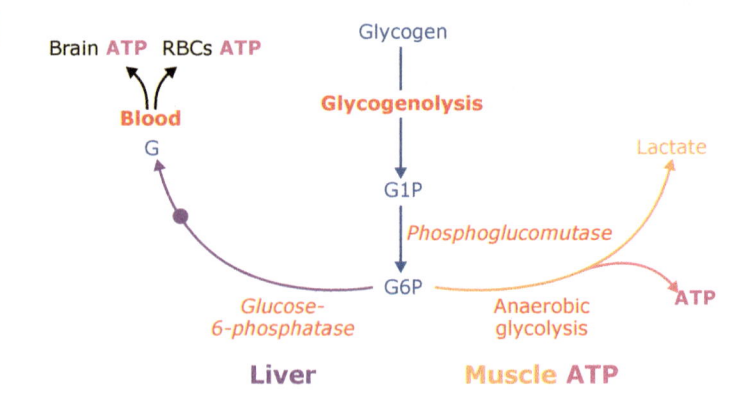

▲ Figure 11-2.2 Fate of Hepatic and Muscle Glycogen

2.3 Role of Lysosomes

- Excess glycogen is removed in lysosomes:
  - α-1,4 glucosidase called acid maltase
  - Unless fasting lasts more than 1 day, stores must be degraded
  - See Pompe disease

2.4 Control of Glycogen Phosphorylase

- Insulin dephosphorylates and inactivates the enzyme
- Glucagon phosphorylates and activates the enzyme
- Local regulation:
  - AMP and Ca^{2+} activate in muscle only
  - AMP does NOT activate hepatic glycogenolysis
  - In muscle, calmodulin is a subunit of phosphorylase kinase

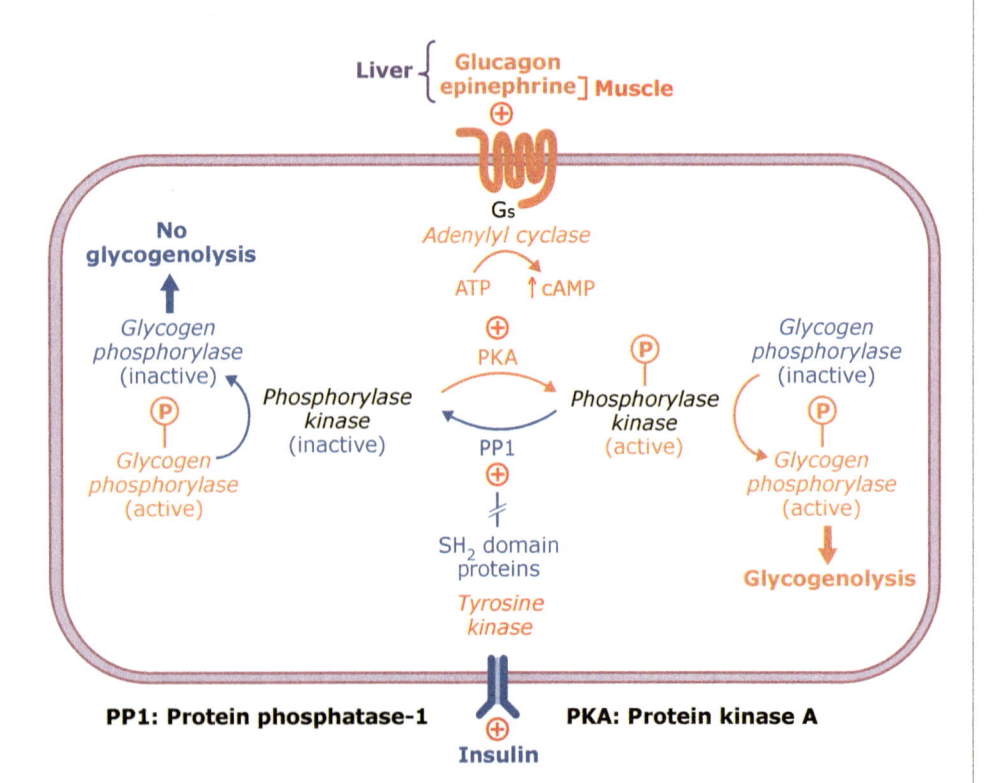

PP1: Protein phosphatase-1   PKA: Protein kinase A

▲ Figure 11-2.4 Hormonal Control of Glycogen Phosphorylase

3 Gluconeogenesis

3.1 Substrates for Gluconeogenesis

- Three important substrates:
  - Lactate:
    —Anaerobic activity in RBCs, muscle
  - Glycerol:
    —HSL activity in adipose
  - 18 out of 20 amino acids:
    —Proteolysis in muscle
- Acetyl-CoA from β-oxidation cannot be converted back to glucose:
  - PDH is irreversible
  - Glucose can be converted to fatty acids (insulin, ↑ ATP)
  - Fatty acids cannot be converted back to glucose during fasting
    —Minor exception with propionyl-CoA from odd-C chains FAs

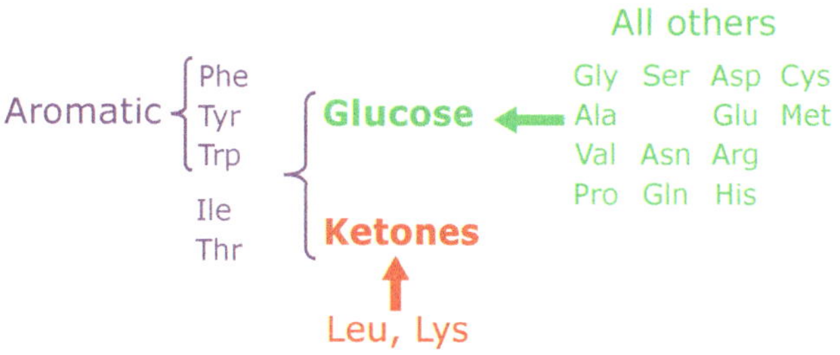

▲ Figure 11–3.1 Glucogenic and Ketogenic Amino Acids

3.2 Circumventing Glycolysis

- Three irreversible steps in glycolysis:
  - Hexokinase/glucokinase
  - PFK-1
  - Pyruvate kinase
- Different enzymes are needed to circumvent these three steps

Table 11-3.2 Circumventing Glycolysis Irreversible Steps

Glycolysis	Gluconeogenesis
Hexokinase/glucokinase	Glucose-6-phosphatase
PFK-1	Fructose-1,6-bisphosphatase
Pyruvate kinase	Pyruvate carboxylase Malate dehydrogenase Phosphoenolpyruvate carboxykinase

Chapter 11 • Gluconeogenesis and Glycogenolysis

- **Hepatocytes require ↑ ATP to carry out gluconeogenesis**
  - Energy comes from β-oxidation of fatty acids
  - A defect in β-oxidation will result in fasting hypoglycemia

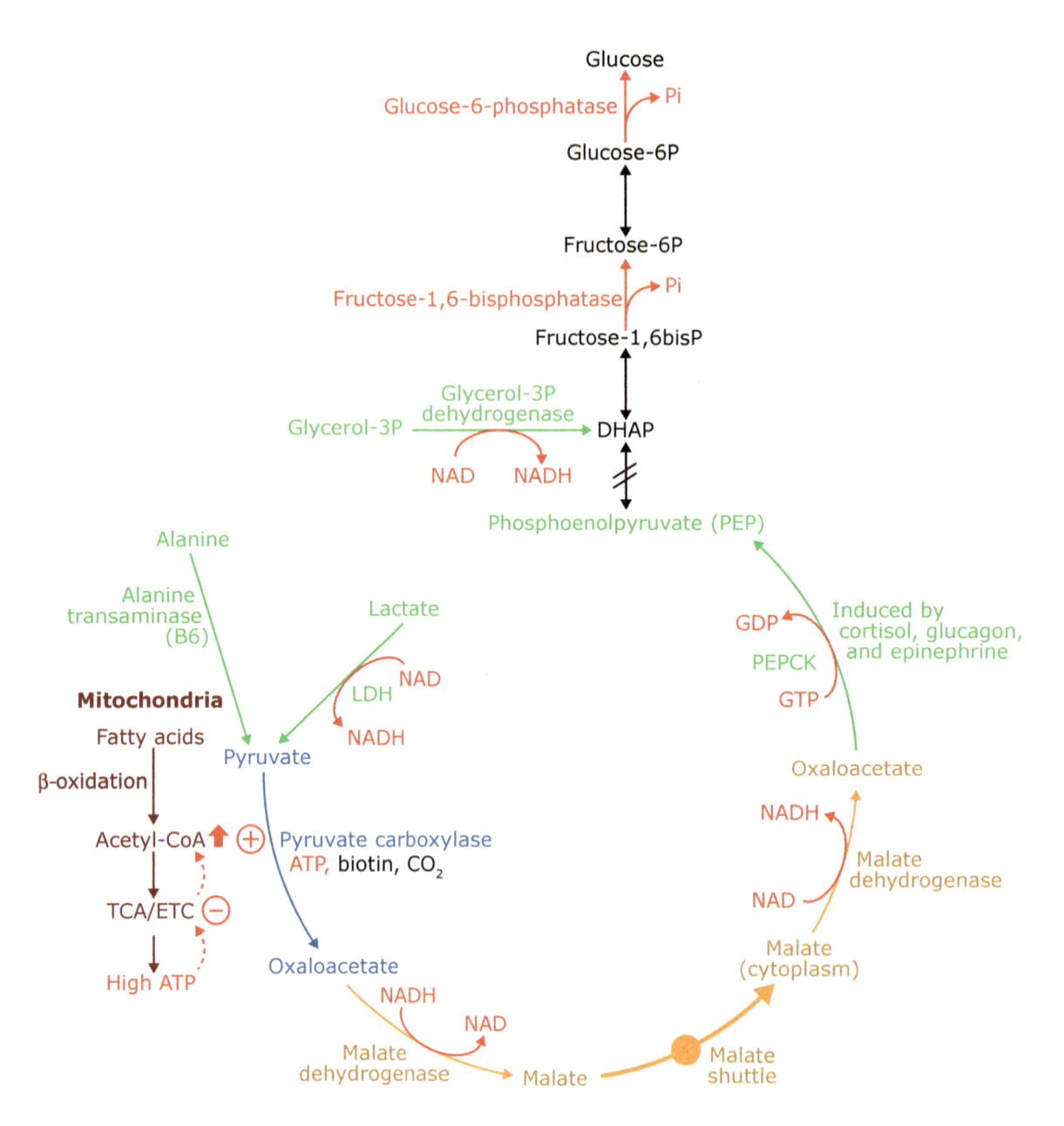

▲ Figure 11-3.2 Gluconeogenesis in Hepatocytes

3.3 Important Enzymes

- **Pyruvate carboxylase:**
  - Mitochondrial
  - Requires ATP, biotin, CO_2 ("ABC" enzyme)
  - Acetyl-CoA is an allosteric activator
- **Phosphoenolpyruvate carboxykinase:**
  - Cytoplasmic
  - Requires GTP
  - Induced by stress hormones
- **Fructose-1,6-bisphosphatase**
  - Cytoplasmic
  - Rate-limiting
  - Opposite regulation from PFK-1

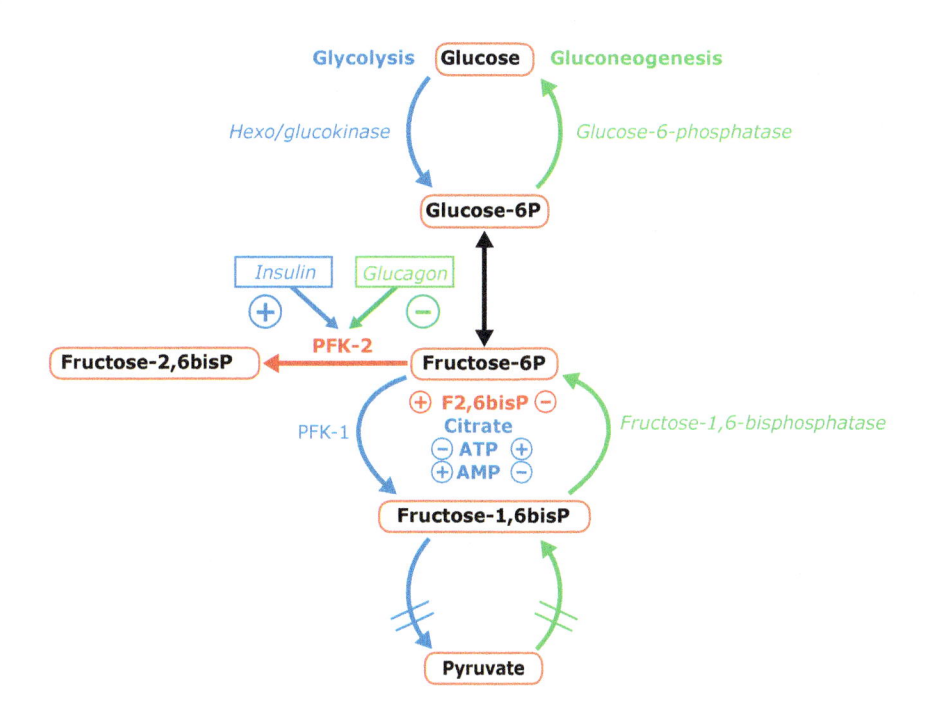

▲ **Figure 11-3.3** Glycolysis vs. Gluconeogenesis

- **Glucose-6-phosphatase (G6Pase):**
  - Final step for liver glycogenolysis and gluconeogenesis
  - Primarily expressed in hepatocytes:
    —Allows release of newly synthesized glucose in blood
  - Expression in renal cortex:
    —Allows reabsorption of existing filtered glucose
  - G6Pase is located in ER membrane:
    —Active site is in lumen of ER
    —Glucose is exocytosed by ER fusion with cell membrane

4 Cori and Alanine Cycles

- Hepatic gluconeogenesis recycles metabolites from RBCs and muscle:
  - In doing so, hepatocytes provide glucose back to these tissues

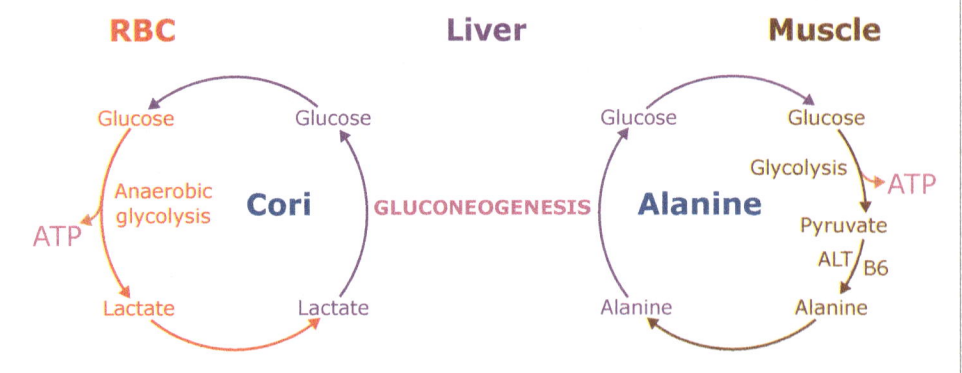

▲ Figure 11–4.0 Cori and Alanine Cycles

5 Clinical Relevance

5.1 Glycogen Storage Diseases
- Also known as dextrinoses
- 11 diseases that affect liver, muscle, or other tissues
  - Three are most important:
    - von Gierke: Type I
    - McArdle: Type V
    - Pompe: Type II

5.1.1 von Gierke Disease
- Glucose-6-phosphatase deficiency:
  - Affects liver and kidney
  - Autosomal recessive:
    - Type Ia = enzyme deficiency
    - Type Ib = microsomal G6P transport deficiency
  - Characterized by severe fasting hypoglycemia:
    - Hepatocytes cannot release glucose in the blood upon fasting
    - Seizures, developmental delay
  - Hyperlipidemia:
    - Low blood glucose ↓ insulin, ↑ glucagon, epinephrine
    - Results in ↑ HSL and lipid mobilization
  - Lactacidemia:
    - ↑ Lactate from disruption of Cori cycle

- **Hyperuricemia:**
  - Phosphate trapping ↓ purine salvage by PRTases
- **Hepatomegaly, cirrhosis, and liver failure:**
  - ↑ G6P and lactate contribute to osmotic and pH-induced damages
  - Abdominal protuberance
- **Fanconi syndrome:**
  - Renal PCT get damaged by ↑ G6P
  - U/S: Enlarged kidneys

■ Diagnosis:
  - If severe, infant dies after overnight fast
  - If mild, symptoms are precipitated by prolonged fasting:
    - Child with gastroenteritis
    - Seizures, severe hypoglycemia after 2–3 days

■ Rx:
  - Frequent feeding
  - Diet high in carbohydrates
  - Liver transplant in most severe cases

5.1.2 McArdle Disease

■ **Muscle glycogen phosphorylase deficiency:**
  - Only affects skeletal muscle:
    - Fast twitch, type II fibers
    - Use glycogen as source of glucose for anaerobic glycolysis
    - No hypoglycemia

■ **Weakness, cramping at onset of exercise:**
  - Second wind when slow twitch, type I fibers take over
  - Type I fibers use fatty acids for aerobic metabolism
  - Possible **myoglobinuria:**
    - From rhabdomyolysis after intense exercise

■ Autosomal recessive:
  - Generally late diagnosis
  - Muscle fatigue after excess exercise in older child, young adults

■ Rx:
  - Aerobic exercise and appropriate diet (carbs, proteins) prior to exercise

5.1.3 Pompe Disease

- **Lysosomal α-1,4 glucosidase deficiency:**
  - Also known as acid maltase
  - Degrades excess glycogen
- **Multiple organs affected:**
  - Liver
  - Heart
  - Skeletal muscle
  - CNS
- Death from **restrictive cardiomyopathy:**
  - Cardiorespiratory failure: Death < 2 years
  - A late onset form is described with minimal cardiac involvement
- **Rx:**
  - Enzyme replacement therapy

Table 11-5.1 Glycogenoses

Eponym	Type	Enzyme Deficiency	Tissue	Key Point
von Gierke	I	Glucose-6-phosphatase	Liver	Severe fasting hypoglycemia
Pompe	II	α-1,4 glucosidase	Heart Muscle Liver CNS	Restrictive cardiomyopathy
Cori	III	Debranching enzyme	Muscle Liver Heart	Short outer branches (limit dextrinosis)
Andersen	IV	Branching enzyme	Liver Heart Muscle	Long linear glycogen
McArdle	V	Glycogen phosphorylase	Muscle	Muscle weakness Onset of exercise No hypoglycemia
Hers	VI	Glycogen phosphorylase	Liver	Mild hypoglycemia
Tarui	VII	PFK	Muscle RBC	Muscle weakness Hemolytic anemia

5.2 Chronic Alcoholism and Hypoglycemia

- Ethanol metabolism yields ↑ NADH, ↑ ATP in hepatocytes
- ↑ NADH reverses dehydrogenases of gluconeogenesis:
  - LDH:
    —Favors pyruvate conversion to lactate
    —Lactic acidosis
    —Hyperuricemia and gout:
    - Lactate competes with urate for excretion
  - Cytoplasmic malate dehydrogenase:
    —Favors oxaloacetate conversion back to malate
  - Glycerol-3P dehydrogenase:
    —Favors DHAP conversion to glycerol-3-phosphate
    —↑ Glycerol-3P
    - Combines with unoxidized free fatty acid
    - Results in abnormal build up of TGLs
    - Macrovesicular steatosis
- Results in chronic fasting hypoglycemia
- ↑ ATP from ethanol metabolism ↓ β-oxidation of fatty acids

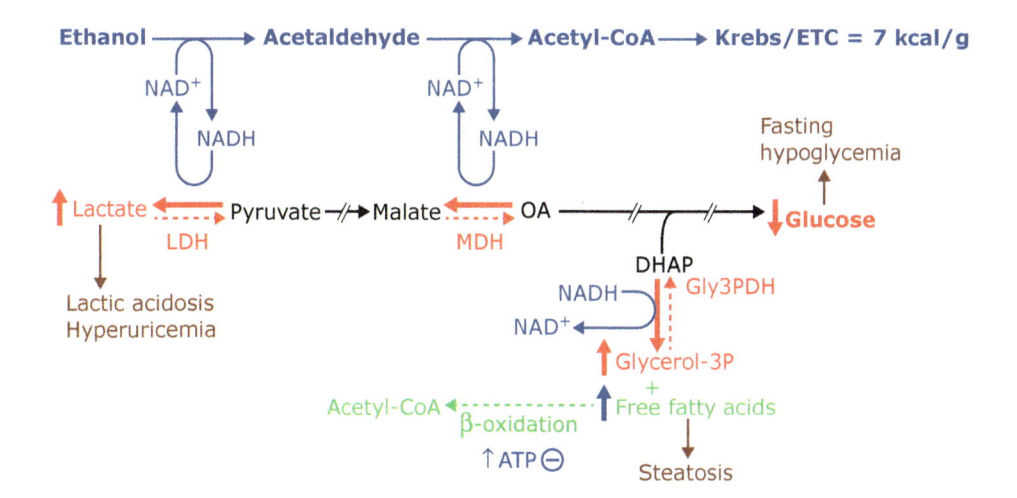

▲ Figure 11–5.2 Alcoholism and Gluconeogenesis

Protein World

Unit 5

CHAPTER 12: Protein Digestion and Ammonia Detoxification

1 Overview

- Stomach and pancreatic proteases:
  - Digest dietary proteins into small peptides
- Intestinal peptidases:
  - Convert peptides into individual amino acids
- Amino acid transport:
  - Na$^+$-dependent
  - Na$^+$-independent
- Amino acids can be catabolized to produce energy
  - 10%–35% of total calorie intake
  - 4 kcal/g
- Amino acids are required for translation
- Amino acids are precursors of important products:
  - Glucose (gluconeogenesis)
  - Neurotransmitters
  - Heme
  - Nucleotides
  - Creatine
  - Sphingosine
- Metabolism of amino acids releases ammonia:
  - Toxicity:
    —Associated with encephalopathy
  - Liver detoxification:
    —Urea cycle
  - Renal elimination:
    —Urea
    —Ammonium chloride

USMLE® Key Concepts

For Step 1, you must be able to:

- Describe the process of protein digestion.
- Understand the role of the urea cycle in detoxification of ammonia.
- Discuss urea cycle enzyme deficiencies.

Chapter 12 • Protein Digestion and Ammonia Detoxification — Biochemistry

2 Dietary Protein Digestion and Absorption

2.1 Digestion

- Denaturation by stomach acid
- Pepsin:
  - Gastric chief cells produce pepsinogen:
    - Located in fundus
    - Base of glands
  - Parietal cells release HCL:
    - Activates pepsinogen into pepsin
  - Gastrin and PANS stimulate chief and parietal cells
- Pancreatic zymogens:
  - Trypsinogen:
    - Activated by gut enteropeptidase
  - Chymotrypsinogen, proelastase, procarboxypeptidases:
    - Activated in gut by trypsin
- Intestinal peptidases:
  - Aminopeptidases:
    - Brush border
    - Cleave one amino acid at a time

2.2 Absorption

- Absorption of dietary amino acids
  - Na^+-cotransport:
    - Secondary active
  - Facilitated diffusion
  - Same transporters in renal epithelium
  - Similar to carbohydrate transport

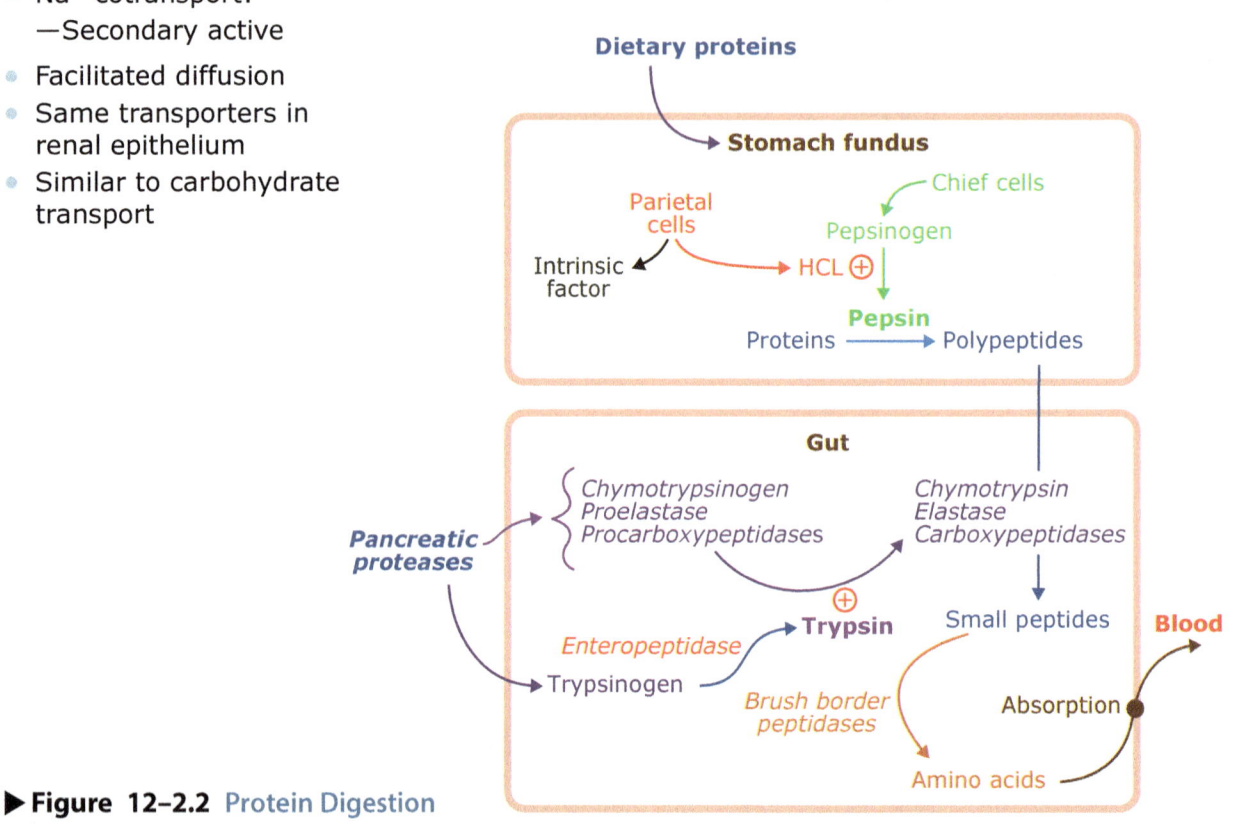

▶ Figure 12-2.2 Protein Digestion

3 Detoxification of Amino Acid Nitrogen

- Glutamate plays a key role:
  - Transaminations
  - Glutamate dehydrogenase
  - Glutamine synthetase
  - Glutaminase
- Glutamine and alanine carry nitrogen from periphery to liver

3.1 Transamination Reactions

- Transaminases transfer an amino group to a ketoacid
  - Ketoacid becomes an amino acid
  - The original amino acid becomes a ketoacid

Amino acid ⇌ Ketoacid (B6)
Ketoacid ⇌ Amino acid

Amino acid ⇌ Ketoacid (B6)
α-ketoglutarate ⇌ Glutamate

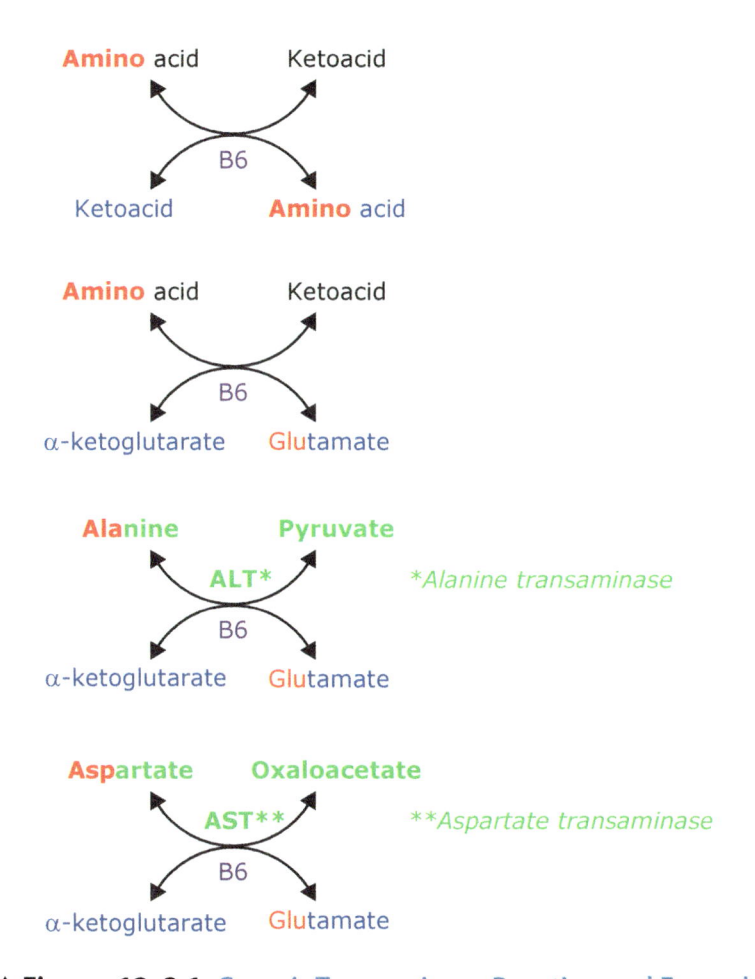

Alanine ⇌ Pyruvate (ALT*, B6)   *Alanine transaminase
α-ketoglutarate ⇌ Glutamate

Aspartate ⇌ Oxaloacetate (AST**, B6)   **Aspartate transaminase
α-ketoglutarate ⇌ Glutamate

▲ Figure 12-3.1 Generic Transaminase Reaction and Examples

- All amino acids except lysine and threonine undergo transaminations
- Most reactions use α-KG and glutamate
- All transaminases require pyridoxal phosphate (PLP):
  - Derived from vitamin B6
- Aspartate can enter the urea cycle

3.2 Glutamate Dehydrogenase

- Found in mitochondria of most cells
- Reversible
- Can incorporate ammonia from deaminations
- In liver can release ammonia into urea cycle

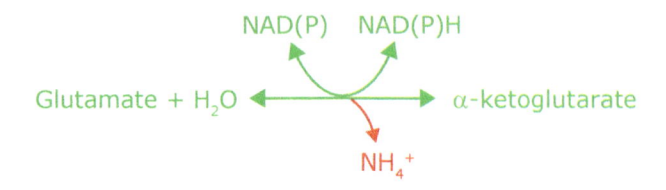

Glutamate + H_2O ⇌ α-ketoglutarate
(NAD(P) → NAD(P)H; NH$_4^+$)

▲ Figure 12-3.2 Glutamate Dehydrogenase

3.3 Glutamine Synthetase

- Found in cytoplasm of all cells
- Glutamate accepts ammonia to become glutamine
- Requires ATP
- Glutamine safely takes ammonia to liver

Glutamate → Glutamine → To liver
(NH$_4^+$; ATP → ADP)

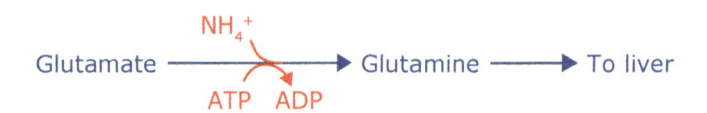

▲ Figure 12-3.3 Glutamine Synthetase

3.4 Glutaminase

- Liver glutaminase:
  - Releases NH_4^+ into urea cycle
- Kidney glutaminase:
  - Releases NH_4^+ in urine
  - Excreted as NH_4Cl
  - Important form of acid excretion:
    — Non-titratable acid
- Intestinal glutaminase:
  - Releases NH_4^+ in gut
  - Portal circulation delivers NH_4^+ to liver
  - Enters urea cycle

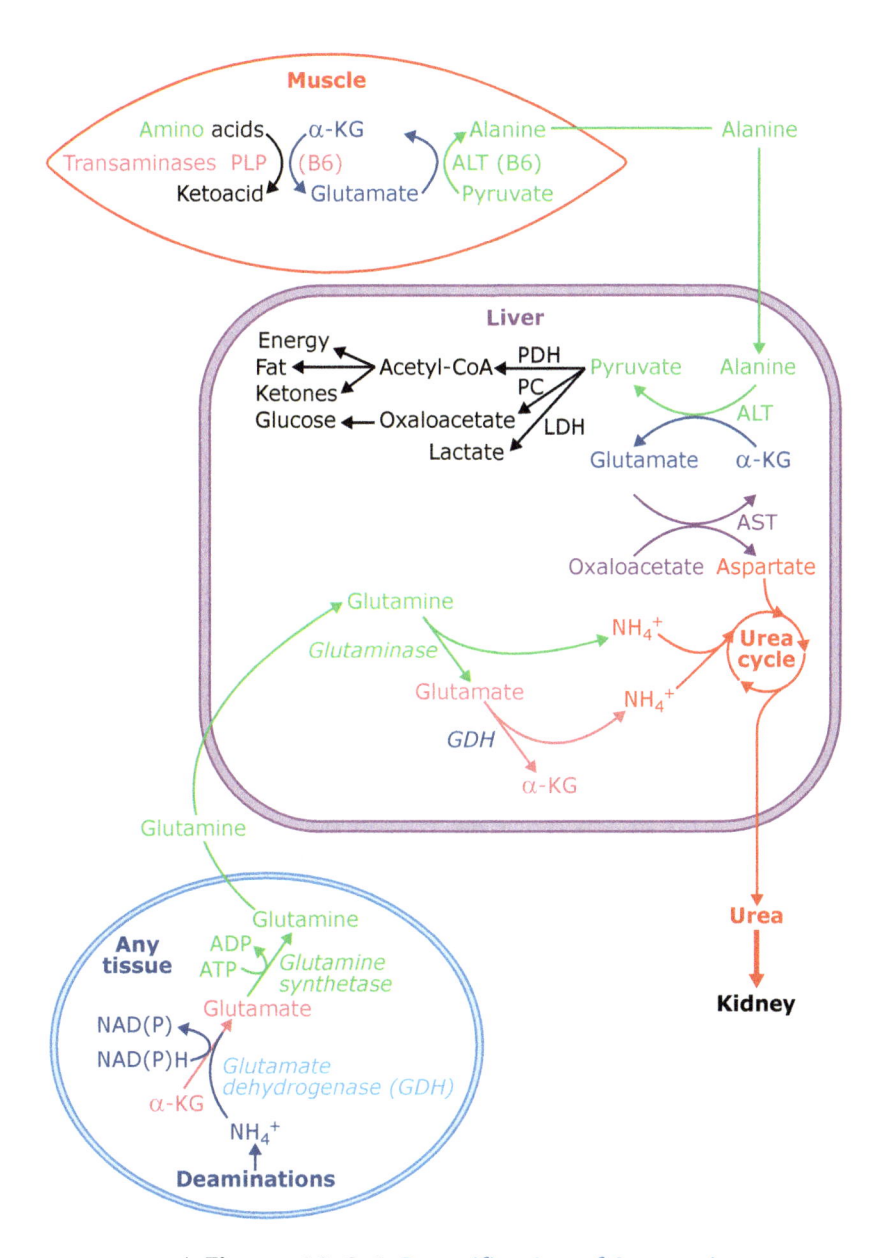

▲ Figure 12-3.4 Detoxification of Ammonia

Chapter 12 • Protein Digestion and Ammonia Detoxification — Biochemistry

4 Urea Cycle

- Four-step cycle
  - Spans mitochondria and cytoplasm
  - Only occurs in liver
  - Requires energy
- Two points of entry for nitrogen:
  - NH_4^+ as carbamoyl phosphate
  - Aspartate from AST
- Two products of the urea cycle:
  - Urea
  - Fumarate

Mitochondria

Deaminations / GI/liver glutaminase / Glutamate dehydrogenase → $NH_3 + H^+ + HCO_3^-$ ← CO_2, H_2O — Krebs cycle, ETC

N-acetylglutamate ⊕ → Carbamoyl P synthetase I (CPS I) — 2ATP → 2ADP + P_i

↓

Carbamoyl Phosphate

Ornithine transcarbamoylase (OTC)

Ornithine ← → Citrulline

Ornithine translocase

Cytoplasm

Ornithine ← Citrulline

Transaminations / AST, B6

Urea ← Arginase ← Arginine ← Argininosuccinate lyase ← Argininosuccinate ← Argininosuccinate synthetase ← Citrulline

H_2O, Aspartate, ATP → AMP

Fumarate

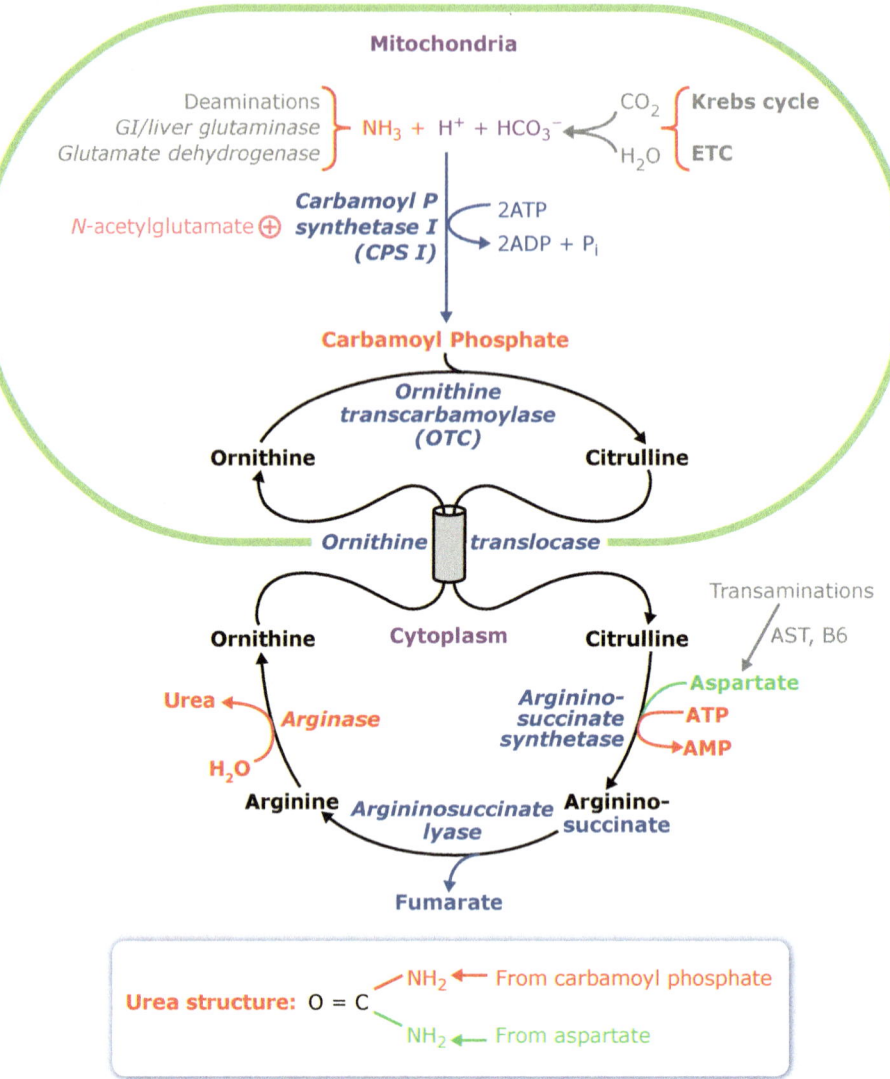

Urea structure: $O=C \begin{array}{l} NH_2 \leftarrow \text{From carbamoyl phosphate} \\ NH_2 \leftarrow \text{From aspartate} \end{array}$

▲ Figure 12–4.0A Urea Cycle

- Regulation of urea cycle:
  - N-acetylglutamate (NAG)
  - Allosteric activation of CPSI
  - NAG synthase is ⊕ by arginine
  - All enzymes in the urea cycle are also induced in a high-protein diet or in prolonged starvation:
    —Conditions ↑ requirement for protein breakdown

Glutamate + Acetyl-CoA — NAG Synthase ⊕ Arginine → N-acetylglutamate

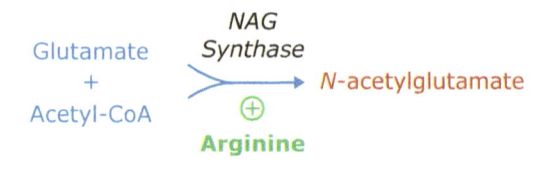

▲ Figure 12–4.0B N-Acetylglutamate (NAG) Production

5 Clinical Relevance: Urea Cycle Enzyme Deficiencies

- Six disorders
- All cause ↑ ammonia, ↑ glutamine, ↓ urea in blood:
- Ammonia is toxic to the nervous system:
  - All cause encephalopathy:
    - —Ammonia → osmotic swelling
      - Brain edema, seizures
    - —Ammonia and high glutamine damage membranes
      - Including mitochondrial membrane
    - —↓ CNS glutamate as it becomes glutamine
      - ↓ Neural activity
      - Lethargy, coma
- Treatment:
  - All benefit from low-protein diet
  - Glycerol phenylbutyrate:
    - —Triglyceride with N_2-binding capacity
    - —Prodrug
    - —Traps ammonia
    - —Urine excretion
  - Arginine therapy:
    - —High amounts of arginine lead to more ornithine made

Chapter 12 • Protein Digestion and Ammonia Detoxification

- **Differential diagnosis:**
  - Based on intermediate/metabolite accumulation

$$NH_4^+ + HCO_3^-$$

Glu + Acetyl-CoA ⟶ **NAG** ⊕

NAG synthetase deficiency
- AR
- Fatal
- Dx: DNA sequencing
- Rx: Supportive and carbamylglutamate

CPSI deficiency
- Rare
- AR
- No orotic acid
- ↑ Ammonia
- Fatal in infancy

Carbamoyl P

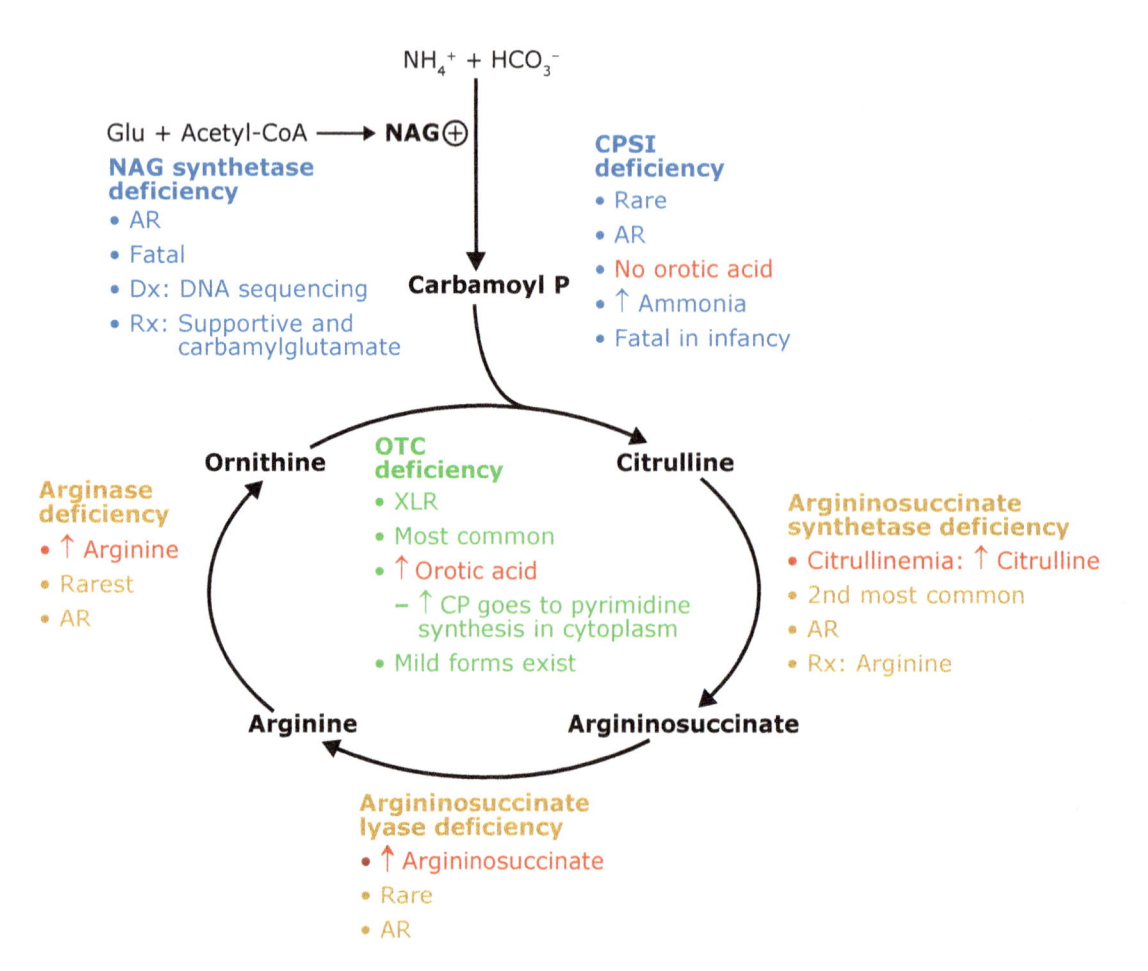

Ornithine → Citrulline → Argininosuccinate → Arginine → Ornithine (cycle)

OTC deficiency
- XLR
- Most common
- ↑ Orotic acid
  - ↑ CP goes to pyrimidine synthesis in cytoplasm
- Mild forms exist

Arginase deficiency
- ↑ Arginine
- Rarest
- AR

Argininosuccinate synthetase deficiency
- Citrullinemia: ↑ Citrulline
- 2nd most common
- AR
- Rx: Arginine

Argininosuccinate lyase deficiency
- ↑ Argininosuccinate
- Rare
- AR

▲ **Figure 12-5.0** Urea Cycle Enzyme Deficiencies

CHAPTER 13: Amino Acid Metabolism and Special Products

1 Overview

- Half of 20 amino acids are essential:
  - Must be provided by diet
- Glycolysis and Krebs cycle intermediates provide source for synthesis
- Degradation:
  - Substrates for gluconeogenesis and ketogenesis
    - Conversion to pyruvate
    - Conversion to Krebs cycle intermediates
- Multiple enzyme deficiencies of amino acid metabolism exist
- Specialized products include:
  - Neurotransmitters
  - Ceramide for sphingolipids
  - Creatine
  - Heme
  - Purines and pyrimidines

USMLE® Key Concepts

For Step 1, you must be able to:

- Describe the families of amino acids based on their side chains.
- Identify major metabolic features of amino acids.
- Discuss selected enzyme deficiencies in amino acid metabolism.
- Discuss specialized products from amino acids, their roles, and relevance to drugs and diseases.

2 Amino Acids

- 20 different amino acids in proteins:
  - Differ through side-chain R
  - Classified in five groups
- At physiologic pH:
  - Amino group is ⊕
  - Carboxyl group is ⊖
  - Some side chains add a ⊕ or ⊖ charge

2.1 Classification

Ionized/Charged
- Negative:
  Glutamate (Glu, E)
  Aspartate (Asp, D)
- Positive:
  Arginine (Arg, R)
  Lysine (Lys, K)
  Histidine (His, H)

Aromatic
- Nonpolar:
  Phenylalanine (Phe, F)
- More polar:
  Tyrosine (Tyr, Y)
  Tryptophan (Trp, W)

Polar/Uncharged
Glutamine (Gln, Q)
Asparagine (Asn, N)
Serine (Ser, S)
Threonine (Thr, T)

Sulfur Containing
Cysteine (Cys, C)
Methionine (Met, M)

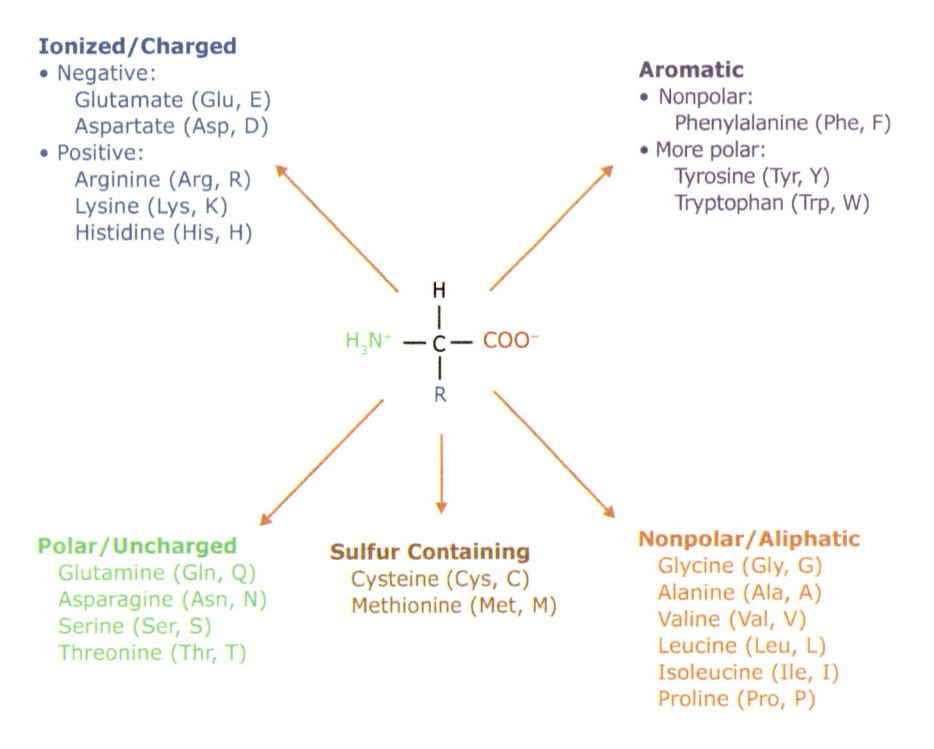

Nonpolar/Aliphatic
Glycine (Gly, G)
Alanine (Ala, A)
Valine (Val, V)
Leucine (Leu, L)
Isoleucine (Ile, I)
Proline (Pro, P)

▲ **Figure 13–2.1** Classification of Amino Acids

- Ionized:
  - Give charge to proteins
  - Negatively charged:
    - Glu, Asp are also excitatory amino acids
    - Glu is the precursor of GABA
    - Glu can be γ-carboxylated to allow Ca^{2+}-binding
  - Positively charged:
    - His is precursor of histamine
    - His is a buffer at physiologic pH (e.g., Hb)
    - Lys and Arg are plentiful in DNA-binding proteins (e.g., histones)
    - Arg is precursor of nitric oxide

- Aromatic:
  - Phe is a precursor of tyrosine:
    - Phenylalanine hydroxylase
    - Deficient in phenylketonuria
  - Tyr is an important precursor:
    - Catecholamines
    - Thyroid hormones
    - Melanin
    - Can be phosphorylated by tyrosine kinases
    - Has a phenol group
  - Trp is a precursor of:
    - Serotonin
    - Melatonin
    - Niacin:
      - Mild pellagra in Hartnup disease
      - Deficiency in Trp transport
- Nonpolar/aliphatic:
  - Gly is smallest (R = H):
    - Disrupts α-helices
    - Every third amino acid in collagen
    - Inhibitory neurotransmitter
  - Val, Leu, and Ile are branched chain amino acids:
    - Accumulate in maple syrup urine disease
    - Branched chain ketoacid dehydrogenase deficiency
  - Pro has a cyclized side chain:
    - Disrupts α-helices
- Sulfur-containing:
  - Cys has –SH (sulfhydryl groups):
    - Can form disulfide bonds
    - *N*-acetylcysteine is an analog used in acetaminophen hepatotoxicity
    - Active moiety in glutathione (GSH)
  - Met has –S-CH$_3$:
    - Initiation codon
    - Used for methylation as S-adenosyl methionine (SAM)
- Polar, uncharged:
  - Asn, Gln can be N-glycosylated
  - Gln carries ammonia from periphery to liver
  - Ser, Thr have –OH, hydroxyl groups:
    - O-glycosylation
    - O-phosphorylation

2.2 Essential Amino Acids

Table 13-2.2 — Essential Amino Acids

Classification	Amino Acids	Notes
Aromatics	Phe, Trp	Tyr becomes essential in PKU
Branched chain	Val, Leu, Ile	
Positively charged	His, Arg, Lys	Arg is essential in period of ⊕ nitrogen balance (growth)
Other	Met, Thr	

- Kwashiorkor:
  - Selective dietary protein deficiency
  - Lack of essential amino acids
  - Generalized edema
- Marasmus:
  - Total caloric deficiency
  - No edema

3 Amino Acid Synthesis

- Three important cofactors for synthesis and degradation:
  - Pyridoxal phosphate (PLP) from vitamin B6
  - Tetrahydrofolate (FH$_4$) from folic acid (B9)
  - Tetrahydrobiopterin (BH$_4$), synthesized from GTP
- Four amino acids come from glycolysis:
  - Ala, Gly
  - Ser, Cys
- Six amino acids come from Krebs cycle intermediates:
  - Glu, Gln
  - Asp, Asn
  - Pro, Arg
- Tyr from Phe
- Others are all essential

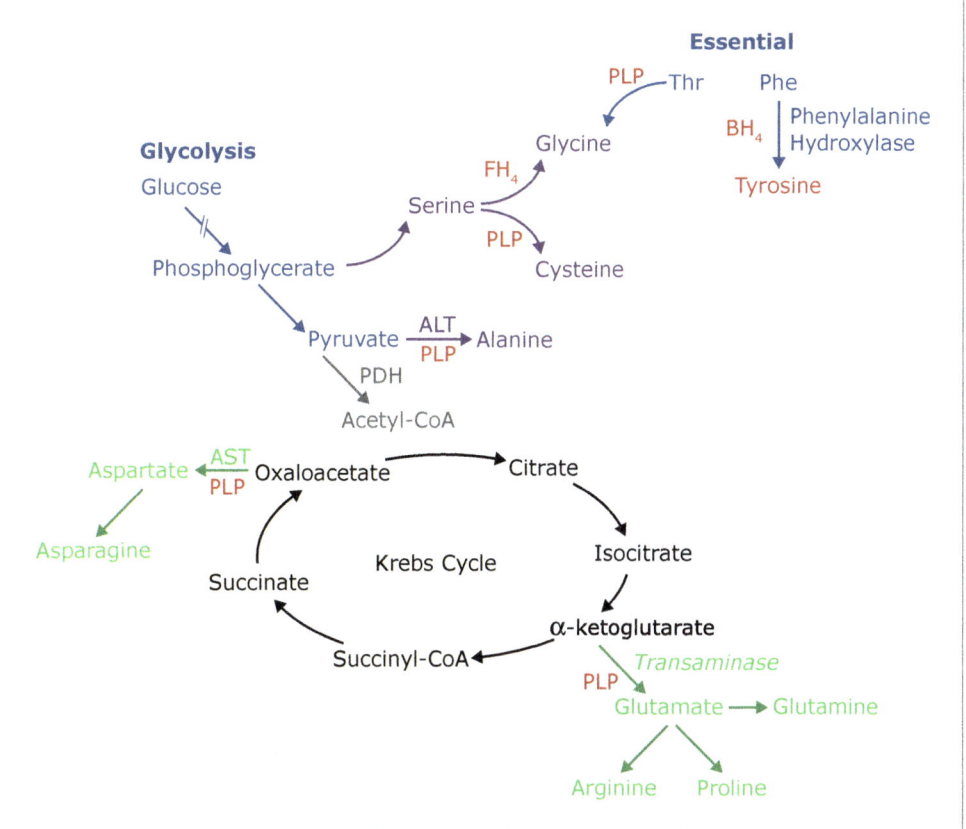

▲ Figure 13-3.0 Synthesis of Nonessential Amino Acids

4 Amino Acid Degradation

- Recall that Leu and Lys are strictly ketogenic
- All other amino acids are glucogenic
- Aromatic amino acids, Ile and Thr, are both ketogenic and glucogenic

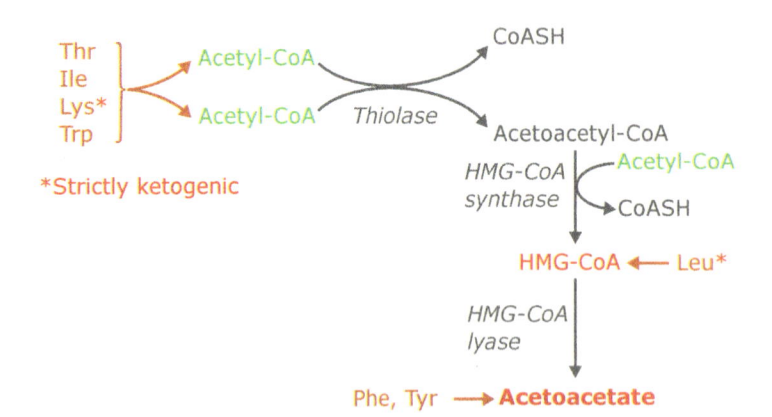

```
Thr ⎫
Ile ⎬ → Acetyl-CoA ⎫           CoASH
Lys*⎪   Acetyl-CoA ⎭ Thiolase ↗
Trp ⎭                          ↘ Acetoacetyl-CoA
                                     ⎪  ← Acetyl-CoA
*Strictly ketogenic          HMG-CoA
                             synthase → CoASH
                                  ↓
                               HMG-CoA ← Leu*
                                  ⎪
                               HMG-CoA
                                lyase
                                  ↓
                    Phe, Tyr → Acetoacetate
```

▲ **Figure 13-4.0A** Degradation of Ketogenic Amino Acids

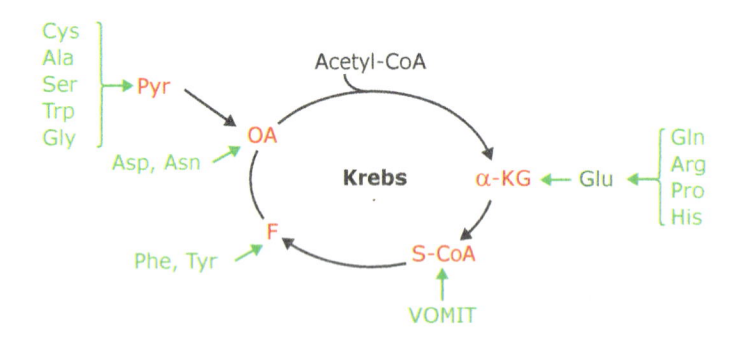

```
Cys ⎫
Ala ⎪         Acetyl-CoA
Ser ⎬→ Pyr ↘    ↓                    ⎧ Gln
Trp ⎪       OA                        ⎪ Arg
Gly ⎭    ↗       \                    ⎨ Pro
   Asp, Asn     Krebs   α-KG ← Glu    ⎩ His
              /           ↑
             F           S-CoA
       Phe, Tyr ↗           ↑
                          VOMIT
```

▲ **Figure 13-4.0B** Degradation of Glucogenic Amino Acids

4.1 Phenylalanine and Tyrosine Catabolism

- Relevant for two genetic disorders
  - Phenylketonuria
  - Alkaptonuria

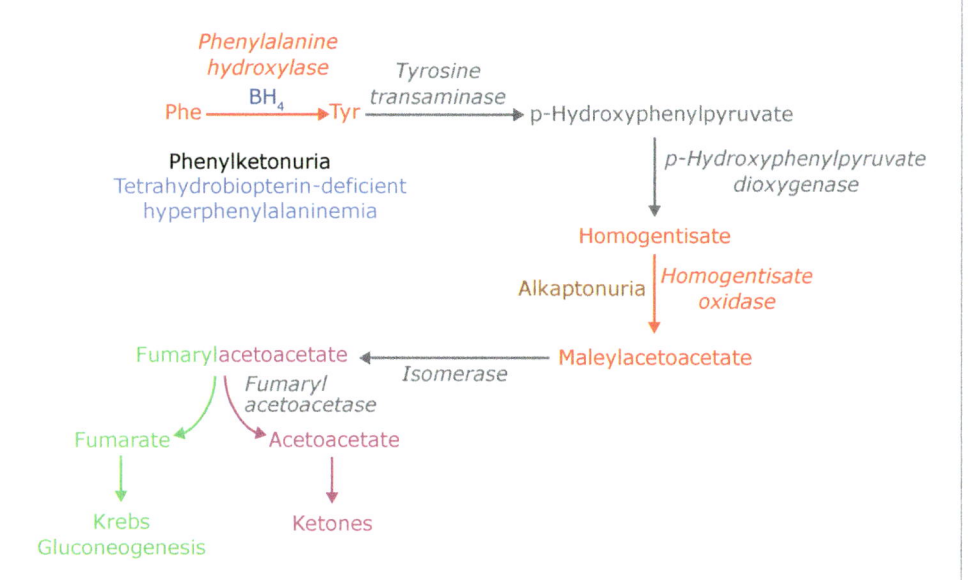

▲ Figure 13-4.1A Phe and Tyr Catabolism and Clinical Relevance

4.1.1 Phenylketonuria (PKU)

- Autosomal recessive:
  - 1/25,000 in U.S.
  - More common in Caucasians and Asians
- *PAH* gene is on chromosome 12:
  - > 500 different mutations, missense most common (62%)
- Fair skin and hair:
  - ↓ Tyr results in ↓ melanin
- Musty or mousy odor:
  - ↑ "Aromatic" amino acid/metabolites
- CNS manifestations include:
  - Intellectual disability:
    - Most common finding in PKU
    - Due to toxic Phe levels:
      - Dietary restriction a few weeks after birth improves outcome
      - Strong correlation between IQ and blood Phe levels
    - Due to decreased levels of catecholamines:
      - Parkinsonism: ↓ Tyr leads to ↓ dopamine
  - Epilepsy

- Dx: Blood levels of phenylalanine by tandem mass spectrometry
  - Replaces the Guthrie test (neonatal heel prick)
    — Based on Phe and phenylketones allowing *Bacillus subtilis* growth when a minimal-medium agar plate is used.
- Rx: Dietary restriction of Phe
  - Supplementation of Tyr
    — Tyr becomes essential in PKU
  - Avoidance of aspartame
    — Methyl ester of an Asp/Phe dipeptide (NutraSweet®)
  - Supplementation of essential amino acids, vitamins, and minerals
  - Rx of pregnant PKU patients is critical:
    — Microcephaly
    — Intellectual disability
    — IUGR
    — Congenital heart diseases:
      - Coarctation of aorta
      - Hypoplastic left ventricle

4.1.2 Tetrahydrobiopterin Deficiency

- BH_4 deficient-hyperphenylalaninemia
- Grouped with PKU:
  - Several enzyme deficiencies:
    — BH_4 is not a vitamin
    — BH_4 is synthesized from GTP
- BH_4 is essential for aromatic amino acid hydroxylases
- Presentation is similar to PKU with prominent neurobehavioral defects

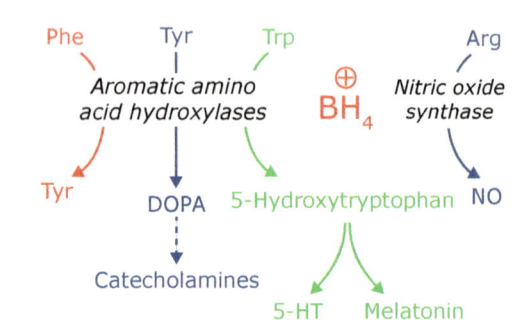

▲ Figure 13–4.1B Roles of Tetrahydrobiopterin (BH_4) as a Cofactor

4.1.3 Alkaptonuria

- Urine turns black when left standing:
  - Hallmark of the disease
  - Due to oxidation by air of homogentisic acid
- Homogentisate is also deposited in cartilage:
  - Ochronosis
    — Slate-blue discoloration in sclerae or ear cartilage
  - Causes osteoarthritis-like symptoms
  - Affects hips, knees, intervertebral joints, shoulder
  - Occurs in early adulthood
    — Third decade of life
- Autosomal recessive

4.2 Branched Chain Amino Acids Catabolism
- Relevant for maple syrup urine disease
- Val, Leu, and Ile
- Make up one quarter of the average protein content:
  - Used to generate energy:
    —Particularly important for muscle
  - Val and Ile are also a source of succinyl-CoA:
    —Part of the VOMIT pathway
  - Leu gives acetoacetate and is strictly ketogenic

4.2.1 Maple Syrup Urine Disease
- Branched chain α-ketoacid dehydrogenase deficiency
- Urine has odor of maple syrup or burnt sugar:
  - Due to isoleucine
- Accumulation of ketoacids:
  - Neurological complication
  - Ketoacidosis
  - Primarily due to leucine
  - Death within first months of life
- Enzyme requires the same cofactors as PDH:
  - Thiamine pyrophosphate
  - Lipoic acid
  - CoASH
  - FAD
  - NAD
- Rare autosomal recessive disorder:
  - 1/180,000 in the U.S.
- Dx: Detection of alloisoleucine in plasma
  - Molecular diagnostic: Genetic testing
- Rx: Dietary restriction of Val, Leu, and Ile

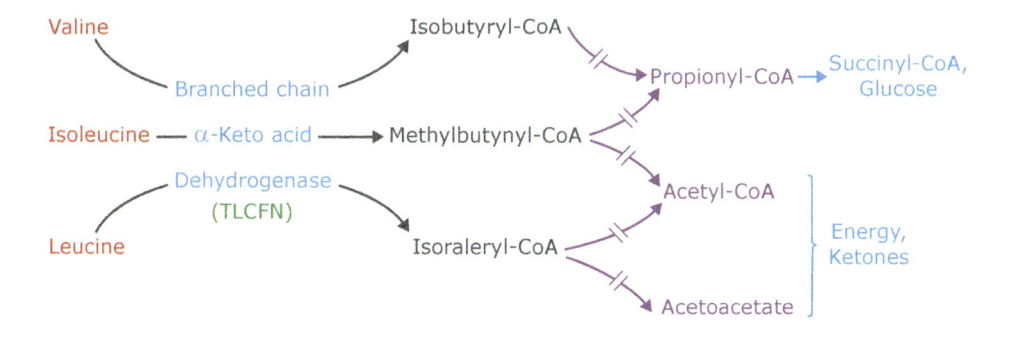

▲ Figure 13–4.2 Metabolism of Branched Chain Amino Acids

4.3 The VOMIT Pathway

- Valine, methionine, isoleucine, threonine:
  - All four are essential in the diet
- Odd C-chain fatty acids
- Relevance:
  - VOMIT ends with succinyl-CoA
  - Last step uses vitamin B12
  - Several enzyme deficiencies
  - Role of vitamins B6, B12, and folate
  - Homocysteine metabolism

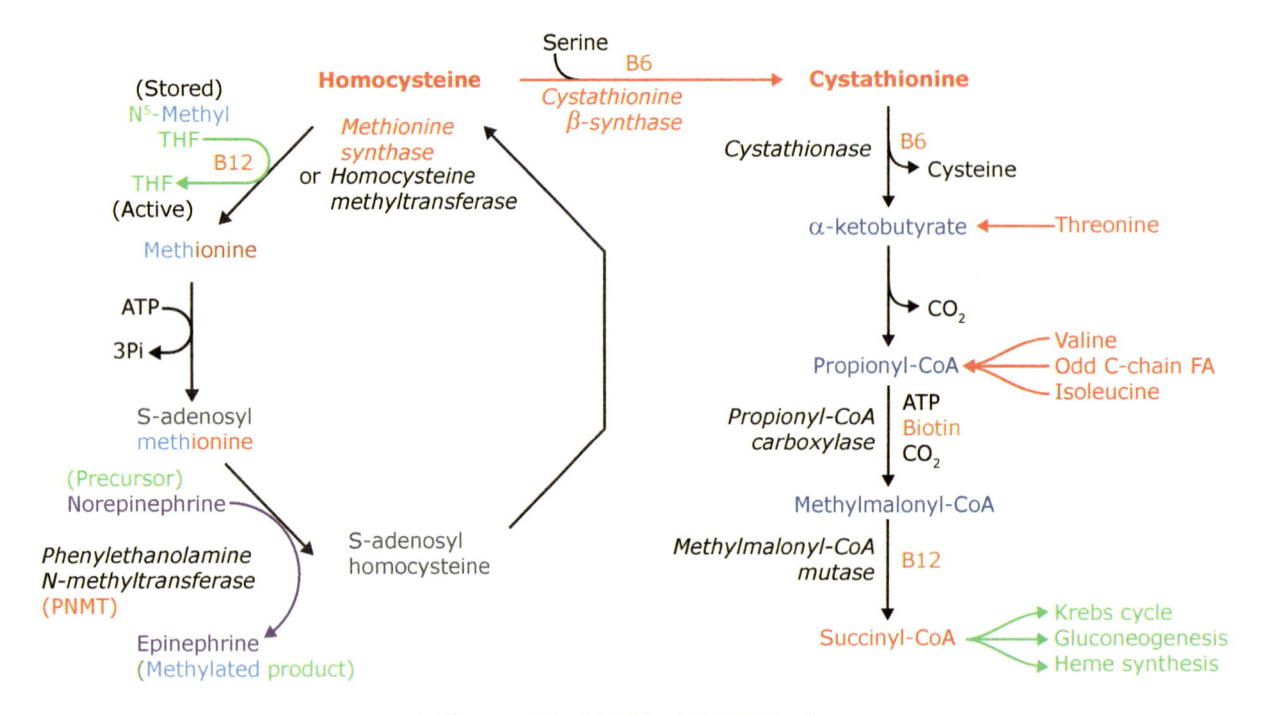

▲ Figure 13-4.3 The VOMIT Pathway

4.3.1 Homocystinuria

- Familial homocystinuria:
  - Autosomal recessive
  - Cystathionine β-synthase deficiency
  - Marfan-like habitus:
    - Tall, thin, long extremities
    - High-arched feet
    - Ectopia lentis:
      - Downward dislocation
      - Marfan syndrome is upward
  - Intellectual disability
  - Vascular disease:
    - Atherosclerosis
    - Thromboembolic disease
  - Dx: Elevated plasma/urine homocysteine
  - Rx: Restrict methionine in diet:
    - Betaine: Promotes conversion of homocysteine to methionine
    - Vitamin B6
- Methionine synthase deficiency also results in similar findings:
  - Rx must supply methionine in diet
- Acquired homocysteinemia:
  - Deficiency of B6, B12, or folate
  - Elevated homocysteine is a risk factor for CV disease
    - Homocysteine damages vascular proteins
    - Degrades cysteine disulfide bonds

4.3.2 Folate and B12 Deficiencies

- Both cause macrocytic megaloblastic anemia
- B12 deficiency also causes subacute combined degeneration of the spinal cord
- Both result in homocysteinemia
- B12 deficiency also causes methylmalonic aciduria

Table 13-4.3 — Folate vs. B12 Deficiencies

	Folate (B9)	B12
Source	Diet: • Dark green leafy vegetables • Poultry, meat, eggs • Beer, grains	Microorganisms: • Gut flora • Animal products • Bacteria in food supply
Role	Methyl donor: • dUMP → dTMP through thymidylate synthetase • Synthesis of A, G (purines) • Synthesis of serine from glycine • Synthesis of methionine from homocysteine	Contains cobalt: • Cofactor of methylmalonyl-CoA mutase • Untraps N^5-methyl THF: 　– Makes methionine 　– Places folate back into active pool
Deficiency	1. Dietary: 　– Takes months 　– Elderly, malnutrition 2. ↑ Demand: 　– Pregnancy 　– Neural tube defects 3. Drugs: 　– DHF reductase inhibitors 　– Anticonvulsants	1. Rarely dietary: 　– Takes years 　– Strict vegan 2. Malabsorption: 　– Atrophic gastritis type A (pernicious anemia) 　– Chronic pancreatitis 　– Intestinal parasites 　– Bacterial overgrowth 　– Terminal ileal resection (Crohn disease) 　– Bariatric surgery 3. Drugs: 　– Metformin 　– Nitrous oxide abuse 　– Long-term PPIs or H_2 blockers
Symptoms	1. Megaloblastic anemia: 　– Pallor 　– Tachycardia 　– Fatigue 　– Weakness 2. GI upset: 　– Weight loss 　– Glossitis	1. Megaloblastic anemia: 2. Sensory and motor neuropathies: 　– Proprioception defects 　– Ataxia 　– Paresis and abnormal reflexes 3. GI upset: 　– ↓ Cell turnover 　– Weight loss 　– Diarrhea/constipation 　– Glossitis
Laboratory Diagnosis	• Serum folate • Serum homocysteine ↑ • No ↑ in methylmalonic acid	• Serum cobalamin • Serum homocysteine ↑ • ↑ Methylmalonic acid
Treatment	Folate PO	B12 IM (not oral)

5 Special Products Derived From Amino Acids

5.1 Neurotransmitters

- Decarboxylation of amino acids produces amine neurotransmitters

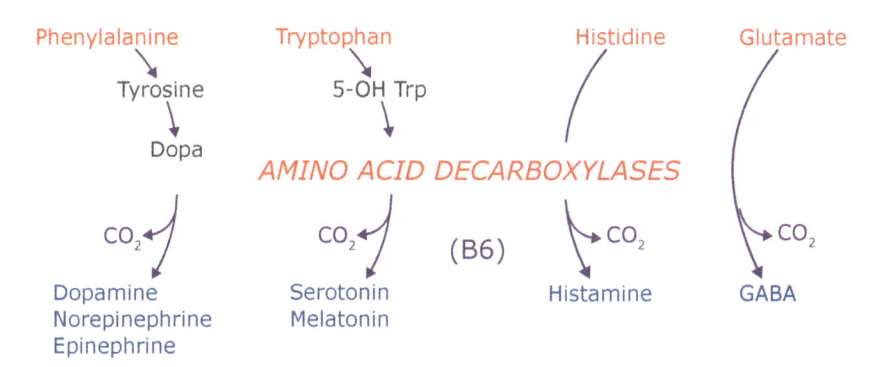

▲ Figure 13-5.1 Amino Acid Precursors of Neurotransmitters

5.2 Creatine

- Produced in kidney and liver from Gly, Arg, and SAM
- Sent to muscle and brain:
  - Phosphorylated by creatine kinases
    - MM: Muscle
    - MB: Heart
    - BB: CNS
  - Smaller reservoir of high-energy phosphate
- Spontaneous cyclization to creatinine
  - Renal elimination
  - Index of GFR

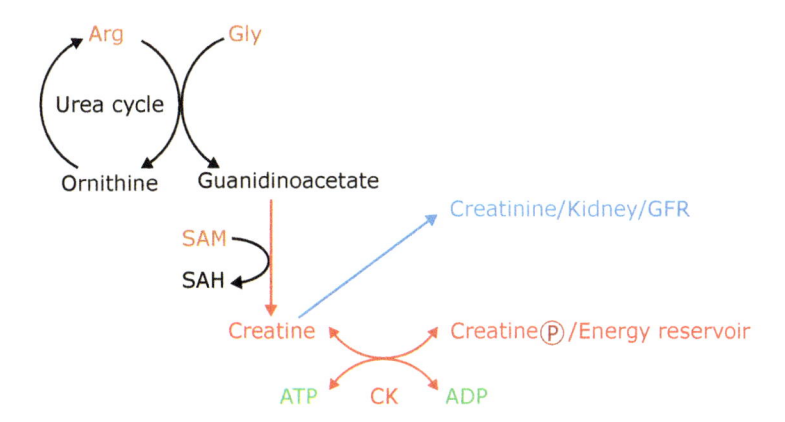

▲ Figure 13-5.2 Creatine Synthesis, Role, and Degradation

5.3 Serine and Sphingolipids

- Sphingolipids are derived from serine rather than glycerol
- Serine + Palmitoyl-CoA: Sphingosine
- Serine + Fatty acyl-CoA: Ceramide
  - Ceramide is the parent of all sphingolipids
- Sphingolipidoses are lysosomal enzyme deficiencies:
  - Decreased catabolism results in neurological and/or reticuloendothelial system dysfunction

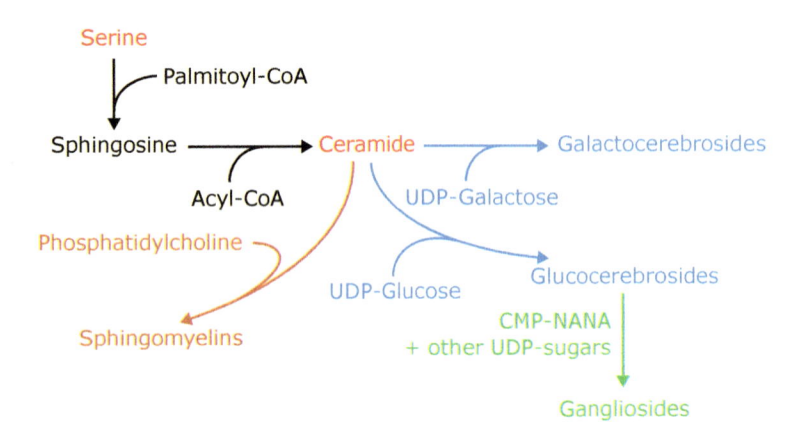

Serine → (Palmitoyl-CoA) → Sphingosine → (Acyl-CoA) → Ceramide
Ceramide + Phosphatidylcholine → Sphingomyelins
Ceramide + UDP-Galactose → Galactocerebrosides
Ceramide + UDP-Glucose → Glucocerebrosides
Glucocerebrosides + CMP-NANA + other UDP-sugars → Gangliosides

Abbrev.: NANA: N-acetylneuraminic acid, a sialic acid

▲ Figure 13-5.3A Synthesis of Major Sphingolipids

Chapter 13 • Amino Acids Metabolism and Special Products — Biochemistry

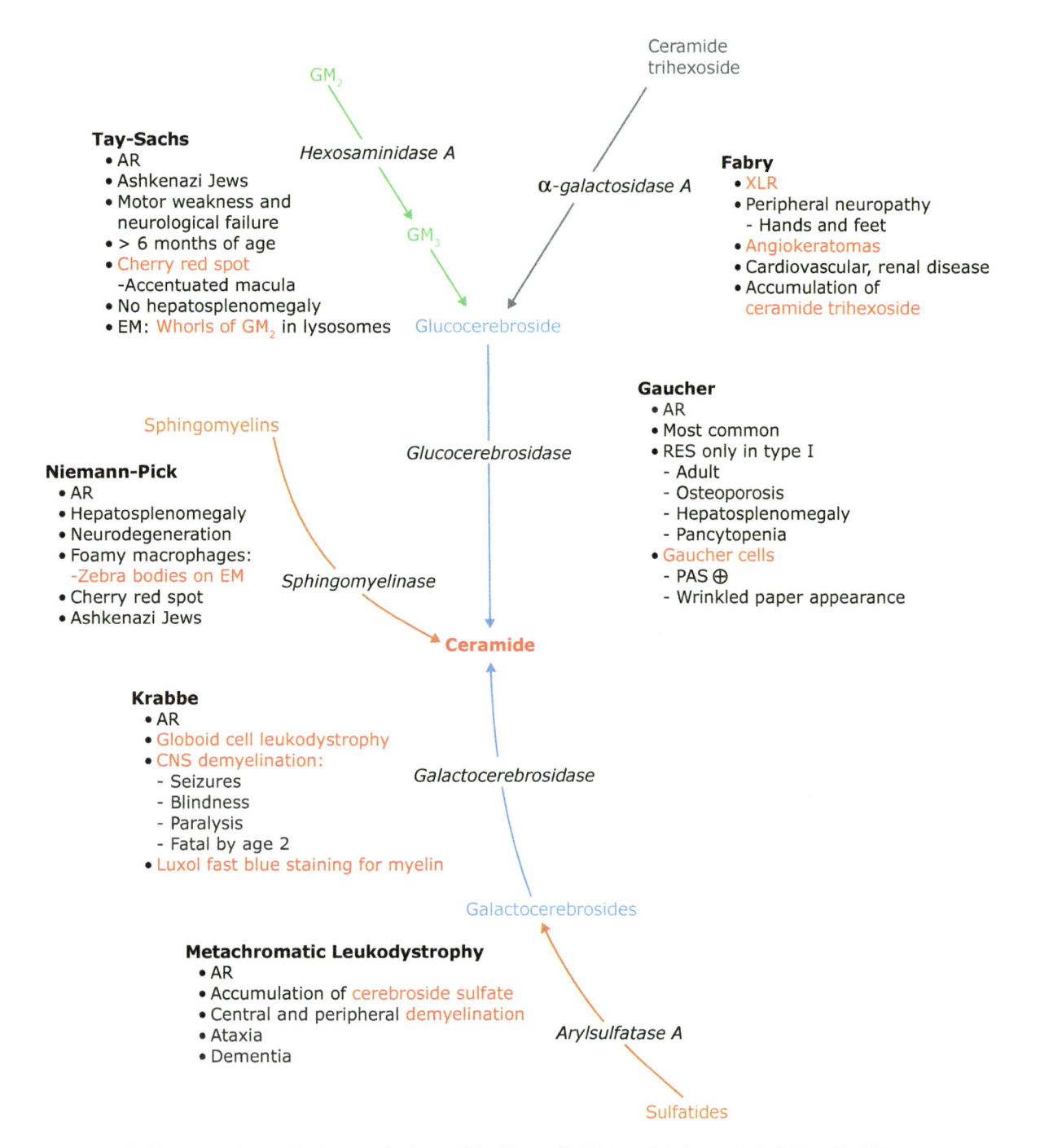

Tay-Sachs
- AR
- Ashkenazi Jews
- Motor weakness and neurological failure
- > 6 months of age
- Cherry red spot
  - Accentuated macula
- No hepatosplenomegaly
- EM: Whorls of GM$_2$ in lysosomes

GM$_2$ → (Hexosaminidase A) → GM$_3$ → Glucocerebroside

Ceramide trihexoside → (α-galactosidase A) → Glucocerebroside

Fabry
- XLR
- Peripheral neuropathy
  - Hands and feet
- Angiokeratomas
- Cardiovascular, renal disease
- Accumulation of ceramide trihexoside

Glucocerebroside → (Glucocerebrosidase) → Ceramide

Niemann-Pick
- AR
- Hepatosplenomegaly
- Neurodegeneration
- Foamy macrophages:
  - Zebra bodies on EM
- Cherry red spot
- Ashkenazi Jews

Sphingomyelins → (Sphingomyelinase) → Ceramide

Gaucher
- AR
- Most common
- RES only in type I
  - Adult
  - Osteoporosis
  - Hepatosplenomegaly
  - Pancytopenia
- Gaucher cells
  - PAS ⊕
  - Wrinkled paper appearance

Krabbe
- AR
- Globoid cell leukodystrophy
- CNS demyelination:
  - Seizures
  - Blindness
  - Paralysis
  - Fatal by age 2
- Luxol fast blue staining for myelin

Galactocerebrosides → (Galactocerebrosidase) → Ceramide

Metachromatic Leukodystrophy
- AR
- Accumulation of cerebroside sulfate
- Central and peripheral demyelination
- Ataxia
- Dementia

Sulfatides → (Arylsulfatase A) → Galactocerebrosides

▲ **Figure 13–5.3B** Degradation of Sphingolipids and Selected Sphingolipidoses

5.4 Heme Synthesis and Degradation

- **Glycine** and **succinyl-CoA** are required to build heme
- Heme is the prosthetic group of multiple proteins:
  - Hemoglobin
  - Myoglobin
  - Cytochromes
  - Soluble guanylyl cyclase
  - NO synthase
  - Catalase
  - Peroxidase
- **B6 deficiency, lead poisoning,** and **porphyria** affect heme synthesis
- Heme is catabolized to bilirubin, which is excreted by the liver
- Increased bilirubin leads to **jaundice**

5.4.1 Heme Synthesis

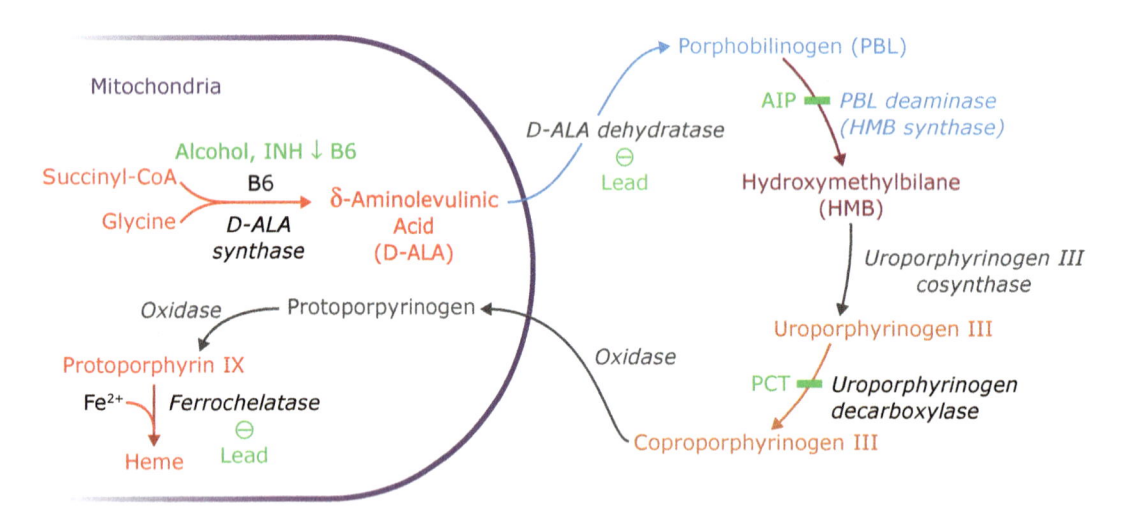

▲ **Figure 13-5.4A** Heme Synthesis

B6 Deficiency

- Active form is pyridoxal phosphate (PLP)
- Required for decarboxylation
  - Decarboxylases of neurotransmitter synthesis
- Required for transamination
  - All transaminases
- Cofactor for cystathionine synthase
- Plants and animal products contain B6
- Chronic alcoholism and isoniazid (iatrogenic) are the most common causes of deficiency

↓ Heme Synthesis
- Sideroblastic Anemia
  - Microcytic
  - ↑ Ferritin, ↓ TIBC
  - ↑ Serum iron, ↑ % saturation
  - Bone marrow sideroblasts
    (Prussian blue staining)
  - Rx: Oral or IV B6

Chronic Alcohol
Isoniazid
↓ B6

Skin Manifestations
- Seborrheic dermatitis
- Atrophic glossitis
- Cheilosis
- Likely due to ↓ Trp to niacin conversion

Neurological Symptoms
- Neuropathy
- Somnolence
- Confusion
- Likely due to ↓ sphingosine synthesis, ↓ neurotransmitters

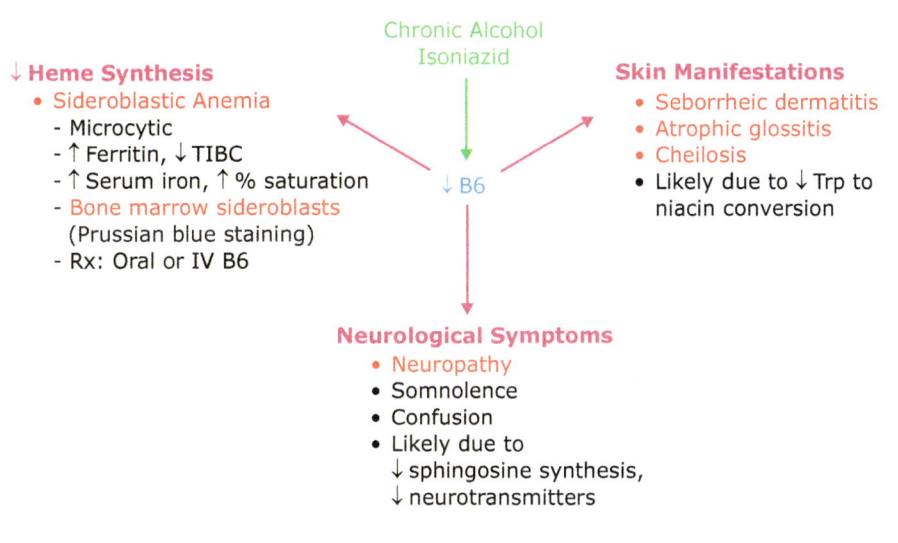

▲ Figure 13–5.4B Effects of Vitamin B6 Deficiency

Lead Poisoning

- Lead inhibits ALA dehydrase and ferrochelatase
- ↑ D-ALA and protoporphyrin IX
- Environmental contamination:
  - Lead pipes: "Old plumbing"
  - Lead paint: "Old houses"
  - Industrial exposure: Batteries, foundries with lead smelters, welding
- Causes CNS, GI, kidney and bone symptoms, as well as sideroblastic anemia
- Dx:
  - Blood lead levels
  - Basophilic stippling in RBCs
    - Due to 5'-nucleotidase inhibition
  - Erythrocyte protoporphyrin levels
  - X-ray fluorescence of bones:
    - Best test to estimate total body burden
    - Lead lines at metaphyses of long bones
- Rx:
  - Removal from source
  - Chelators:
    - EDTA
    - Dimercaprol
    - Oral succimer
    - Oral penicillamine

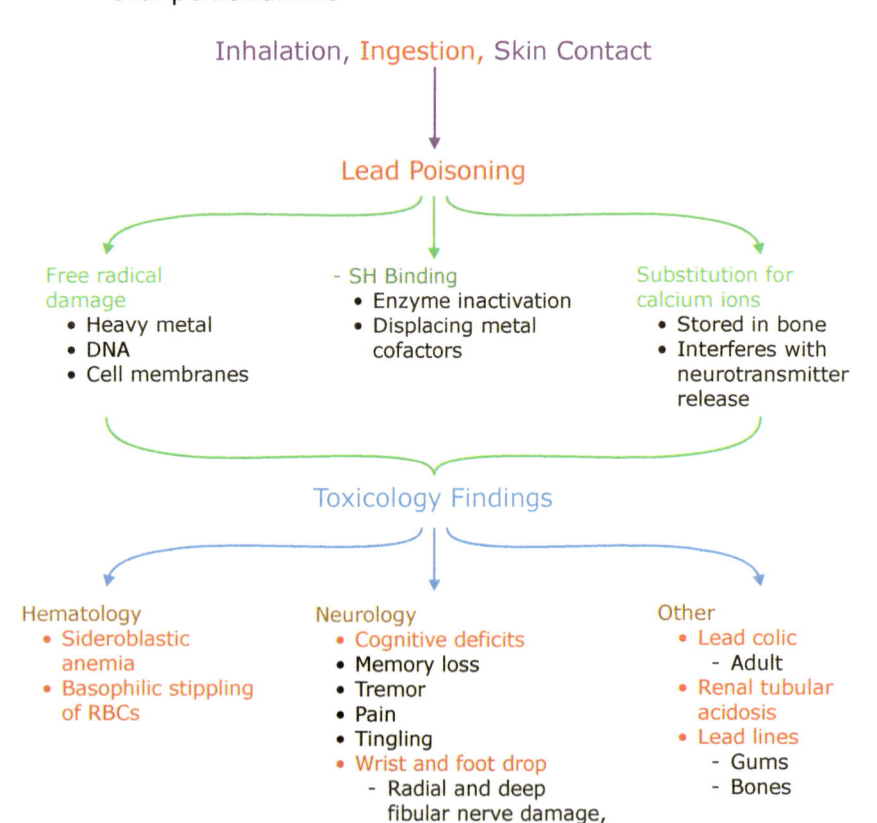

```
Inhalation, Ingestion, Skin Contact
              ↓
        Lead Poisoning
```

Free radical damage	-SH Binding	Substitution for calcium ions
• Heavy metal • DNA • Cell membranes	• Enzyme inactivation • Displacing metal cofactors	• Stored in bone • Interferes with neurotransmitter release

Toxicology Findings

Hematology
- Sideroblastic anemia
- Basophilic stippling of RBCs

Neurology
- Cognitive deficits
- Memory loss
- Tremor
- Pain
- Tingling
- Wrist and foot drop
  - Radial and deep fibular nerve damage, respectively

Other
- Lead colic
  - Adult
- Renal tubular acidosis
- Lead lines
  - Gums
  - Bones

◀ **Figure 13-5.4C** Effects of Lead Intoxication

Porphyria

- Rare autosomal disorders
- Buildup of porphyrinogens:
  - Toxic CNS effects
  - Degraded to porphyrins:
    - Port-wine colored urine
    - Bullous dermatitis with photosensitivity
- Porphyrias are precipitated by CYP450 inducers:
  - Drugs (estrogens, barbiturates, anticonvulsants, etc.)
  - Chronic alcohol use
- A genetic cause of sideroblastic anemia

Glycine + Succinyl-CoA
↓
D-ALA
↓
Porphobilinogen —(Porphobilinogen deaminase / AIP)→ Hydroxymethylbilane → Uroporphyrinogen III
↓ (PCT)
Uroporphyrinogen III decarboxylase
↓
Coproporphyrinogen
↓
Heme

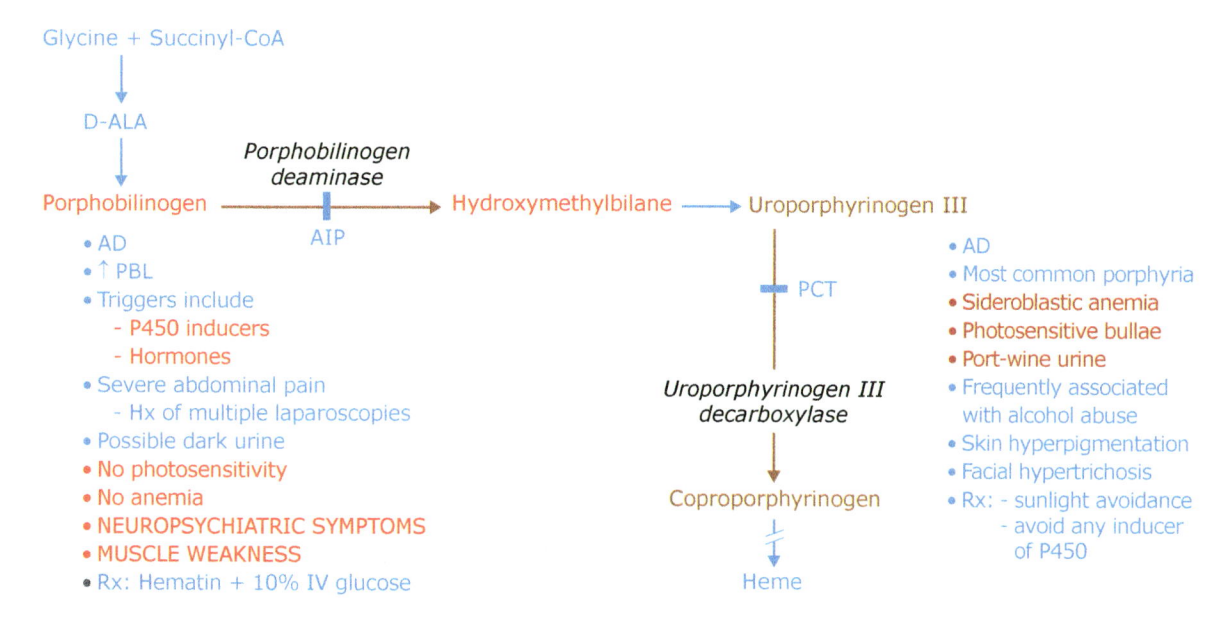

AIP (Porphobilinogen deaminase):
- AD
- ↑ PBL
- Triggers include
  - P450 inducers
  - Hormones
- Severe abdominal pain
  - Hx of multiple laparoscopies
- Possible dark urine
- No photosensitivity
- No anemia
- NEUROPSYCHIATRIC SYMPTOMS
- MUSCLE WEAKNESS
- Rx: Hematin + 10% IV glucose

PCT (Uroporphyrinogen III decarboxylase):
- AD
- Most common porphyria
- Sideroblastic anemia
- Photosensitive bullae
- Port-wine urine
- Frequently associated with alcohol abuse
- Skin hyperpigmentation
- Facial hypertrichosis
- Rx: - sunlight avoidance
  - avoid any inducer of P450

▲ **Figure 13–5.4D** Acute Intermittent Porphyria (AIP) vs. Porphyria Cutanea Tarda (PCT)

5.4.2 Heme Degradation

- Forms bilirubin
- Conjugated bilirubin is excreted through the bile
- Bile pigments give color to urine and feces
- Jaundice is classified based on conjugated or unconjugated bilirubinemia

Hemoglobin
Myoglobin   ① → Heme — *Heme oxygenase* → Biliverdin — *Biliverdin reductase* → Bilirubin
Cytochromes
                    in macrophages of RES

                                    ②
%Bound bilirubin   ⇌   %Free bilirubin
 – Albumin   • Lipid soluble
                          ↓   ↓   ↓
                         Skin   Sclera   CNS
                        jaundice icterus kernicterus

Unconjugated or indirect bilirubinemia

① Chronic hemolytic anemias
② Drug displacement
   ex: sulfonamide
③ Lack of UDP-glucuronosyl transferase activity
   - Neonates
   - Crigler-Najjar (kernicterus)
   - Gilbert

To hepatocytes ④

                UDP-glucuronosyl transferase
Bilirubin ─────────────────→ Bilirubin diglucuronide
                    ③
                                ⑤ Canalicular transport
                                    ↓
                                Into bile ducts
                                    ⑥
                                    ↓
                                   Gut
                            Bilirubin diglucuronide
                               ↙ Bacteria   ↘ Enterohepatic recycling
Blood, urine ← Urobilinogens
                        Oxidation → Stercobilin → Feces

Conjugated or direct bilirubinemia

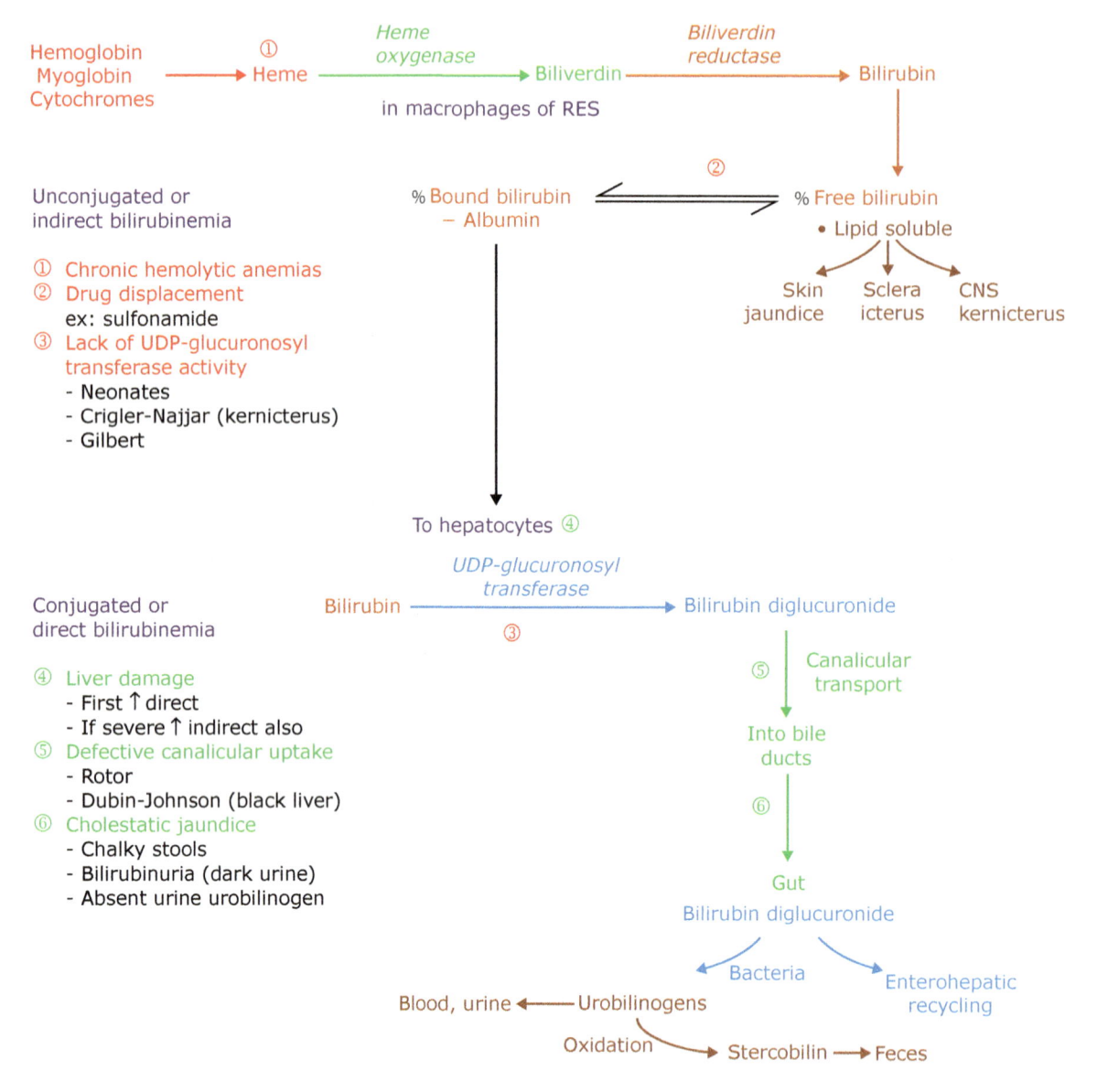

④ Liver damage
   - First ↑ direct
   - If severe ↑ indirect also
⑤ Defective canalicular uptake
   - Rotor
   - Dubin-Johnson (black liver)
⑥ Cholestatic jaundice
   - Chalky stools
   - Bilirubinuria (dark urine)
   - Absent urine urobilinogen

▲ **Figure 13-5.4E** Bilirubin Metabolism and Jaundice

Molecular Biology

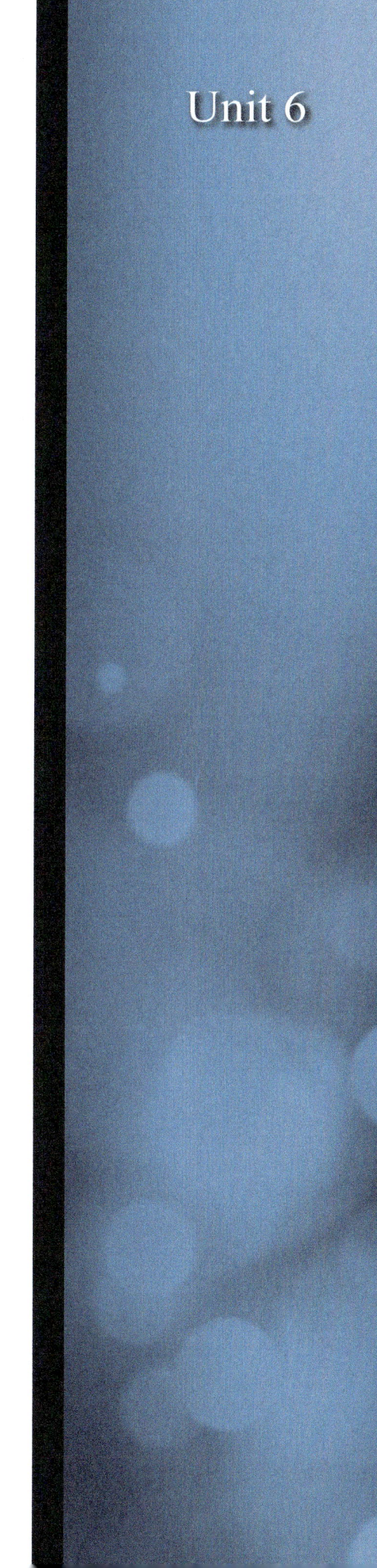

Unit 6

CHAPTER 14: Purines, Pyrimidines, and Nucleotides

1 Overview

- Most purines and pyrimidines used to build nucleotides and nucleic acids are recycled with salvage enzymes
- De novo synthesis mostly occurs in the liver and in the brain

Table 14-1.0 Comparison of De Novo Synthesis of Purines and Pyrimidines

	Purines	Pyrimidines
Amino acid precursor	• Glycine • Glutamine • Aspartate	— • Glutamine • Aspartate
Folate role	• N^{10}-formyl-THF • Building of purine ring structure	• N^5,N^{10}-methylene THF • Methylation of dUMP into dTMP
Rate-limiting step	• Glutamine phosphoribosyl amidotransferase • ⊖ by GMP and AMP	• Carbamoyl phosphate synthetase II • ⊖ by UTP • ⊕ by PRPP
Structure and strategy	• Start with sugar phosphate • Build 2 rings on it	• Start with 1 ring • Attach sugar phosphate
Bases	• Hypoxanthine • Adenine • Guanine	• Orotic acid • Uracil • Cytosine • Thymine

- Degradation of purines and pyrimidines:
    - Purine catabolism yields uric acid
    - Pyrimidine catabolism yields CO_2 and NH_4^+ and has no clinical relevance
    - They do not contribute energy to the cell
- Nucleotides:
    - Base: Purine or pyrimidine
    - Sugar: Ribose or deoxyribose
    - Phosphate: One, two, or three phosphate groups
- Ribonucleotide reductase catalyzes conversion of ribonucleotides to deoxyribonucleotides
- Nucleic acids are DNA or RNA:
    - Polymerases build them
    - Nucleases break them
    - Synthesis is always in 5' to 3' direction
    - Nucleic acid sequence is antiparallel and complementary to a template nucleic acid

USMLE® Key Concepts

For Step 1, you must be able to:

▶ Discuss the clinical relevance of salvage versus de novo synthesis.

▶ Recognize the targets and mechanisms of important drugs.

▶ Identify the structure of purines and pyrimidines.

▶ Describe nucleoside, nucleotide, and nucleic acids.

▶ Understand the meaning of 5' to 3' direction and the relationship between a template and a new strand of a nucleic acid.

2 Salvage Enzymes and Clinical Relevance

- DNA, RNA, nucleotides, and second messengers are recycled rather than catabolized by salvage pathways

Table 14-2.0 Comparison of Salvage Pathways for Purines and Pyrimidines

Purines	Pyrimidines
Three enzymes: • Phosphoribosyltransferases • Purine nucleoside phosphorylases • Deaminases	**Two enzymes:** • Pyrimidine nucleoside phosphorylase • Specific nucleoside kinases

Salvage: Phosphoribosyltransferases (PRT)

Nucleotides → (Nucleotidase) → Nucleosides —PRT— → Base (via Purine nucleoside phosphorylase)

AMP → APRT → Adenosine —Adenosine deaminase (SCID)→ Inosine → Adenine

IMP → HGPRT (Lesch-Nyhan) → Hypoxanthine

GMP → Guanosine → Guanine

Hypoxanthine and Guanine → Xanthine oxidase (⊖ Allopurinol, Febuxostat) → Degradation → Uric acid

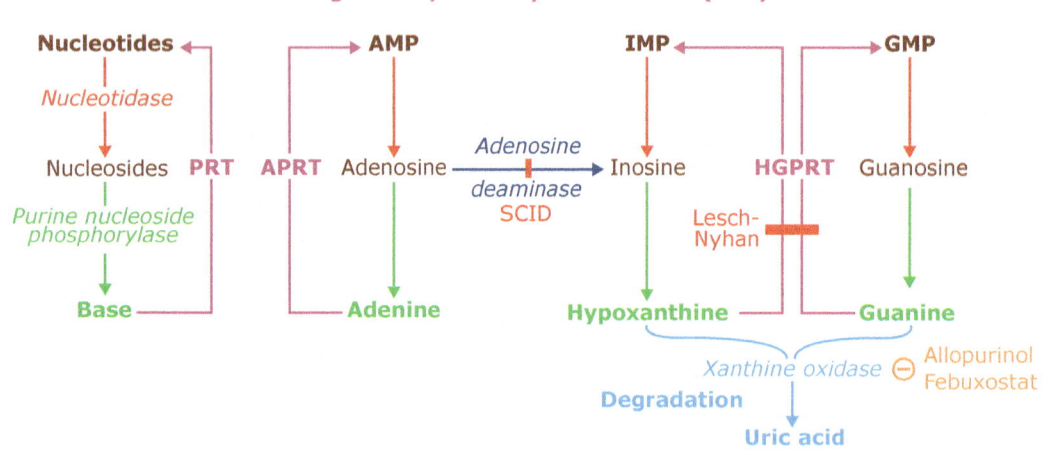

▲ Figure 14–2.0A Purine Salvage Pathway

- Clinical relevance of purine salvage pathway:
  - **Severe combined immunodeficiency syndrome (SCID):**
    - AR, adenosine deaminase deficiency
    - Affects B and T cell functions
    - ↑ Deoxyadenosine in cells:
      - ↑ dATP which ⊖ ribonucleotide reductase
      - No DNA synthesis, no replication
    - ↑ S-adenosylhomocysteine:
      - Toxic to lymphocytes
    - Rx: Bone marrow transplant or gene therapy
    - XLR SCID is more common:
      - Mutation in γ-chain of IL-2 receptor
    - Rarely purine nucleoside phosphorylase deficiency (AR)

- **Lesch-Nyhan syndrome:**
  - XLR, HGPRT deficiency
  - Causes a buildup of uric acid:
    - Severe gout
    - Renal stones
  - Neuromuscular deficits:
    - Basal ganglia: Huntington-like
  - Intellectual disability
  - Self-mutilation
  - Rx: Allopurinol for gout

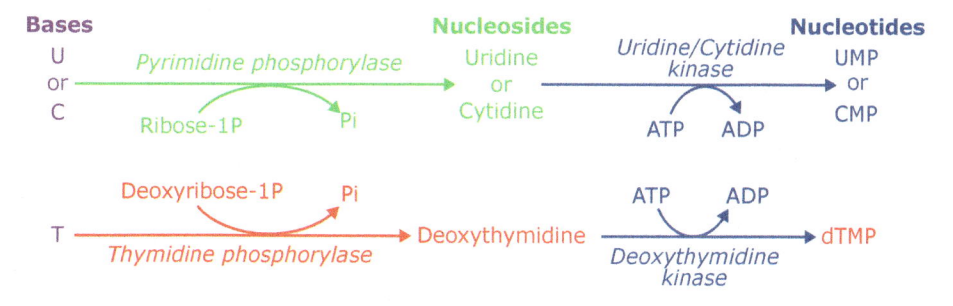

▲ **Figure 14–2.0B** Pyrimidine Salvage Pathway

3 De Novo Synthesis of Purines

- Purines are built on an activated ribose:
  - Phosphoribosylpyrophosphate (PRPP)
- Glutamine, glycine, aspartate, and folate are required
- Hypoxanthine is precursor to adenine and guanine:
  - Hypoxanthine nucleotide is called inosine

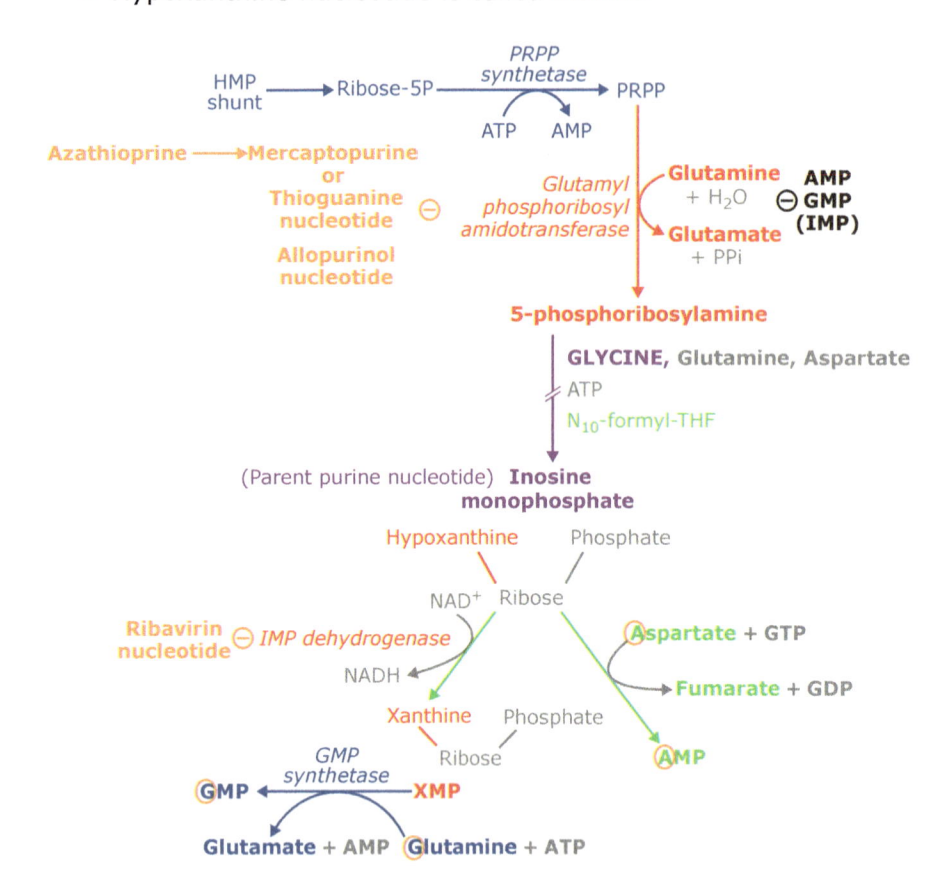

▲ Figure 14–3.0 De Novo Synthesis of Purine Nucleotides

3.1 Drugs Interfering With De Novo Purine Synthesis

- Prodrugs of purine analogs
- Activation to a nucleotide analog
- Mercaptopurine and thioguanine:
  - Anticancer drug
  - S-phase specific
  - Activated by HGPRT
  - ⊖ Glutamyl phosphoribosyl amidotransferase
  - Bone marrow suppression, gastroenteritis, nausea, vomiting
  - Hyperpigmentation of skin
  - Azathioprine is a prodrug of mercaptopurine used as an immunosuppressant

Chapter 14 • Purines, Pyrimidines, and Nucleotides

- **Allopurinol:**
  - Two mechanisms of action:
    - Prodrug of alloxanthine:
      - Alloxanthine is a suicide inhibitor of xanthine oxidase
      - Decreases uric acid synthesis
    - Prodrug of allopurinol nucleotide:
      - ⊖ De novo synthesis of purines
      - ↑ Salvage of purines and ↓ uric acid wasting
  - Prophylaxis of gout
  - Causes hypersensitivity
  - Decreases clearance of mercaptopurine
- **Ribavirin:**
  - Guanosine analog
  - Antiviral
  - Ribavirin monophosphate ⊖ IMP dehydrogenase:
    - ↓ GTP-dependent end-capping of viral mRNA
  - Used in HCV and RSV primarily
  - Causes bone marrow suppression

3.2 Purine Structure

- Nitrogenous base with two rings, double bonds

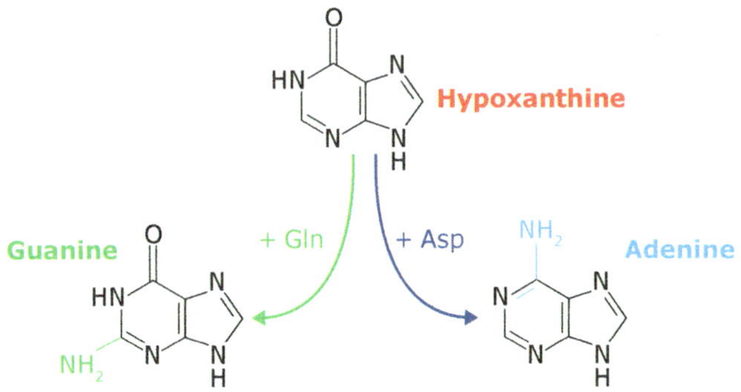

▲ Figure 14-3.2 Purine Structure

- Xanthine and uric acid are purine breakdown products
- **Methylxanthines** are drugs/chemicals with important pharmacology:
  - Theophylline:
    - Used in status asthmaticus
  - Caffeine:
    - Mild stimulant, diuretic
  - Block adenosine receptors:
    - Cause tachycardia
  - Block phosphodiesterases:
    - ↑ cAMP
    - Vasodilate

4 Purine Catabolism

- **Produces uric acid:**
  - ↑ Uric acid causes gout
- **Xanthine oxidase:**
  - Blocked by allopurinol metabolite alloxanthine:
    — Competitive antagonism
  - Requires **molybdenum (Mo):**
    — **Febuxostat** interferes with Mo-pterin site
    — Noncompetitive antagonism
  - Produces H_2O_2:
    — Free radical injury
    — Role in **reperfusion injury** after MI
- **Gout:**
  - Inflammatory arthritis
  - **Metatarsal**-phalangeal joint at base of big toe:
    — Most commonly affected
    — Podagra
  - **Tophi,** urate nephropathy, **renal stones:**
    — Negatively birefringent crystals
    — Needle-shaped
  - Rx:
    — Acute: **Indomethacin,** colchicine
    — Chronic:
      - Allopurinol, febuxostat ↓ synthesis
      - Probenecid ↑ elimination
      - Uricases ↑ degradation into allantoin

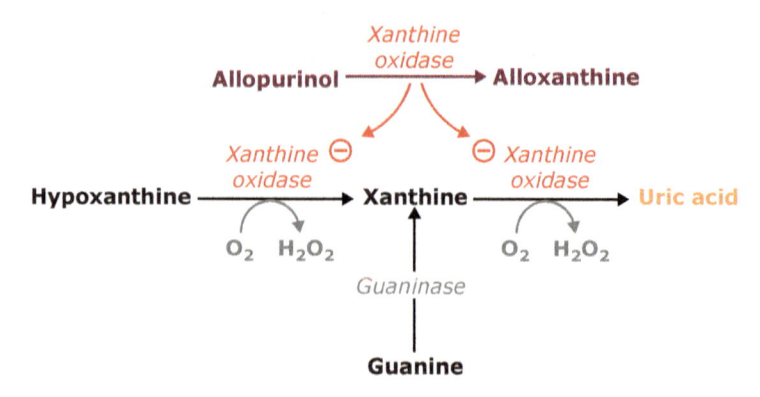

▲ **Figure 14–4.0A** Breakdown of Purines to Uric Acid

Chapter 14 • Purines, Pyrimidines, and Nucleotides

Alcoholism
↑Lactate
Competes with urate

Purine rich diet
- Organ meats
- Meats in general
- Seafood
- Beer

Medications
Thiazides
Loops
Compete with urate for renal tubule access
Salicylates
Cyclosporine
↓Clearance

↑Uric acid and gout

Phosphate trapping or ↑production

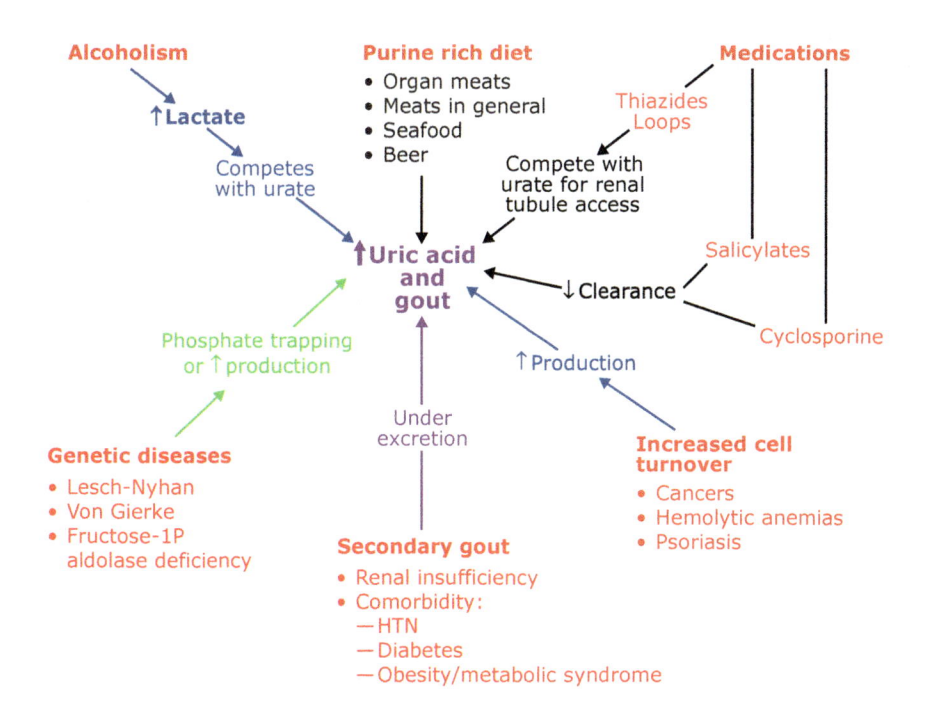

Genetic diseases
- Lesch-Nyhan
- Von Gierke
- Fructose-1P aldolase deficiency

Under excretion

Secondary gout
- Renal insufficiency
- Comorbidity:
  —HTN
  —Diabetes
  —Obesity/metabolic syndrome

↑Production

Increased cell turnover
- Cancers
- Hemolytic anemias
- Psoriasis

▲ **Figure 14–4.0B** Causes of Gout

5 De Novo Pyrimidine Synthesis

- The base is synthesized first
- Ribose phosphate is attached later
- Glutamine, aspartate, and folate are required
- **Orotic acid** is the parent pyrimidine
- The first and rate-limiting step is analogous to **urea cycle:**
  - Catalyzed by **carbamoyl phosphate synthetase II**
  - CPSII is cytoplasmic

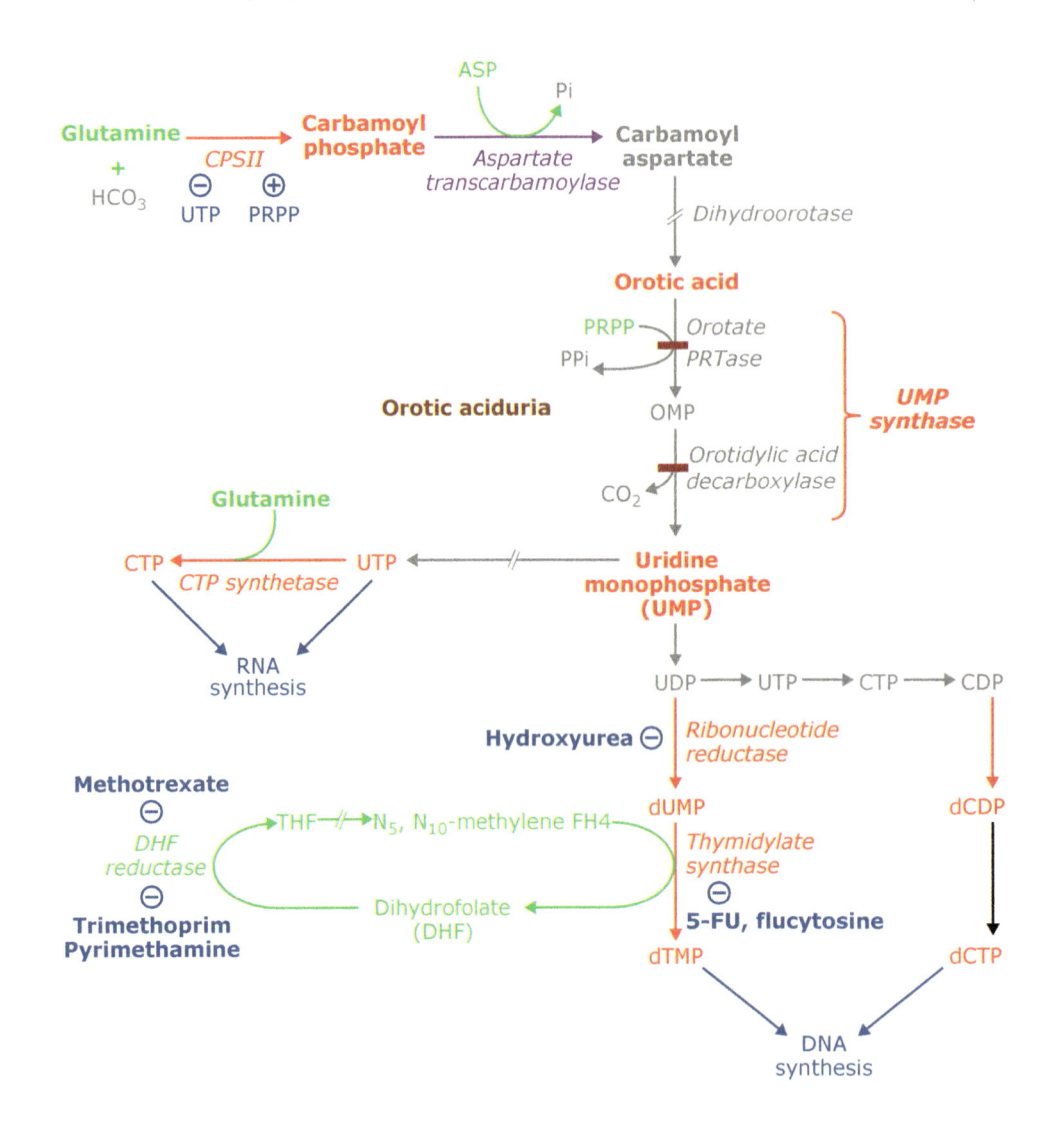

▲ Figure 14–5.0 De Novo Synthesis of Pyrimidines

5.1 Orotic Aciduria

- **Orotate phosphoribosyltransferase** or **orotidylic acid decarboxylase** deficiency
- These enzymes are part of UMP synthase
- AR
- ↑ Orotic acid in blood and urine:
  - Orange crystals in diapers
- Megaloblastic anemia:
  - ↓ Pyrimidines impair DNA/RNA synthesis
- Intellectual and physical disability:
  - ↓ Cell division and differentiation
- Rx: Uridine as a source of pyrimidine

UMP synthase deficiency
- AR
- No effect on urea

→ **Orotic aciduria**
- Ornithine transcarbamoylase deficiency
  - ↓BUN, ↑ammonia
  - XLR

→ **Megaloblastic anemia**
- Folate, B12 deficiency
  - Acquired

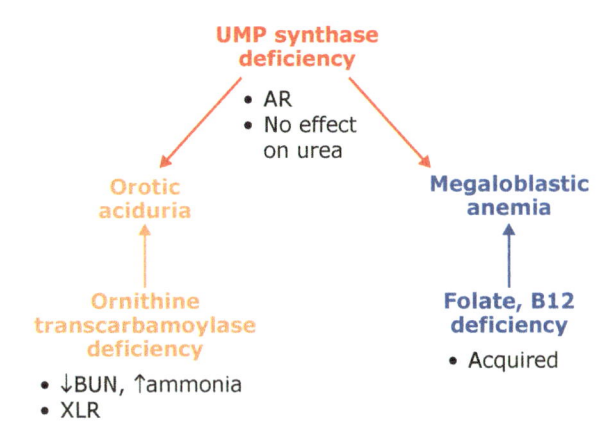

▲ **Figure 14–5.1** Differential Diagnosis of Orotic Aciduria and Megaloblastic Anemia

5.2 Drugs and Pyrimidine Synthesis

- Hydroxyurea ⊖ ribonucleotide reductase:
  - ↓ Deoxyribonucleotides, ↓ DNA
  - S-phase specific
  - Anticancer drug
  - Used in sickle cell anemia to ↑ HbF and ↓ sickling
- DHF reductase inhibitors:
  - Methotrexate:
    - —S-phase specific antimetabolite
    - —↓ Synthesis of A, G, and T, as well as serine and methionine
    - —Anticancer and immunosuppressant
  - Trimethoprim (TMP) and pyrimethamine (PYR):
    - —Synergy with sulfonamides
    - —TMP-sulfamethoxazole:
      - DOC in *Haemophilus*, *Nocardia*, and *Pneumocystis*
    - —PYR-sulfadiazine:
      - DOC in *Toxoplasma*

- **Thymidylate synthase inhibitors:**
  - **5-fluorouracil (5-FU):**
    - —Prodrug of 5-FdUMP
    - —S-phase specific
  - **Flucytosine:**
    - —Prodrug of 5-FU
    - —Used as antifungal
    - —Synergy with amphotericin B

5.3 Pyrimidine Structure

- Nitrogenous base with one ring, double bonds

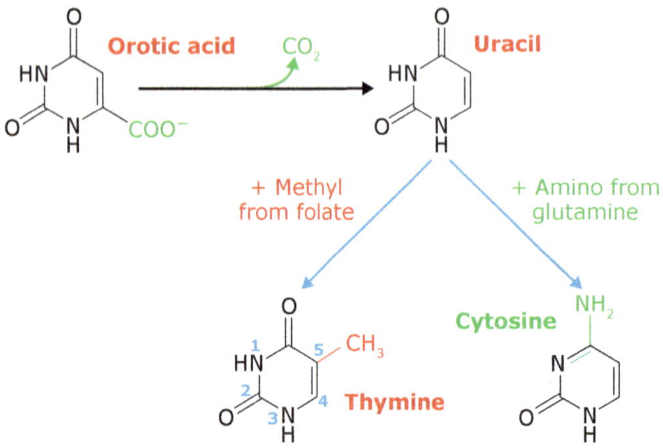

▲ Figure 14-5.3 Pyrimidine Structure

Chapter 14 • Purines, Pyrimidines, and Nucleotides

6 Nucleic Acid Chemistry

- Nucleic acids are polymers of nucleotides

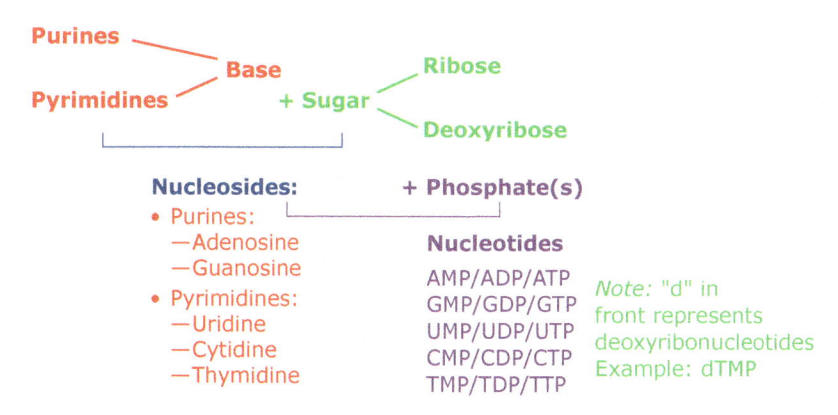

▲ Figure 14–6.0A Nucleotides

- Five-carbon sugar is central to nucleotide structure

▲ Figure 14–6.0B Ribose vs. Deoxyribose

5': • Attach 1–3 phosphates
 • 2,3 ℗ confers high energy
 • ℗ gives negative charges to DNA/RNA

1': Attach base

2': Check for ribose (–OH)/RNA or deoxyribose (no –OH)/DNA

3': Attach to 5' phosphate of next nucleotide with phosphodiester bond (polymerases)

▲ Figure 14–6.0C Key Sugar Positions

- Phosphodiester bonds:
  - Link nucleotides to form nucleic acids
  - Polymerases make them
  - Give two distinct ends:
    — 5' phosphate at the beginning
    — 3' hydroxyl at the end
    — Called polarity
  - Polymerases copy a template:
    — Read it from 3' end to 5' end
    — Make a complementary and antiparallel sequence

- Convention: Read, write, and understand in 5' to 3' direction
- Nucleases break them:
  - —Exonucleases release single nucleotides:
    - 5' and 3' exonucleases
  - —Endonucleases release nucleic acid fragments:
    - Cut within nucleic acids
    - Restriction endonucleases:
      - –Recognize palindromes
      - –Release restriction fragments
      - –Used in molecular technologies

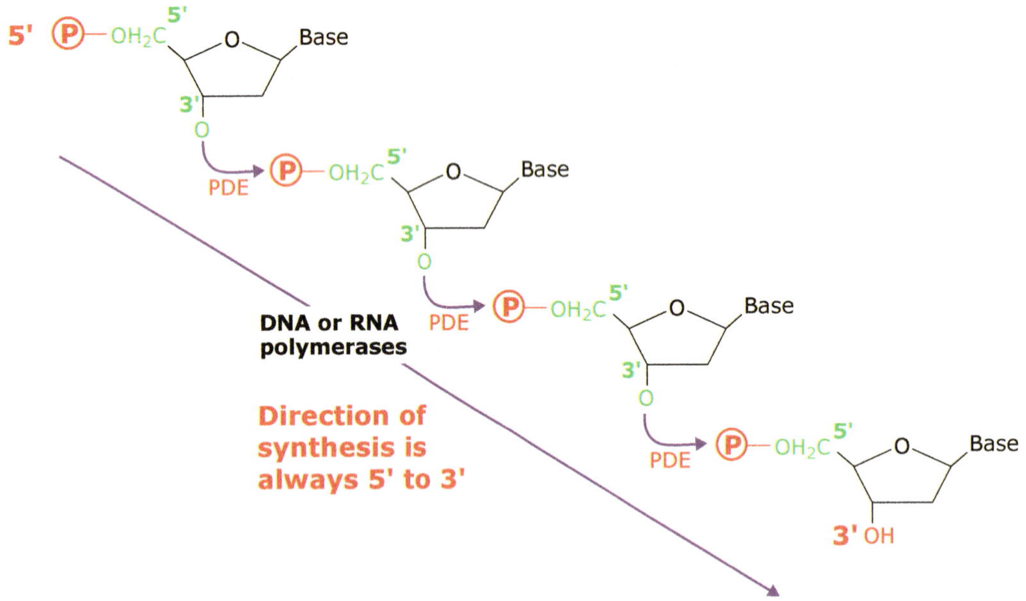
5'
P
OH2C
5'
O
Base
3'
O
PDE
DNA or RNA polymerases
Direction of synthesis is always 5' to 3'
3' OH

▲**Figure 14–6.0D** Phosphodiester Bonds (PDE) and Polarity

Chapter 14 • Purines, Pyrimidines, and Nucleotides

Figure 14-6.0E Synthesis is Complementary and Antiparallel to Template

Figure 14-6.0F Action of Nucleases on a DNA Strand

- Most DNA is double stranded; most RNA is single stranded:
  - Hydrogen (H) bonds are weak bonds
  - Allow base pairing between complementary and antiparallel strands
  - In dsDNA (or dsRNA in viruses), % purines = % pyrimidines
    —Known as Chargaff rule

Chargaff Rule
- % purines = % pyrimidines
- % A = % U or % T
- % G = % C

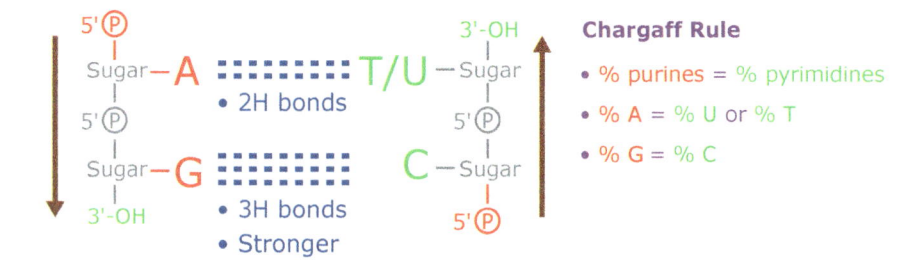

Figure 14-6.0G Base Pairing and Chargaff Rule

- DNA double helix:
  - Spiral staircase
  - Contains grooves:
    —Allow DNA binding proteins to bind
  - Three forms of double helix:
    —B-DNA is most common

Table 14-16.0 — The DNA Double Helix

Type of Helix	Direction	Remarks
B-DNA	Right-handed	• Predominant in vivo • 10.4 base pairs/turn • Bases inside
A-DNA	Right-handed	• Predominant in DNA/RNA hybrids • 11 base pairs/turn, more compact • Bases inside
Z-DNA	Left-handed	• Bases on periphery • 12 base pairs/turn • Correlates with regions of high transcription

- In A and B DNA, bases are hidden inside the molecule:
  - The sugar phosphate backbone is protecting the base sequence
- RNA also can take unique, telltale structures:
  - Cloverleaf shape of tRNA
  - Stem-and-loop to terminate bacterial transcription
- Further packaging of DNA requires histones and other proteins:
  - See Chapter 15 on replication

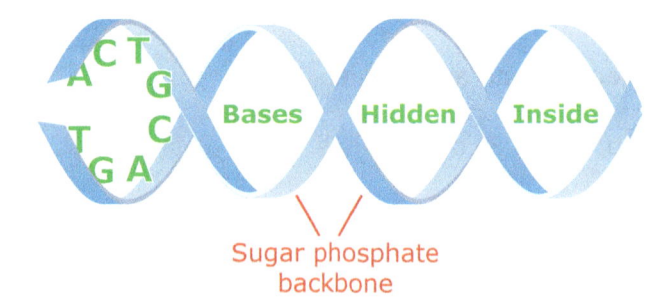

▲ Figure 14–6.0H Structure of A and B DNA

CHAPTER 15 — DNA Replication

1 Overview

- Cell division requires DNA synthesis to produce two daughter cells with identical DNA
- DNA replication occurs exclusively in the S phase of the cell cycle
- DNA is double stranded: Both strands serve as templates
- DNA replication occurs at replication forks:
  - DNA polymerases synthesize the new DNA:
    - Synthesis is in the 5' → 3' direction
    - New strand is antiparallel and complementary to the template
    - Requires deoxyribonucleoside triphosphates (dNTPs)
    - Requires a primer: A free 3'-OH to attach to
- Accessory enzymes include:
  - Helicases
  - Topoisomerases
  - Nucleases
  - Ligases
  - Telomerase (eukaryotes only)
- Cancers result from uncontrolled replication due to errors or mutations
- Multiple anticancer drugs interfere with the process of replication
- Certain antibacterial and most antiviral medications also do so

USMLE® Key Concepts

For Step 1, you must be able to:
- Describe the phases of the cell cycle.
- Describe replication step-by-step in prokaryotes and eukaryotes.
- Understand the mechanisms of action of important antibiotics.
- Discuss DNA damage and repair strategies.

2 Cell Cycle Concepts

- Five phases:
  - S phase: DNA replication
    - Eukaryote cells are diploid (except gametes, haploid)
    - Diploid = 2N DNA with N = 1 copy each of 22 autosomes and 1 sex chromosome (X or Y)
    - At the end of S-phase, DNA content is 4N
  - M phase: Mitosis
    - Prophase: DNA condensation and nuclear membrane dissolution
    - Metaphase: Sister chromatids line up in center on metaphase plate
    - Anaphase: Migration to opposite poles of cell
    - Telophase: Chromosomes decondense, nuclear membrane forms
    - Cytokinesis: Two daughter cells are created with identical DNA content
  - Gap phases:
    - Preparative phases
    - G_1: Preparation for S-phase entry:
      - Expression of cyclins, cyclin-dependent kinases
      - Specific transcription factors
      - Enzymes of replication
      - Entry into S phase is the committed step of cell cycle
    - G_2: Preparation for M-phase
      - Mismatch repair by specialized endonucleases
      - Expression of required proteins for mitosis
    - G_0: Resting phase
      - No cell division takes place

- Three types of cells:
  - Permanent
  - Stable
  - Labile

- Interphase:
  - G_0, G_1, S, G_2
  - Gene expression occurs

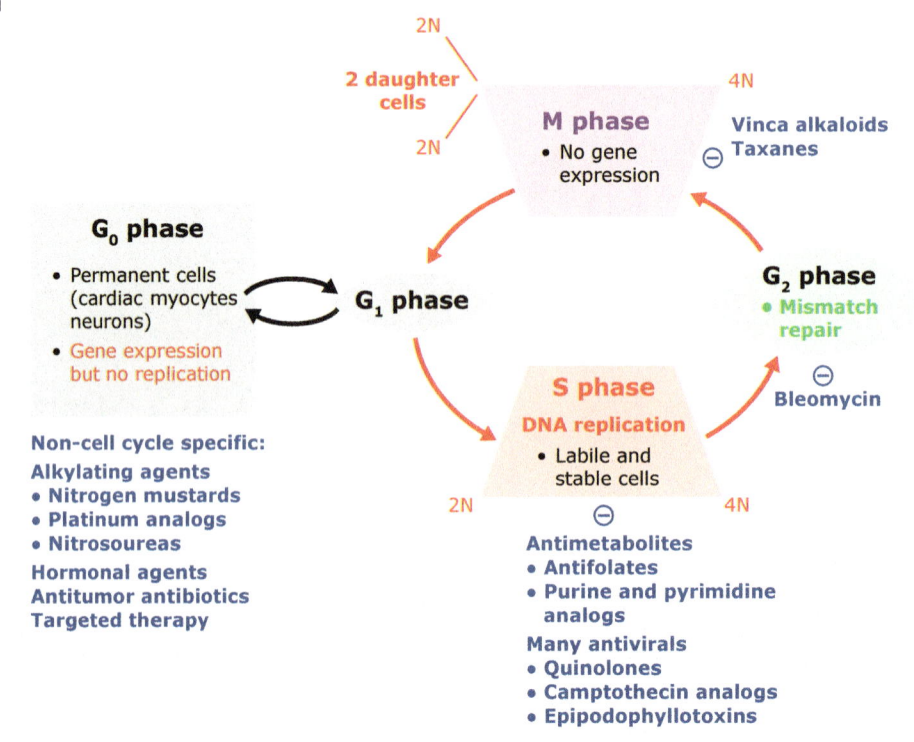

G₀ phase
- Permanent cells (cardiac myocytes, neurons)
- Gene expression but no replication

Non-cell cycle specific:
Alkylating agents
- Nitrogen mustards
- Platinum analogs
- Nitrosoureas

Hormonal agents
Antitumor antibiotics
Targeted therapy

M phase
- No gene expression

Vinca alkaloids
Taxanes

G₂ phase
- Mismatch repair

Bleomycin

S phase
DNA replication
- Labile and stable cells

Antimetabolites
- Antifolates
- Purine and pyrimidine analogs

Many antivirals
- Quinolones
- Camptothecin analogs
- Epipodophyllotoxins

▶ Figure 15-2.0
Cell Cycle

3 DNA Replication

- Initiation:
  - ORI: Origin of replication
  - Unwinding
  - Stabilization of separated templates
- Elongation:
  - Need for RNA primers
  - DNA polymerases
  - Topoisomerases
  - Nucleases
  - Ligases
- Termination:
  - Entire DNA must be copied to the end
  - Telomerase in eukaryotes
- DNA replication in prokaryotes and eukaryotes are similar
- Process is semiconservative and bidirectional

Bidirectional

Parent ds DNA
5' ATCGATCGATCG 3'
             ← 5'
5' →
3' TAGCTAGCTAGC 5'

Semiconservative

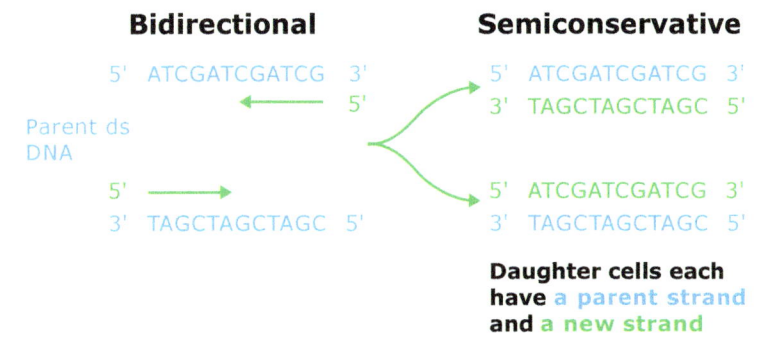

5' ATCGATCGATCG 3'
3' TAGCTAGCTAGC 5'

5' ATCGATCGATCG 3'
3' TAGCTAGCTAGC 5'

Daughter cells each have a parent strand and a new strand

▲ Figure 15-3.0 DNA Replication

3.1 Initiation

- Origins of replication ORI:
  - Specific DNA sequences found in prokaryotes, eukaryotes, and ds viruses
  - High AT content:
    —Easier to separate
  - Pre-replication complex binds to ORI
  - Eukaryotes have many ORI sequences:
    —Multiple linear chromosomes (3 billion base pairs)
    —Spaced 30 to 300,000 base pairs away
  - Prokaryotes have a single ORI:
    —Circular chromosome
    —Smaller (4 to 5 million base pairs)
    —ORI is bound by DNA_A protein

- Eukaryotic pre-replication complex (pre-RC):
  - Complex of proteins
  - Mini-chromosome maintenance (MCM):
    - Hexamer of MCM proteins
  - Cdc6 and Cdt1:
    - Cell division cycle 6 is an ATP-binding protein
    - Cdc6 and Cdt1 help MCM binding
  - Pre-RC identifies ORIs to initiate replication process

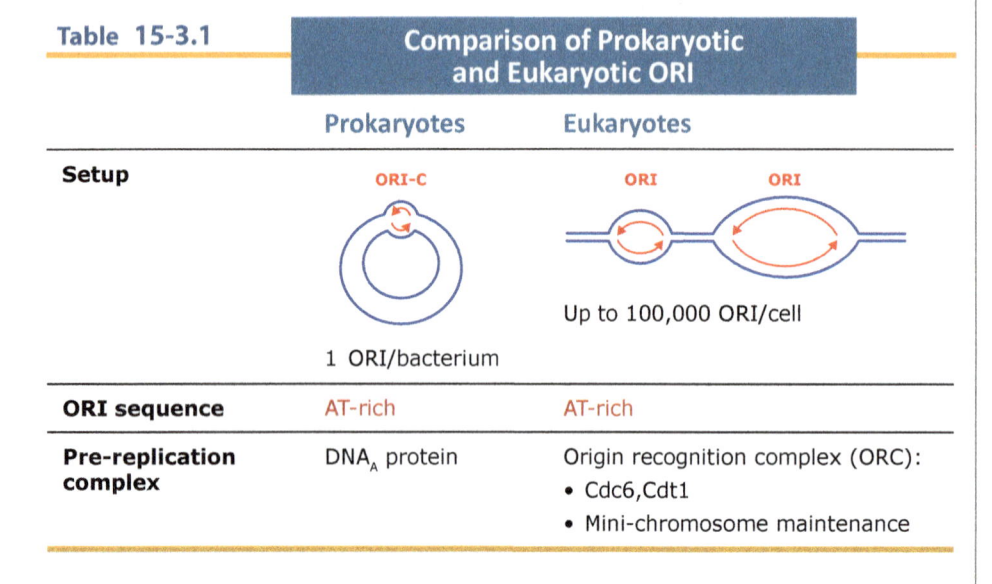

Table 15-3.1 Comparison of Prokaryotic and Eukaryotic ORI

	Prokaryotes	Eukaryotes
Setup	ORI-C 1 ORI/bacterium	ORI, ORI Up to 100,000 ORI/cell
ORI sequence	AT-rich	AT-rich
Pre-replication complex	DNA_A protein	Origin recognition complex (ORC): • Cdc6, Cdt1 • Mini-chromosome maintenance

- Unwinding:
  - DNA helicases:
    - Break H bonds at ORI sites
    - Require ATP
    - Are used by prokaryotes and eukaryotes
- Template stabilization:
  - Single-stranded DNA binding proteins (SSBPs)

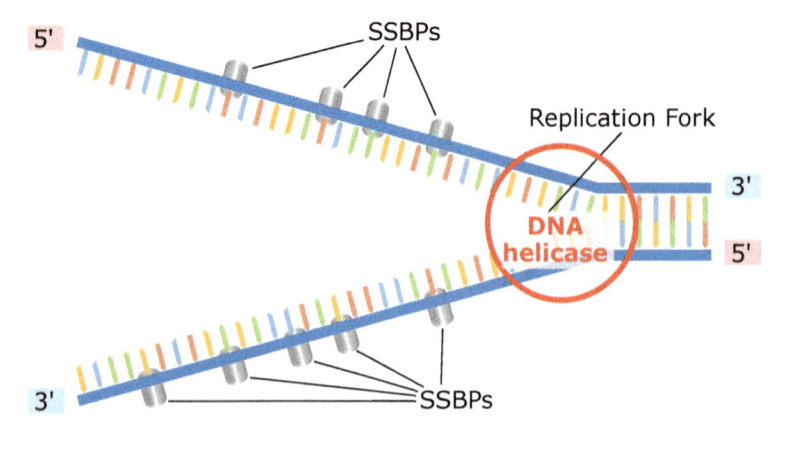

▲ **Figure 15–3.1** Unwinding Parent DNA

Chapter 15 • DNA Replication

3.2 Elongation
- Replication enzyme complex moves into the forks
- Process causes overwinding ahead, positive supercoils:
  - DNA topoisomerase I relaxes supercoils
  - DNA topoisomerase II introduces negative supercoils:
    — Negative supercoils = Unwinding
    — Requires ATP
    — Called DNA gyrase in bacteria
  - Various anticancer drugs and quinolones block topoisomerases

Tensed DNA	Relaxed DNA	Tensed DNA
⊖ Supercoils	Coils	⊕ Supercoils

Topoisomerase II ← ⊖ ← Etoposide / Teniposide / Quinolones
Replication transcription →
Topoisomerase I →
Topoisomerase I ← ⊖ ← Irinotecan / Topotecan

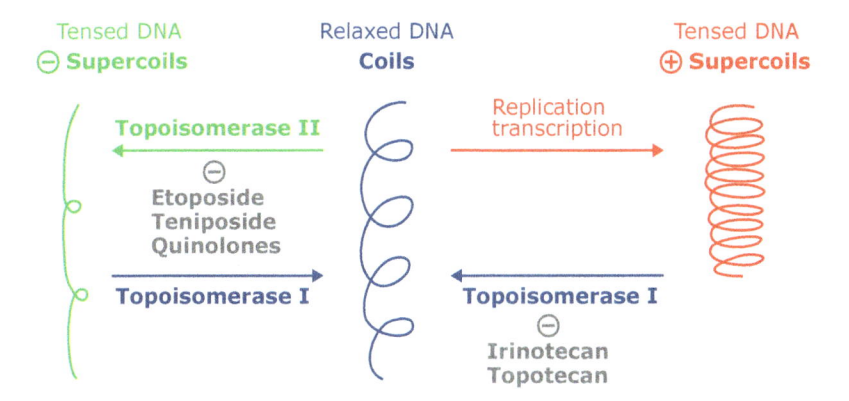

▲ Figure 15–3.2A DNA Coils, Supercoils, and Role of Topoisomerases

3.2.1 RNA Primer Synthesis
- DNA polymerases cannot initiate synthesis without a primer
  - Requires a free 3'-OH to attach to
- Primers consist of short pieces of RNA
  - Can be DNA in repair processes
- RNA primase makes an 8–12 base pairs long RNA
  - Needed in prokaryotes and eukaryotes

3.2.2 DNA Synthesis
- DNA polymerases:
  - Attach to 3'-OH of RNA primer
  - Use NTPs:

$$\text{NTP} \xrightarrow{\text{DNA polymerase}} \text{NMP in DNA} + \text{PPi}$$

  - Requires energy
  - Makes PDE bonds
  - New strand is made in 5' → 3' direction
    — Complementary, antiparallel to template strand

- **Leading strand:**
  - Continuous
  - Grows into fork
  - Single RNA primer
- **Lagging strand:**
  - Discontinuous
    —Okazaki fragments
    —About 150 base pairs long
    —Each has an RNA primer
  - Grows away from fork
- DNA polymerases differ in function and cell type

Table 15-3.2A — DNA Polymerases in Prokaryotes

DNA Polymerase	Function
Pol III	• Replication • Proofreading – 3' → 5' exonuclease activity
Pol I	• Has 5' → 3' exonuclease activity • Removes RNA primers • Replaces with DNA • Proofreading
Pol II	• DNA repair • Proofreading

Table 15-3.2B — DNA Polymerases in Eukaryotes

DNA Polymerase	Function

Pol α	• DNA primase complex
	  – RNA primer first
	    • PRIM1 and PRIM2 subunits
	  – Elongation by ~20 nucleotides
	    • POLA1 and POLA2 subunits

Pol ε	• Leading strand • Proofreading
Pol δ	• Lagging strand • Proofreading
Pol β	• DNA repair
Pol γ	• Mitochondrial DNA • Proofreading • Repair

Chapter 15 • DNA Replication

3.2.3 Removal of RNA Primers

- RNA primers are removed by 5' → 3' exonucleases
- In prokaryotes Pol I removes the RNA primers:
  - Has intrinsic 5' → 3' exonuclease activity
  - Uses RNase H also
  - Replaces RNA with DNA
- In eukaryotes, Pol δ removes the RNA primers:
  - Displaces 5' end of primer into a ssRNA flap
  - Endonuclease 1 cleaves RNA flap
  - Pol δ replaces RNA with DNA
  - Another possibility involves coating flap with SSBPs and cleavage with DNA 2 nuclease

3.2.4 Ligation of Okazaki Fragments

- Performed by DNA ligases:
  - Create a PDE bond
- Require NADH
- Prokaryotes and eukaryotes

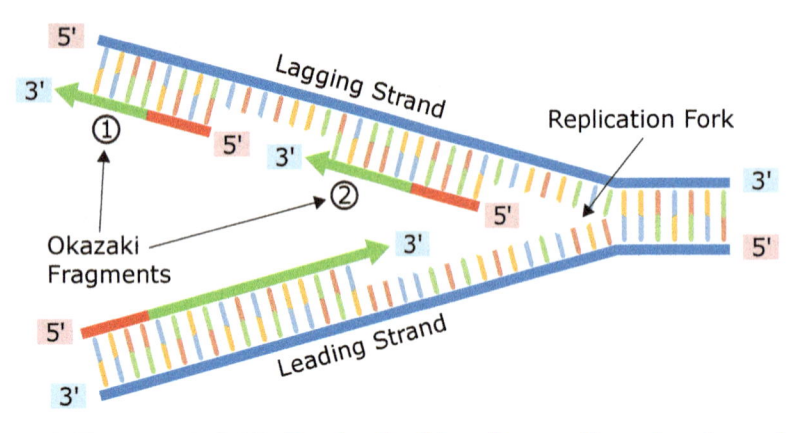

▲ Figure 15-3.2B Synthesis of Leading and Lagging Strand

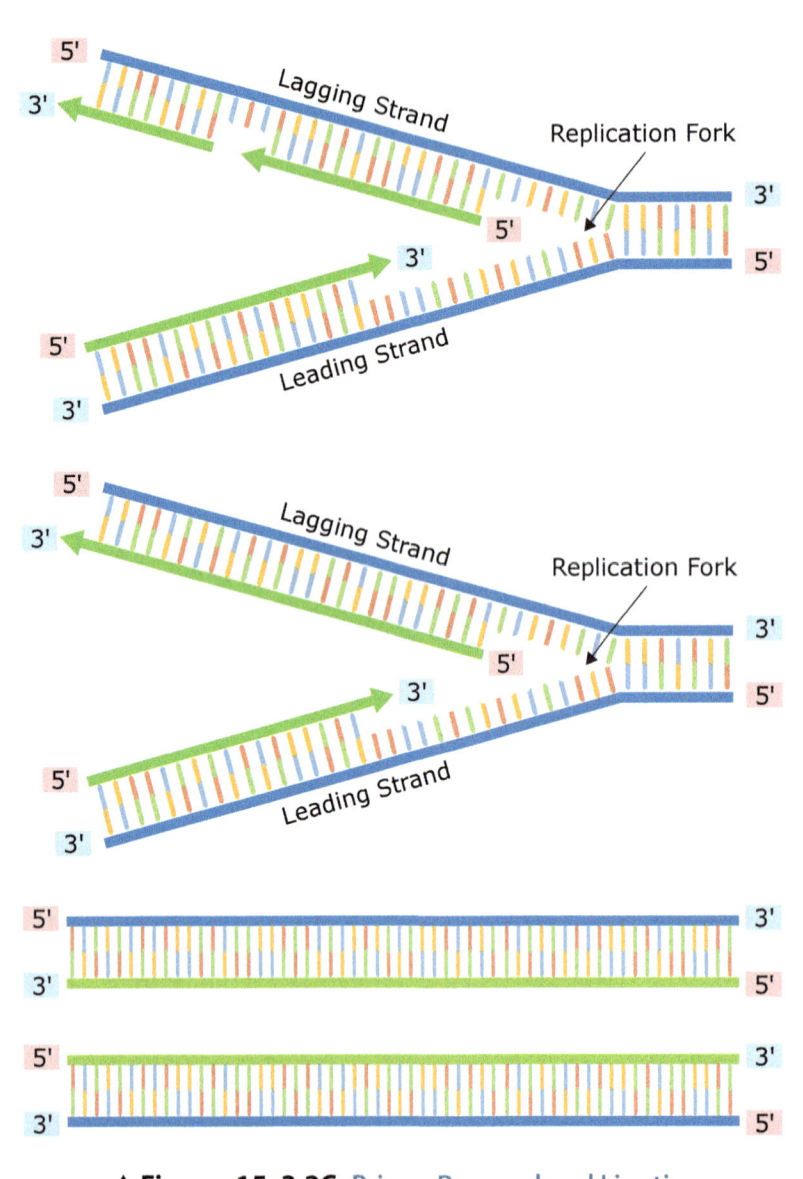

▲ Figure 15-3.2C Primer Removal and Ligation

3.3 Termination

- Prokaryotes:
  - Termination occurs when replication forks meet each other

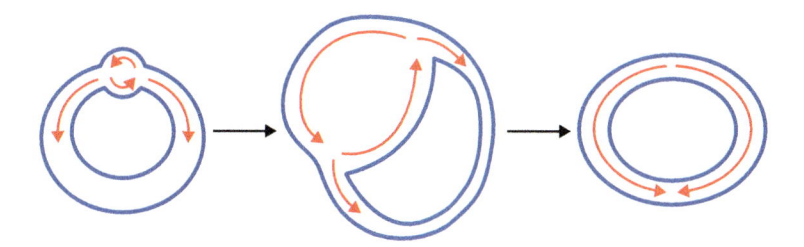

▲ Figure 15–3.3 Terminations

- Tus protein:
  - Termination utilization substance
  - Acts as counter-helicase
  - Halts DNA polymerase movement
  - An example of Ter protein (DNA replication termination site-binding protein)
- Eukaryotes:
  - Replication forks meet and terminate at many points along chromosome
  - Ends at telomere regions

3.4 Eukaryotic Telomeres and Telomerase

- Telomeres are TTAGGG sequences:
  - Repeated 2,500 times in humans
  - Protect end of chromosomes
  - Are not replicated all the way to the end:
    - Shortening telomeres correlate with cell aging and death
    - Telomerase can build telomeres
- Telomerase complex:
  - ↑ Activity in germ cells, some stem cells, and cancer cells
  - Human reverse transcriptase:
    - TERT: Telomerase reverse transcriptase
      - hTERT gene is on chromosome 5
      - Deleted in cri-du-chat syndrome
    - TERC: Telomerase RNA component
      - Serves as template for TTAGGG sequence
  - Oncogenesis:
    - Deregulation of TERT expression in somatic cells plays a role

4 DNA Proofreading

- DNA polymerases make mistakes:
  - Rate of 1 in 10^5 base pairs
  - Human genome 2 × 3 billion nucleotides to copy
  - 60,000 errors
- Most are corrected during replication:
  - 3' → 5' exonuclease activity of Pol ε and δ and Pol I → III in prokaryotes
  - Only correct mismatches as they occur
  - Reduces errors to ~600

S Phase: Proofreading

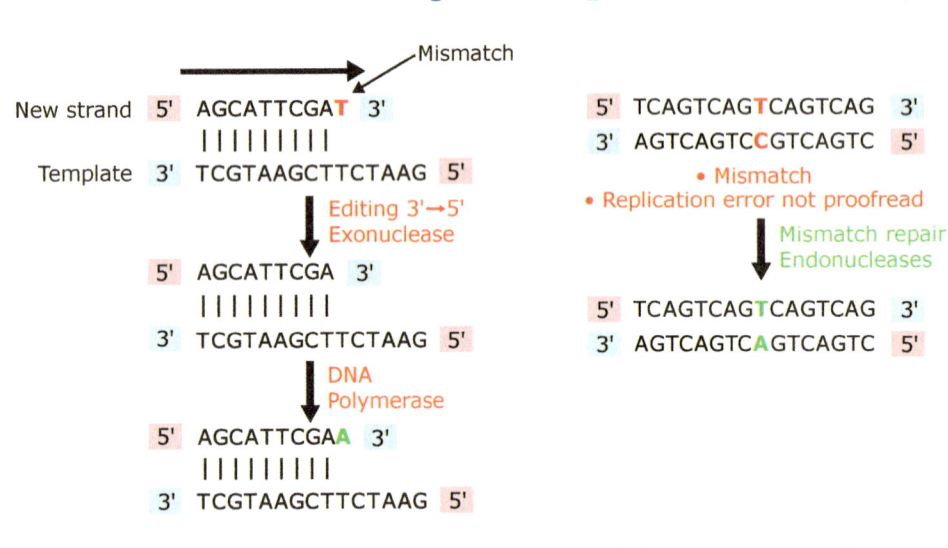

New strand 5' AGCATTCGA**T** 3' (Mismatch)
Template 3' TCGTAAGCTTCTAAG 5'

↓ Editing 3'→5' Exonuclease

5' AGCATTCGA 3'
3' TCGTAAGCTTCTAAG 5'

↓ DNA Polymerase

5' AGCATTCGA**A** 3'
3' TCGTAAGCTTCTAAG 5'

G₂ Phase: Mismatch Repair

5' TCAGTCAG**T**CAGTCAG 3'
3' AGTCAGTC**C**GTCAGTC 5'

- Mismatch
- Replication error not proofread

↓ Mismatch repair Endonucleases

5' TCAGTCAG**T**CAGTCAG 3'
3' AGTCAGTC**A**GTCAGTC 5'

▲ **Figure 15-4.0** DNA Editing: High-Fidelity DNA Synthesis

- Remaining replication errors are removed during G_2 phase:
  - Mismatch repair endonucleases
  - Final error rate ~6 per cell division
  - Hereditary nonpolyposis colorectal cancer (HNPCC)
    —Defect in $hMSH_2$ (60%) and $hMLH_1$ (30%)
    - Leads to microsatellite instability (MSI)
    - Most alter the length of CA repeats
    —AD: 2%–7% of diagnosed CRC yearly
    —Right-sided, poorly differentiated adenocarcinoma
    —↑ Risk of endometrial, ovarian, stomach, hepatobiliary, brain, and skin cancers as well
    —Known also as Lynch syndrome

5 DNA Polymerase Inhibitors

- Nucleoside analogs
- Used in cancer and viral infections
- Interrupt DNA replication
- Prodrugs requiring kinases:
  - Activation to nucleotide analogs
- Two strategies:
  - Different sugar: Cytarabine

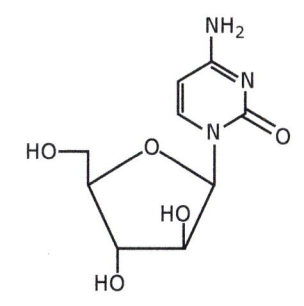

▲ Figure 15-5.0A Cytarabine

- Chain terminators:
  — Lack 3'-OH
  — Inserted in growing DNA
  — No further elongation possible
  — Include anti-herpes medications (acyclovir, ganciclovir) and all nucleoside reverse transcriptase inhibitors (NRTIs)

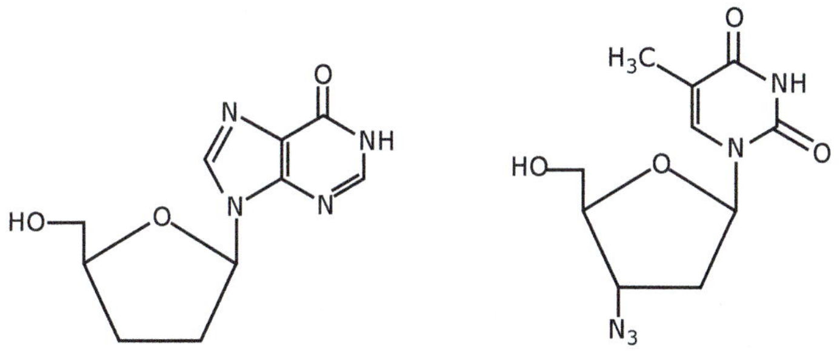

Dideoxyinosine (dDI)   **Azidothymidine (AZT)**

▲ Figure 15-5.0B Two Chain Terminators Used in HIV

6 DNA Repair

- Damage can be caused by DNA replication errors as seen previously in topic 4, DNA Proofreading
- Environmental damage:
  - Heat causes loss of bases:
    — Apurination or apyrimidation
    — Called AP site
  - Nitrites, nitrosamines, and heat cause deamination:
    — C → U
    — 5-Methylcytosine → T
    — G → Xanthine
    — A → Hypoxanthine
  - UV causes pyrimidine dimers
  - Ionizing radiation, alkylating agents modify nucleotides and break bonds
- Mechanism of repair:
  - Specific endonuclease recognizes damage:
    — Excises area to be repaired
  - Repair enzymes include:
    — DNA polymerase β:
      - Can utilize DNA as primer
    — DNA ligase

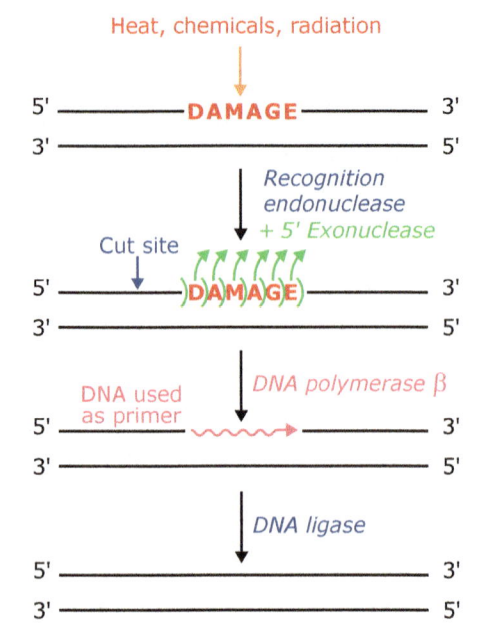

▲ Figure 15–6.0 Steps in DNA Repair

Table 15-6.0	DNA Damage and Specific Recognition Endonucleases		
DNA Damage	**Cause**	**Recognition Enzyme**	**Remarks**
AP site	• Heat	• AP endonuclease	

Deamination C → U	• Nitrites
	• Nitrosamines
		• Uracil glycosylase
		  – Removes U
		  – Leaves AP site
		• AP endonuclease
			• These chemicals are used as food preservatives
			• ↑ Risk of esophageal and gastric cancers

Thymine dimers	• UV light	• UV excinuclease	• Deficiency in xeroderma pigmentosum • Autosomal recessive
Mismatch repair	• Replication errors	• Mismatch repair endonucleases	• Occurs in G_2 phase • Deficient in HNPCC and Lynch syndrome
DNA strand breaks	• Ionizing radiation • X-rays	• Multiple systems: – BRCA1 and BRCA2	• BRCA1 and BRCA2 are part of ds breaks repair • 5%–10% of breast/ovarian tumors have mutated BRCAs • Also factors in certain colon, pancreas, and prostate cancers
		– ATM	• Ser/thr kinase recruited and activated by ds breaks in DNA • Mutated in ataxia telangiectasia

CHAPTER 16 — Gene Expression: Transcription and Control

1 Overview

- DNA is made of expressed and non-expressed sequences of nucleotides:
  - Genes are expressed DNA or coding DNA:
    — They can be transcribed to an RNA molecule
    — If the RNA is a messenger RNA (mRNA), they can be further translated into a protein
  - Non-expressed DNA:
    — Also called spacer DNA or intergenic spacer, or non-coding DNA
    — Comprises the majority of our genome (> 98%)
    — Controls gene expression:
      - Where?
      - When?
      - How much?
- RNA polymerases transcribe dsDNA from a gene into an ssRNA:
  - RNA is complementary and antiparallel to the template strand of the gene
- Promoter and terminator regions bracket a gene:
  - Promoters allow RNA polymerase to recognize where a gene starts:
    — Promoters are not transcribed
    — Impose which of the two gene strands is used as the template
  - Terminators allow RNA polymerase to recognize where a gene ends:
    — Eukaryotic terminators are not well characterized
- Transcription requires factors:
  - General transcription factors allow RNA polymerase to start:
    — Bind to promoters
  - Specific transcription factors allow fine control of expression:
    — Bind to enhancers or silencers
  - All transcription factors bind to specific DNA sequences in intergenic DNA
- There are significant differences between prokaryotes and eukaryotes
- Several types of RNA molecules are transcribed by various RNA polymerases:
  - Each type serves a different function in gene expression

USMLE® Key Concepts

For Step 1, you must be able to:

▶ Describe the structure of a gene and its relationship to intergenic DNA.

▶ Contrast prokaryotic and eukaryotic transcription.

▶ Understand the role of packaging DNA in the control of gene expression.

▶ Describe general and specific transcription factors.

Chapter 16 • Gene Expression: Transcription and Control Biochemistry

2 Gene Structure

- Genes are double-stranded DNA:
  - Contain a template to generate the RNA
  - Begin at a transcription start
  - Transcription start is arbitrarily given +1 as a location marker:
    — Nucleotides to be transcribed are downstream and sequentially numbered (+2, +3, +4, etc.)
    — Nucleotides that are upstream are NOT TRANSCRIBED and are negatively numbered (−1, −2, −3, etc.)
    — Promoters are always immediately upstream from +1

A. Gene Organization

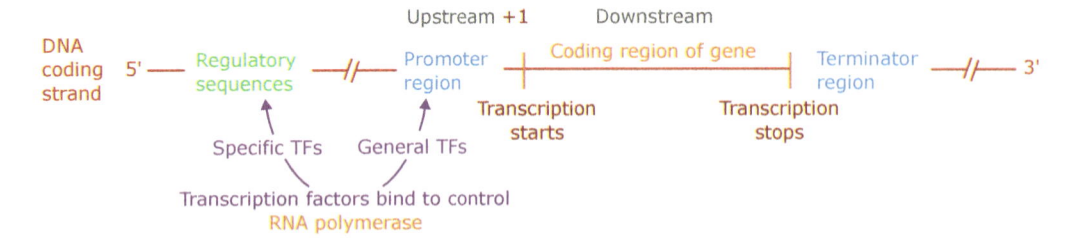

DNA coding strand 5'— Regulatory sequences —//— Promoter region | Coding region of gene | Terminator region —//— 3'

Upstream +1 Downstream
Transcription starts — Transcription stops

Specific TFs, General TFs — Transcription factors bind to control RNA polymerase

B. Template Versus Coding Strand

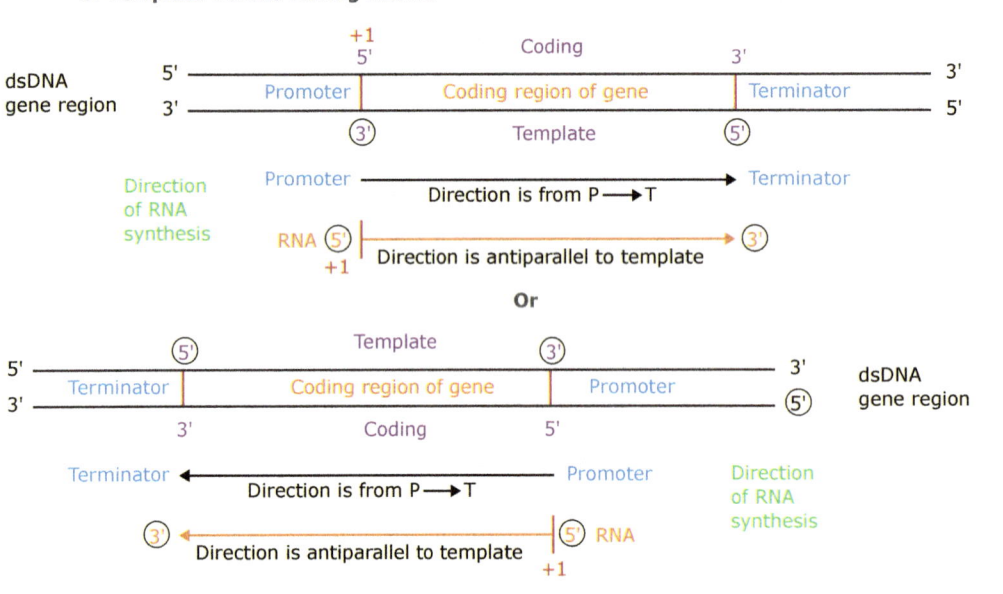

dsDNA gene region:
5'— Promoter | Coding region of gene | Terminator —3'
3'— (3') Template (5') —5'
+1 5' Coding 3'

Direction of RNA synthesis: Promoter → Terminator
Direction is from P → T
RNA 5' +1 — 3' Direction is antiparallel to template

Or

5'— Terminator | Coding region of gene | Promoter —3' dsDNA gene region
3'— (5') Template (3') —5'
3' Coding 5'

Terminator ← Promoter Direction of RNA synthesis
Direction is from P → T
3' ← RNA 5' +1 Direction is antiparallel to template

C. Relationship Between DNA Coding, Template, RNA, and Protein Sequence

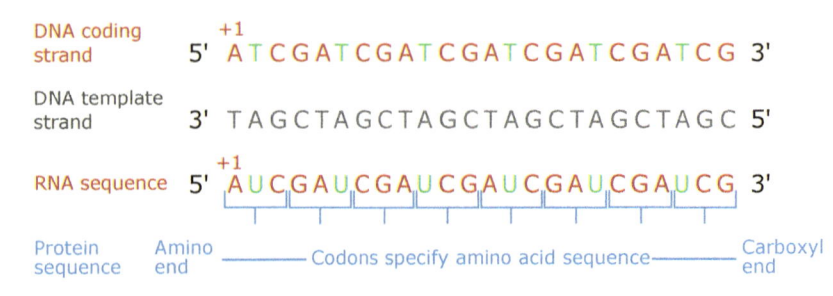

DNA coding strand   5' ATCGATCGATCGATCGATCGATCG 3'
                         +1
DNA template strand   3' TAGCTAGCTAGCTAGCTAGCTAGC 5'

RNA sequence   5' AUCGAUCGAUCGAUCGAUCGAUCG 3'
                         +1

Protein sequence: Amino end ——— Codons specify amino acid sequence ——— Carboxyl end

- Coding DNA and RNA sequence is identical except T/U
- Proteins are translated from amino to carboxyl end by reading RNA from 5' to 3' direction

◀ **Figure 16–2.0**
Gene Structure

- Convention:
    1. **Gene sequences are given as coding sequences:**
        — If template strand is given instead, it would have to be specified
    2. **When writing DNA/RNA sequences:**
        — No numbering is needed if written as in English (left to right):
            5'TCAG3' is TCAG
        — Numbering is required if written backward:
            TCAG but 3'GACT5'

2.1 Promoters

- **Immediately upstream** from +1 transcription start:
  - Promoters extend to about −100
  - Other regulatory regions are distal to promoters
- **On/off switch** for transcription
- First bound to by **general transcription factors (TFs)**
- Once general TFs label the promoter, **RNA polymerase can start at +1:**
  - At least 6 TFs are required
  - Labeled A, B, D, E, F, and H
- Promoters contain **boxes:**
  - Boxes are unique DNA sequences recognized by general TFs
  - Boxes function as "receptors" for general TFs to bind to
  - Boxes have specific locations within the promoter regions
  - Boxes are also known as **response or recognition elements (REs)**
- Prokaryotic and eukaryotic promoter regions are different

Table 16-2.1 — Transcription Factors and Binding Sites in Promoters

Cell Type	DNA-Binding Site	Sequence	Transcription Factors
Prokaryote	−35 consensus sequence	TTGACA	σ-70
	−10 TATA box (Pribnow)	TATAAT	σ-70
Eukaryote	−25 TATA box (Hogness)	TATAAA or TATATA	TATA binding protein (TBP), a subunit of TFIID
	−35 TFIIB recognition element (BRE)	GC-rich region	TFIIB
	−70 CAT box	CCAAT	NF-Y

A. Bacterial Promoters

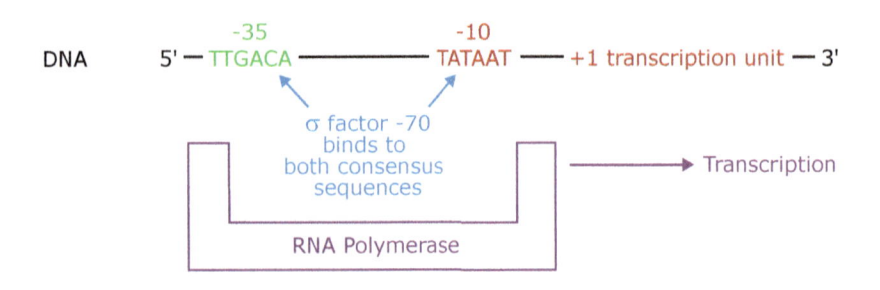

DNA 5' — TTGACA ———— TATAAT —— +1 transcription unit — 3'
         -35   -10

σ factor -70 binds to both consensus sequences → RNA Polymerase → Transcription

B. Eukaryotic Promoters

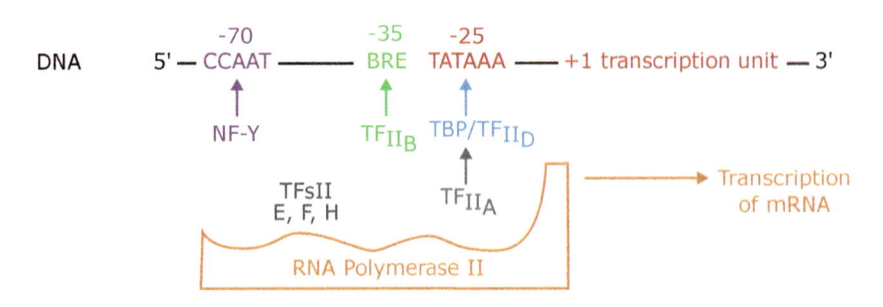

DNA 5' — CCAAT ———— BRE — TATAAA —— +1 transcription unit — 3'
         -70   -35   -25

- NF-Y binds CCAAT
- TF_{IIB} binds BRE
- TBP/TF_{IID} binds TATAAA
- TF_{IIA}, TFsII E, F, H with RNA Polymerase II → Transcription of mRNA

*Note: TF_{IIH} has ATPase and helicase activity to make transcription bubble

▲ **Figure 16-2.1** Upstream Promoter Elements in Prokaryotes and Eukaryotes

- Clinical relevance:
  - Mutations in promoter regions result in altered expression of genes
  - In Gilbert syndrome, mutations in TATA box of UGT1A1 gene on chr. 2 ↓ expression by 70%–80%
  - Somatic TERT promoter mutations resulting in reactivation of telomerase in:
    - —43% of CNS tumors
    - —59% of bladder cancers
    - —29% of melanomas
    - —10% of follicular thyroid carcinomas (Vinagre, et al., Nature Communications, 2013; 4:2185.)

2.2 Transcription Units

- Start at +1 and end at termination signal
- Contains various sequences:
  - 5' untranslated region (5'UTR)
  - Exons
  - Introns
  - 3'UTR
- Prokaryotes have no introns:
  - 5'UTR
  - Coding sequence for protein
  - 3'UTR

Table 16-2.2 — Comparison of Prokaryote and Eukaryote Transcription Units

Cell Type	DNA Region	Location	Description
Prokaryote	5'UTR	• +1 to coding region	• Short • Contains ribosome binding site: – Shine-Dalgarno sequence – AGGAGGT
	Protein coding sequence	• Downstream from 5'UTR	• Starts with ATG • Ends with TGA, TAG, or TAA • Continuous
	3'UTR	• Downstream from coding region	• Contains termination signal: – ρ-factor dependent or – ρ-factor independent • ρ-factor independent: – GC-rich hairpin loop (or stem-and-loop followed by a series of Us in RNA
Eukaryote	5'UTR	• +1 to first exon	• Long (100s to 1,000s of nucleotides) • Contains cap site (Pyr-A-Pyr) • Contains regulatory sequences for translation: – Upstream open reading frames (uORF) – Contains its own upstream initiation codon (uAUG) and termination codon – Can be translated as a leader peptide – Leader peptide regulates translation of main protein sequence
	Kozak consensus sequence	• End of 5'UTR and beginning of first exon	• Ribosome binding sequence: – ACCATGG – Contains initiation codon ATG
	Exon 1	• First exon: Downstream from 5'UTR	• Starts with ATG
	Splice donor site	• 3' end of exon and 5' end of intron	• AGGT sequence • Spliceosome first cuts here to remove introns
	Introns	• In between exons • Bordered by splice sites: – Donor, 5' end – Acceptor, 3' end	• Removed by splicing: – Not translated • Contain regulatory regions: – Alternative splicing – Intron-mediated enhancement (IME) – ↑ Expression of gene
	Splice acceptor site	• 3' end of intron and 5' end of next exon	• AGGT sequence • Spliceosome cuts and removes intron as a lariat
	Last exon	• Upstream from 3'UTR	• Ends with TGA, TAG, or TAA
	3'UTR	• Downstream from last exon	• Contains polyadenylation signal: – AATAAA – Used to attach poly(A) tail on RNA

Chapter 16 • Gene Expression: Transcription and Control

A. Prokaryotes

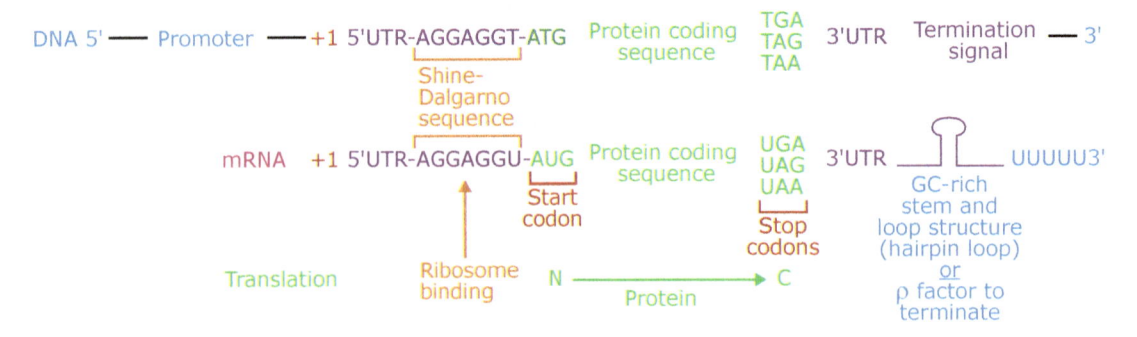

DNA 5' — Promoter — +1 5'UTR-AGGAGGT-ATG Protein coding sequence TGA/TAG/TAA 3'UTR Termination signal — 3'

Shine-Dalgarno sequence

mRNA +1 5'UTR-AGGAGGU-AUG Protein coding sequence UGA/UAG/UAA 3'UTR GC-rich stem and loop structure (hairpin loop) or ρ factor to terminate UUUUU3'

Start codon — Stop codons

Translation — Ribosome binding — N → Protein → C

B. Eukaryotes

DNA 5' — Promoter — +1 5'UTR ACC ATGG Exon 1 AGGT Intron 1 AGGT Exon 2 TGA/TAG/TAA 3'UTR AATAAA — 3'

Cap site — Kozak consensus sequence — Splice sites — Polyadenylation signal

hnRNA (pre-mRNA) +1 5'UTR ACC AUGG Exon 1 AGGU Intron 1 AGGU Exon 2 UGA/UAG/UAA 3'UTR AAUAAA — 3'

Start codon — Splice donor site — Splice acceptor site — Stop codon

Processing to mRNA prior to translation

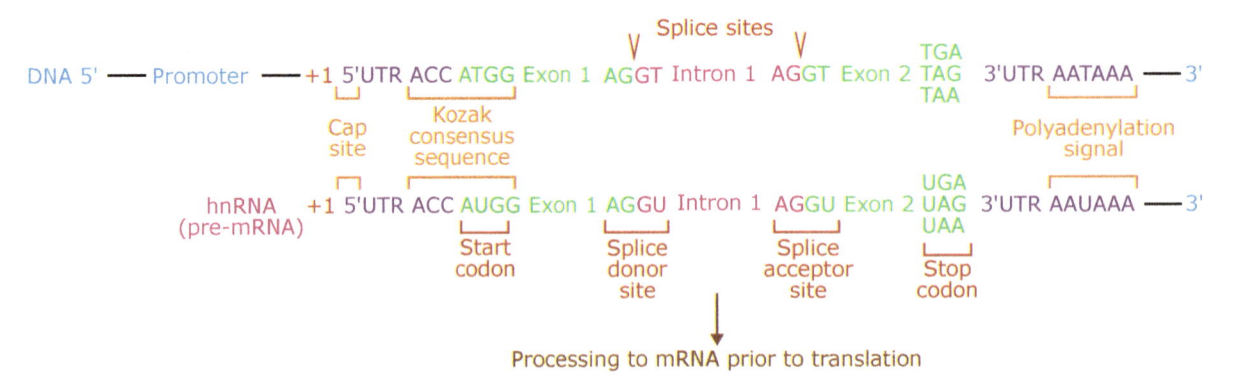

▲ **Figure 16–2.2** Prokaryotic and Eukaryotic Transcription Units

2.3 Terminators

- Mark the end of a gene (3'UTR)
- Mediate termination of transcription:
    - Require termination factors
- Prokaryotes have Rho-dependent or ρ-independent termination signals:
    - ρ factor causes RNA polymerase dissociation from template
    - ρ-independent uses hairpin loops, which cause steric hindrance
- Eukaryotes have a polyadenylation (poly(A) polymerase) signal:
    - Poly(A) sequence is transcribed (AAUAAA)
    - Termination factors CPSF (cleavage and poly(A) specificity factor) and CstF (cleavage stimulation factor) help free RNA from the DNA template within a few kilobases from the poly(A) site

3 RNA Processing

- Prokaryotes transcribe mRNA, which can be immediately translated:
  - No processing
  - Translation and transcription occur simultaneously
- Eukaryotes transcribe hnRNA (heterogeneous RNA):
  - Processing to mRNA (messenger RNA) is required
  - Transcription and translation DO NOT occur simultaneously
    - —Transcription and processing are nuclear events
    - —Translation is a cytoplasmic event

3.1 Co-Transcriptional Capping of RNA

- Occurs at 5' end as hnRNA is being transcribed
- 5'–5' triphosphate linkage between 7-methylguanosine residue and 5' end of hnRNA:
  - Added by mRNA guanylyltransferase
- Protects from degradation by 5' exonuclease of RNases
- Recognition site for ribosome binding
- Helps in nuclear export of mRNA
  - Regulated by cap binding complex (CBC)
  - Nuclear pore complex recognizes CBC on cap

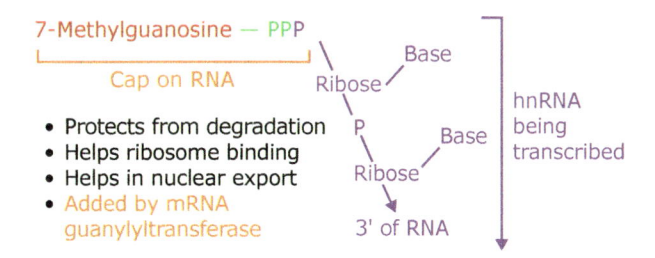

▲ Figure 16-3.1 Capping the hnRNA in Eukaryotes

3.2 Posttranscriptional Poly(A) Tail Addition

- Poly(A) signal sequence AAUAAA is transcribed
- CPSF cleaves 10–20 nucleotides downstream with the help of CstF
- Polyadenylate polymerase (PAP) adds on ~250 A's to 3' end
- Poly(A) tail protects from degradation by 3' exonucleases
- Poly(A) tail helps export mRNA from nucleus to cytoplasm
- Histone mRNA do not have poly(A) tails:
  - They have stem-and-loop followed by a purine-rich sequence

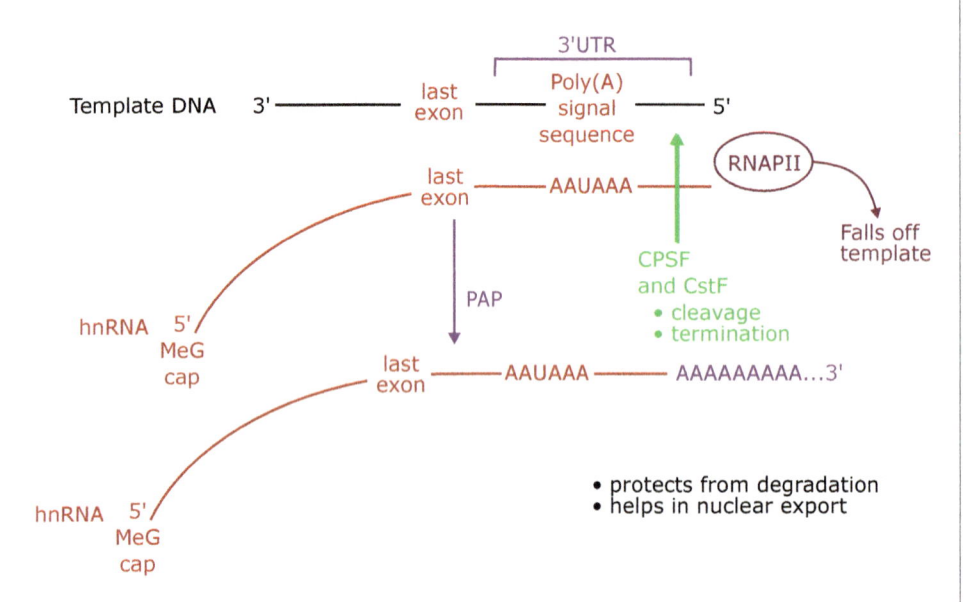

▲ Figure 16–3.2 Poly(A) Tail Addition in Eukaryotes

3.3 Posttranscriptional Intron Splicing

- Genes may contain up to 50 or so introns
- Introns are removed by the spliceosome:
  - Complex of small nuclear RNAs (snRNAs) and proteins called SNRNPs (small nuclear ribonucleoproteins), or "snurps"
  - Remove introns from pre-mRNA
  - Ligates exons back together
  - Converts hnRNA to mRNA
- Splice sites contain invariant AGGU sequence:
  - Splice donor site:
    - —5' end of intron always has GU ("give up")
  - Splice acceptor site:
    - —3' end of intron always has AG ("accept gratefully")
- snRNAs are called U_1, U_2, U_4, U_5, and U_6:
  - U_1 binds first to splice donor site (exon/intron junction):
  - U_2 binds within intron to an A
  - U_4, U_5, and U_6 bind to the complex and form a loop called a lariat
  - Cleavage of intron
  - Ligation of exon

- **Clinical relevance:** Antinuclear antibodies (ANAs)
  - Several autoimmune disorders are diagnosed or monitored following ANA titers
  - In Sjögren syndrome:
    —SS-A (Ro)
    —SS-B (La, also found in SLE)
    —Anti-ribonucleoproteins
  - In mixed connective tissue disease:
    —Anti-U1RNP (also found in SLE)
  - In systemic lupus erythematosus (SLE):
    —Anti-Sm (Smith antigen)
    —Sm proteins are part of snRNP complexes

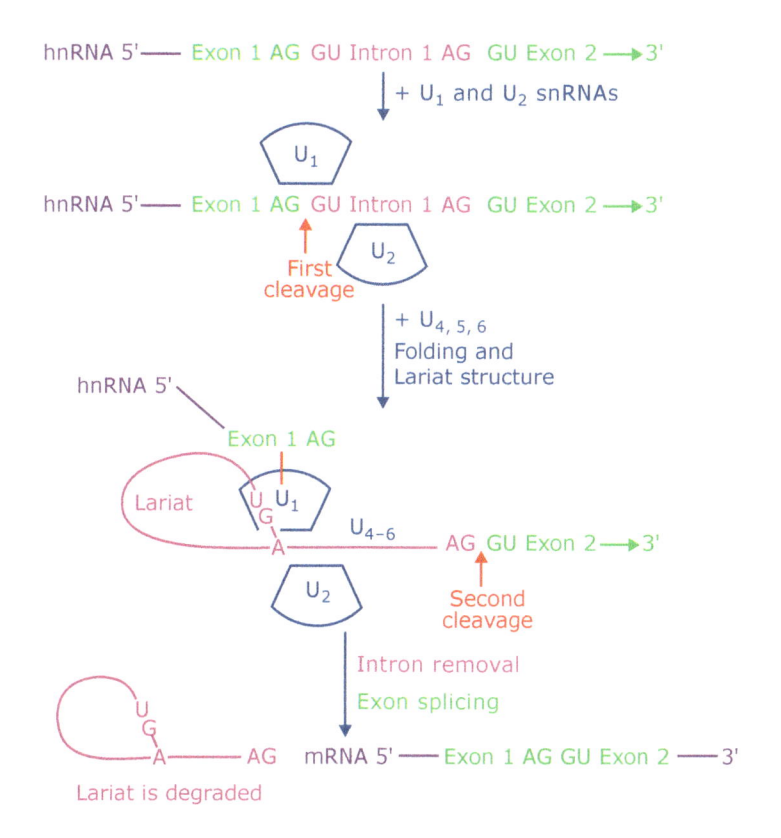

▲ Figure 16-3.3 Intron Removal by Spliceosome

3.4 Alternative Splicing

- Regulated process:
  - Some exons may be excluded or included in final mRNA
  - Called exon skipping
  - Is tissue specific
  - Single gene can code for multiple proteins with different functions
  - ~95% of genes with multiple exons are alternatively spliced

- Requires specific transcription factors:
  - Called splicing factors
  - Splicing factors bind to intronic or exonic splicing silencer sites (ISS or ESS) and act as splicing repressor proteins:
    —Hide splice sites from spliceosome
  - Splicing factors bind to intronic or exonic splicing enhancer site (ISE or ESE) and act as splicing activator proteins:
    —Labeled splice sites for spliceosome

A. Regular Splicing

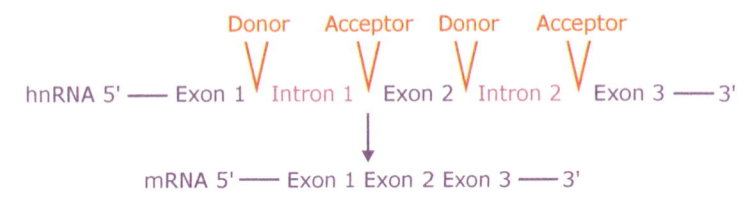

hnRNA 5' — Exon 1 | Intron 1 | Exon 2 | Intron 2 | Exon 3 — 3'
(Donor, Acceptor, Donor, Acceptor)

↓

mRNA 5' — Exon 1 Exon 2 Exon 3 — 3'

B. Alternative Splicing

Splicing repressor proteins bind

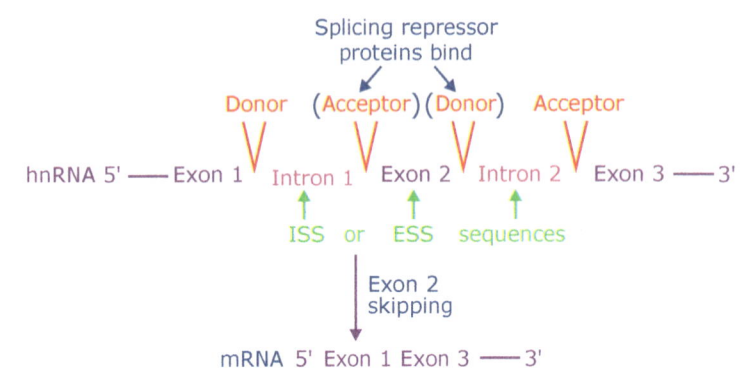

hnRNA 5' — Exon 1 | Intron 1 | Exon 2 | Intron 2 | Exon 3 — 3'
(Donor, (Acceptor), (Donor), Acceptor)

ISS or ESS sequences

Exon 2 skipping

mRNA 5' Exon 1 Exon 3 — 3'

▲ Figure 16–3.4 Alternative Splicing

- Clinical relevance:
  - Mutations affecting splice sites and alternative splicing:
    —30%–50% of mutations that cause human disease affect splicing
    —Abnormal spliced mRNAs are found in many cancer cells
    —Examples include cases of Tay-Sachs, β-thalassemia, TTP, etc.
  - Mutation in exons will be reviewed in a subsequent chapter and include substitution, deletion, and insertion
    —These mutations affect the amino acid sequence of the protein

4 Types of RNA and RNA Polymerases

4.1 Prokaryotic RNA Polymerase

- Prokaryotes have a single RNA polymerase
  - Made of 5 subunits:
    - 2 α subunits:
      - Interact with promoter DNA
    - β and β' subunits:
      - Contain the RNA polymerase active site
    - ω subunit:
      - Helps in assembly and stabilization with template
- Prokaryotes make three types of RNA:
  - Messenger RNA (mRNA):
    - Code for protein sequence
  - Ribosomal RNA (rRNA):
    - Code for ribosomal subunits
  - Transfer RNA (tRNA):
    - Adaptor molecule
    - Link nucleotide sequence with amino acid sequence
- Clinical relevance:
  - Rifampin and rifamycins (rifabutin, rifapentine)
    - Inhibit prokaryotic RNA polymerase:
      - Bind to β subunit
    - Used to treat mycobacteria infections
    - General inducers of CYP450s
    - Red/orange metabolites in body fluids
    - Hepatotoxic

4.2 Eukaryotic RNA Polymerase

- Eukaryotes have three main RNA polymerases:
  - RNAP I
  - RNAP II
  - RNAP III
- Types of RNA:
  - Heterogeneous nuclear (hn)RNA:
    - Initial transcript (pre-mRNA)
  - Messenger (m)RNA
  - Small nuclear (sn)RNA:
    - Part of spliceosomes
  - rRNAs and tRNAs as in prokaryotes

- microRNAs (miRNAs):
  - Small noncoding RNAs:
    - 20+ nucleotides long
    - Can come from introns or have their own genes
    - Single-stranded
  - Function in RNA silencing:
    - Pair with mRNA targets
    - Prevent translation or cause degradation of mRNA
- Small interfering RNAs (siRNAs):
  - Small noncoding RNAs:
    - 20+ nucleotides-long
    - Have their own genes
    - Double-stranded
  - Function in RNA silencing:
    - Cause destruction of mRNA target

- RNA-induced silencing complex (RISC):
  - Multiprotein complex performing RNA interference (RNAi)
  - Uses miRNAs and siRNAs as templates to recognize complementary mRNA transcripts
  - RNase III Dicer help in loading RNAs into RISC
  - Endonuclease called Argonaute cleaves target mRNA
  - Process occurs in cytoplasmic bodies called P-bodies
    - P-bodies are processing bodies
    - Involved in mRNA turnover

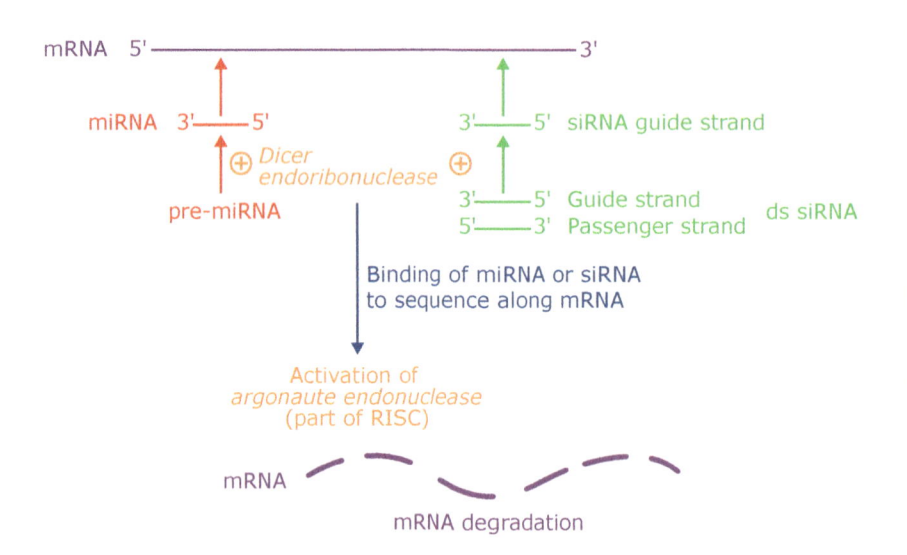

▲ Figure 16–4.2 RNA Interference Pathway in Cytoplasmic P-Bodies

Table 16-4.2 Roles of Eukaryotic RNA Polymerases

RNA Polymerase	Location	Roles
RNAP I	Nucleolus	• rRNA except 5S rRNA
RNAP II	Nucleoplasm	• hnRNA/mRNA • snRNAs • miRNAs • siRNAs
RNAP III	Nucleoplasm	• tRNAs • 5S rRNA

- Clinical relevance of RNA interference:
  - RNA interference is an important part of immune response to viruses
  - RNA interference is a mode of posttranscriptional gene expression control
  - Medical applications:
    — siRNAs are in clinical trials for macular degeneration and RSV infections
    — Potential applications in infectious diseases, cancer treatment
    — Problems with siRNAs therapy include:
      • Delivery to appropriate tissue
      • Specificity of mRNA targeting
- Inhibitors of eukaryotic RNA polymerases
  - Actinomycin D:
    — Dactinomycin
    — Anti-tumor
    — Nonselective inhibitor of RNAP I, II, and III
    — Added to methotrexate in choriocarcinoma treatment
  - α-amanitin:
    — *Amanita phalloides* toxin
    — Selective RNAP II inhibitor
    — No antidote
    — Toxicity:
      • Gastroenteritis
      • Fulminant hepatitis
      • Acute tubular necrosis

5 Control of Gene Expression Through Epigenetic Modifications

- Epigenetic modifications include chromatin modification and DNA methylation

5.1 Chromatin Structure

- Packaging of DNA prevents gene expression
- Histones play a critical role:
  - Positively charged:
    - Rich in Arg and Lys
  - Five types:
    - Two copies each of H_{2A}, H_{2B}, H_3, and H_4 form an octamer
    - DNA binds to octamer forming a nucleosome
    - Each nucleosome is a 10 nm bead
    - Separated by linker DNA:
      - Linker DNA is sensitive to nucleases
    - H_1 binds to linker DNA:
      - Condenses 10 nm chromatin into 30 nm chromatin
      - No longer sensitive to nucleases
  - Further condensation occurs:
    - Euchromatin (loosely packaged) becomes heterochromatin (tightly packaged)
    - Heterochromatin is transcriptionally inactive

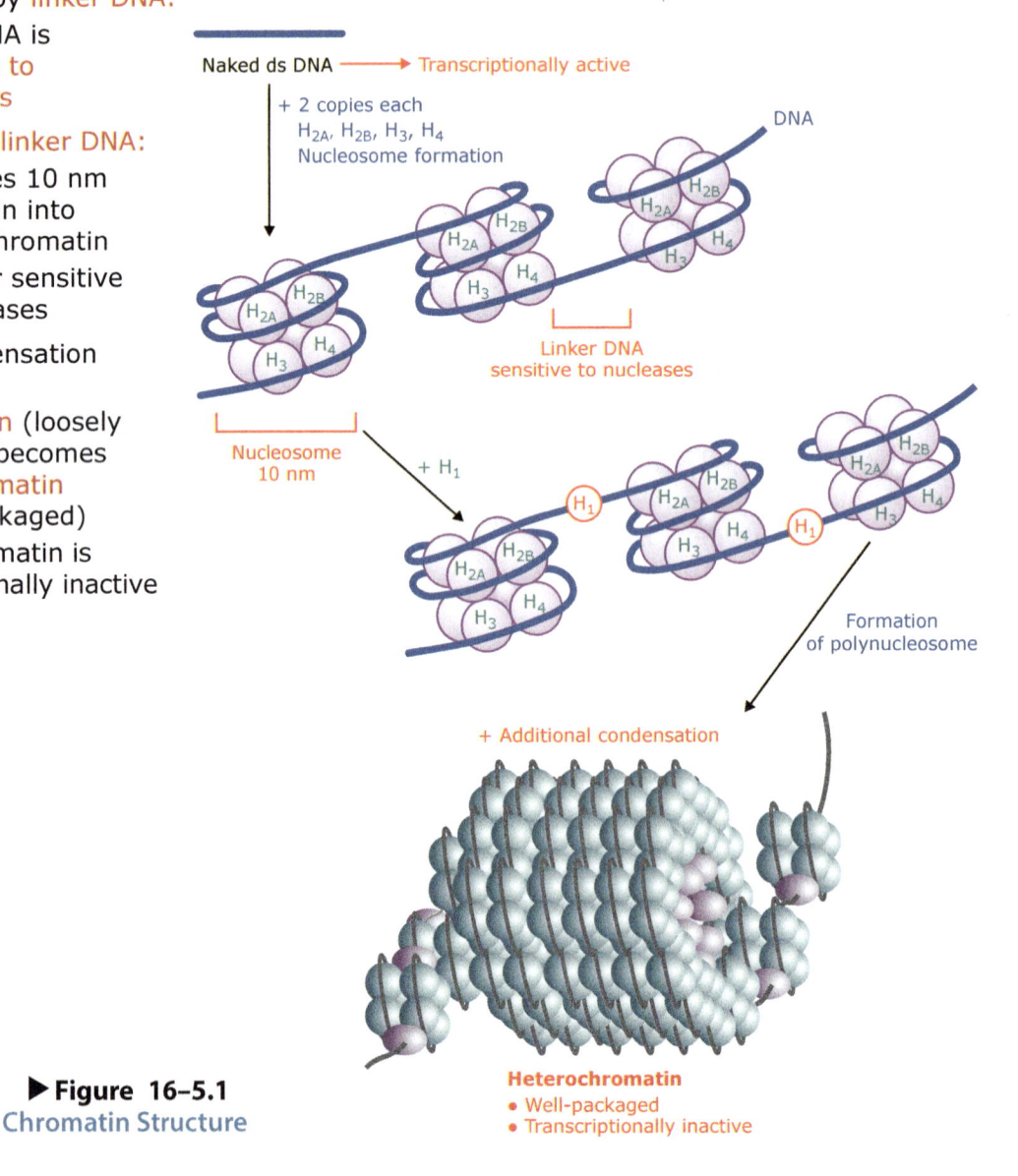

▶ Figure 16-5.1
Chromatin Structure

Heterochromatin
- Well-packaged
- Transcriptionally inactive

5.2 Control of Histone Binding

- Histone acetylases and deacetylases:
  - Alter ⊕ charges and histone-DNA binding
  - Acetylation makes histones negative:
    — Fall off DNA
    — Favor expression
  - Deacetylation makes histones positive:
    — Bind to DNA
    — Prevent expression
- Histone methylation:
  - Alter charges
  - Results vary with methylated amino acid residue
    — May ↑ or ↓ expression

5.3 DNA Methylation

- Suppresses gene expression
- Occurs at CpG sites in eukaryotes:
  - Adjacent CG dinucleotides
  - Methylation is on C only
  - Done by DNA methyltransferase
- Clinical relevance:
  - Silencing of tumor suppressor genes in cancers
  - Silencing of triplet repeat expansion causing diseases
  - Genome imprinting

6 Control of Gene Expression Through Transcription Factors

- General transcription factor binding to promoter regions:
  - On/off switch
- Specific transcription factor binding to enhancer or silencer regions:
  - Modulation switch

6.1 DNA Enhancer and Silencer Regions

- Differ from promoters in location:
  - Can be upstream, downstream, or within introns
  - Can be thousands of nucleotides away from +1:
    —DNA bends can bring enhancer/silencer close to +1
- Bind to specific TFs:
  - Inducers when bound to enhancer regions of DNA
  - Repressors when bound to silencer regions of DNA

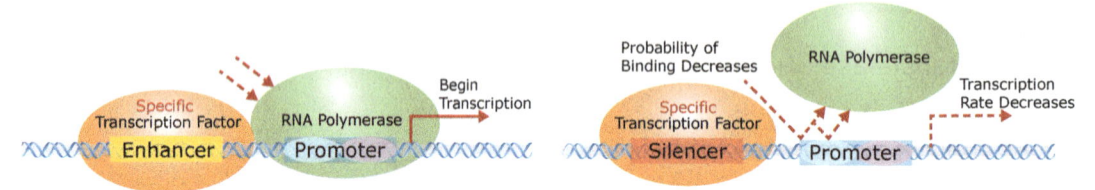

▲ Figure 16–6.1 Interaction of Specific Transcription Factors With DNA Enhancer and Silencer Regions

6.2 Specific Transcription Factors

- Specific TFs are DNA-binding proteins:
  - Bind to enhancers or silencers
- Specific TFs have unique structural features:
  - Zinc fingers:
    —Zinc stabilizes protein folds
    —Zinc binds to Cys and His residues
    —Examples include:
    - All steroid hormone receptors
    - Vitamin A and vitamin D receptors
    - PPARs (peroxisome proliferator activated receptors)
  - Basic leucine zipper (bZIP) domains:
    —Leu is seen every seventh amino acid
    —Consist of dimers of two α-helices
    —Examples include:
    - cAMP response element binding (CREB) protein
    - myc and max oncogenes
  - Basic helix-loop-helix (bHLH):
    —bHLH characterize a large family of TFs
    —c-myc and n-myc have bHLH domains besides Leu zippers

- Rel homology domain (RHD):
  — DNA binding domain of nuclear factor kappa-light-chain-enhancer of activated B cells (NF-κB)
  — RHD are composed of immunoglobulin-like β barrels
    • β barrels are long β-pleated sheets that coil to bind tightly to DNA grooves

Table 16-6.2 Interaction of Specific Transcription Factors With DNA Enhancer and Silencer Regions

Transcription Factor	Enhancer Elements	Examples of Functions
Steroid Receptors (Zinc finger proteins)	HRE (ERE, GRE)	• GRE: – ↑ Transcription of *PEPCK* gene – ↑ Blood glucose
Vitamin D Receptors (VDR) (Zinc finger proteins)	VDE	• Increase Ca^{2+} uptake in intestine and decrease Ca^{2+} excretion • Stimulate osteoblasts, which stimulate preosteoclast differentiation (releases Ca^{2+})
Retinoid and Retinol Receptors (Zinc finger proteins)	RXRE	• Act, with retinoid X receptor (RAX and RAR), as growth regulator in many cells • Growth and differentiation of many cell types • All trans retinoic acid (ATRA) used in AML-M_3 Rx • Force differentiation of promyelocytes • AML-M_3 has t(15,17) • RXR also plays a role in reproduction, cellular differentiation, bone development, hematopoiesis, and pattern formation during embryogenesis
cAMP Response Element Binding Protein (CREB) (Leucine zipper proteins)	CRE	• Modulates transcription based on cAMP levels • PKA phosphorylates and activates CREB • Glucagon and epinephrine induce PEPCK in this manner
Peroxisome Proliferator Activated Receptors (PPARα and PPARγ) (Zinc finger proteins)	PPRE	• Control expression of many genes in lipid and carbohydrate metabolism • Normal ligands are fatty acids or prostaglandins • Fibrates bind PPARα: – Induce LPL – Lower TGLs • Thiazolidinediones (-glitazones): – Bind PPARγ – Stimulate insulin-responsive genes – Used in diabetes
NF-κB (Rel domains)	κB	• Controls cytokine production • Controls cell survival • Roles in: – Inflammation – Autoimmune pathologies – Septic shock – B cell cancers
JAK-STAT STAT: Signal transducers and activators of transcription	Gamma-activated sites (GAS) in promoters of cytokine-inducible genes	• Phosphorylated on tyrosine residues by JAKs (Janus kinases) • Mediates expression of cytokines, interferons • Transduces signal of: – Prolactin – Growth hormone
• *PAX3* • *SHH* • *HOX*		• Control gene expression during development in utero • Loss of function can cause: – Waardenburg syndrome (*PAX3* gene) – Holoprosencephaly (*SHH* gene)

6.2.1 Clinical Relevance

Klein-Waardenburg Syndrome

- Type I and III are mutations in *PAX3* gene:
  - Sensorineural hearing loss:
    - Type I permanent
    - Type III hearing loss over time
  - Pigmentary abnormalities:
    - White forelock (poliosis)
    - Iris heterochromia
    - Patchy skin hypopigmentation
  - Dystopia canthorum
- *PAX3* belongs to the paired box family of genes:
  - Active in neural crest cells during development:
    - Derivatives include melanocytes, iris pigment cells, Schwann cells
    - Association with melanoma
  - Important role in myogenesis:
    - Association with rhabdomyosarcoma

Holoprosencephaly

- Failure of forebrain to separate into two hemispheres:
  - Facial defects
    - Cyclopia
    - Lack of a nose
  - Brain structural and functional defects
  - Generally causes miscarriage or stillbirth
- Mutation in sonic hedgehog gene (*SHH*):
  - Critical for limb patterning
  - Somite differentiation
  - Gut regionalization

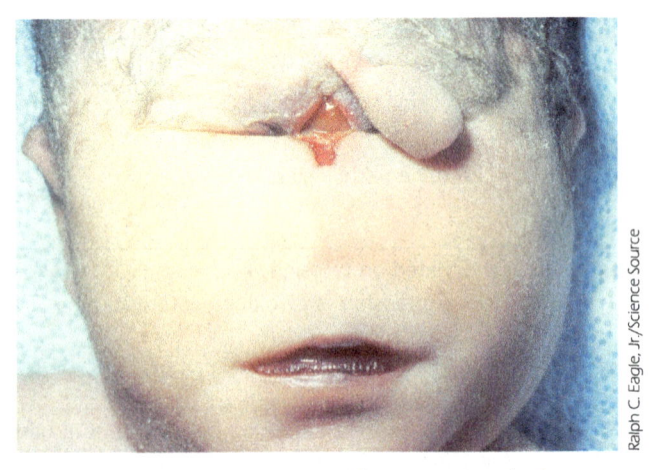

▲ Figure 16-6.2 Holoprosencephaly

CHAPTER 17 — Gene Expression: Translation

1 Overview

- Translation converts mRNA nucleotide sequence into amino acid protein sequence
- Peptidyltransferase makes peptide bonds:
  - Protein synthesis proceeds from N-terminus to C-terminus
  - Ribosomes and activated tRNAs are required
  - 20 amino acids
  - Energy and initiation, elongation, and release factors
- Co- and posttranslational modifications are critical for protein function
- Clinical relevance:
  - Mutations in exons of genes may alter protein sequences, folding, and function
  - Many antibiotics/toxins interfere with bacterial protein synthesis

USMLE® Key Concepts

For Step 1, you must be able to:

- Describe translation in prokaryotes and eukaryotes.
- Relate protein synthesis inhibitors and toxins to steps in translation.
- Discuss and give examples of mutations.
- Describe the targeting of proteins to their appropriate location, using collagen as an example.

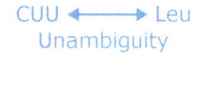

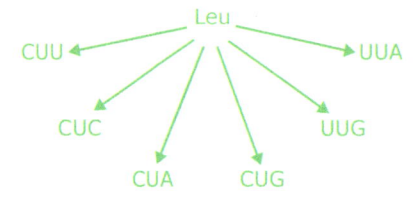

2 The Genetic Code

2.1 Description

- Exon sequences in mRNA are read as codons:
  - Codons are triplets of nucleotides:
    — 4-letter code in 3-nucleotide-long codons:
    - 4 × 4 × 4 = 64 codons
  - Each codon codes for a single amino acid:
    — Genetic code is unambiguous
  - Many amino acids are encoded by more than one codon:
    — Genetic code is degenerate
    — Third position is least conserved
  - 3 stop codons:
    — "Nonsense" codons
    — UAG, UGA, UAA
  - 2 amino acids with a single codon:
    — AUG for methionine
    - Initiation codon
    — UGG for Trp

▲ Figure 17-2.1A The Genetic Code Is Unambiguous but Degenerate

Chapter 17 • Gene Expression: Translation

5'	U		C		A		G		3'
U	UUU	Phe	UCU	Ser	UAU	Tyr	UGU	Cys	U
	UUC		UCC		UAC		UGC		C
	UUA	Leu	UCA		UAA	Stop	UGA	Stop	A
	UUG		UCG		UAG		UGG	Trp	G
C	CUU	Leu	CCU	Pro	CAU	His	CGU	Arg	U
	CUC		CCC		CAC		CGC		C
	CUA		CCA		CAA	Gln	CGA		A
	CUG		CCG		CAG		CGG		G
A	AUU	Ile	ACU	Thr	AAU	Asn	AGU	Ser	U
	AUC		ACC		AAC		AGC		C
	AUA		ACA		AAA	Lys	AGA	Arg	A
	AUG	Met	ACG		AAG		AGG		G
G	GUU	Val	GCU	Ala	GAU	Asp	GGU	Gly	U
	GUC		GCC		GAC		GGC		C
	GUA		GCA		GAA	Glu	GGA		A
	GUG		GCG		GAG		GGG		G

▲ **Figure 17–2.1B** Codon Table

- Codons on mRNA base pair with anticodons on tRNA:
  - Third base pair of codon and first base pair of anticodon wobble:
    —Hypoxanthine in tRNA (I) can pair with A, C, or U
    —G can pair with U
    —Fewer than 61 tRNAs needed

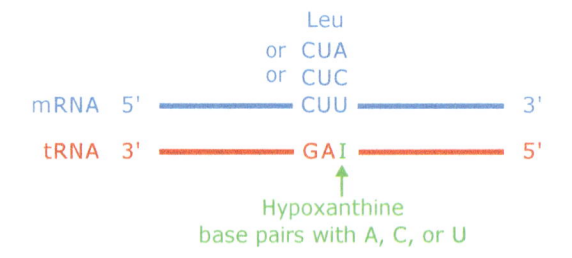

```
                        Leu
                     or CUA
                     or CUC
mRNA  5' ━━━━━━━━━━━ CUU ━━━━━━━━━━━ 3'

tRNA  3' ━━━━━━━━━━━ GAI ━━━━━━━━━━━ 5'
                         ↑
                    Hypoxanthine
                base pairs with A, C, or U
```

▲ **Figure 17–2.1C** Wobble Hypothesis and Role of Hypoxanthine (I)

- Genetic code is universal:
  - Mitochondria (Mt) has three notable exceptions:
    —Mt UGA is for Trp, not stop
    —Mt AUA is for Met, not Ile
    —Mt CUA is for Thr, not Leu
- Reading the code is non-overlapping:
  - Each nucleotide of each codon is only read once
  - Codons are read in sequence from 5' AUG to 3' stop codon
- Primary structure of protein:
  - Order of codons in mRNA = Amino acid sequence in protein

2.2 Mutations Affecting the Genetic Code

- **Mutations:**
  - Permanent change in DNA base sequence of an organism
  - Acquired or inherited
  - Three types:
    — Substitutions
    — Insertions
    — Deletions

2.2.1 Substitutions

- Substitution of a single nucleotide is called a point mutation:
  - Transition:
    — Purine for another purine
    — Pyrimidine for another pyrimidine
  - Transversion:
    — Purine for a pyrimidine
    — Pyrimidine for a purine
- Three types of point mutations affect codons of mRNA:
  - Silent mutations:
    — Specify same amino acid
    — Generally third codon nucleotide
  - Missense mutations:
    — Specify a different amino acid:
      - Conservative:
        - New amino acid has similar property
        - Of little consequence
      - Nonconservative:
        - New amino acid has different property
        - Protein shape/function is altered
  - Nonsense mutations:
    — Produce a stop codon
    — Result in truncated protein

```
5' –AUG CAU UGU GGC AGA CCA– 3'
    Met His Cys Gly Arg Pro

5' –AUG CAU UGC GGG AGA CCA– 3'
    Met His Cys Gly Arg Pro
```
A. Two Silent Mutations

```
5' –AUG CUU UGU GGC AGA CCA– 3'
    Met Leu Cys Gly Arg Pro

5' –AUG GUU UGU GGC AUA CCA– 3'
    Met Val Cys Gly Ile Pro
```
B. Missense Mutations

```
5' –AUG CAU UGU GGC AGA CCA– 3'
    Met His Cys Gly Arg Pro

5' –AUG CAU UGA GGC AGA CCA– 3'
    Met His Stop
```
C. Nonsense Mutations

▲ Figure 17-2.2A Point Mutations

2.2.2 Insertions or Deletions

- Addition or removal of one or more nucleotides in a sequence
  - In-frame:
    - Multiple of three nucleotides
    - Insertion or deletion of amino acid in the sequence
  - Frameshift:
    - Non-multiple of three nucleotides
    - Different amino acid sequence
    - Often shorter than normal

```
5' –AUG CAU GGG UGU CGA CCA– 3'
    Met His Gly Cys Arg Pro

5' –AUG CAU GGG UGU GGC CGA CCA– 3'
    Met His Gly Cys Gly Arg Pro

5' –AUG CAU GGG UGU GGG AGA CCA– 3'
    Met His Gly Cys Gly Arg Pro

5' –AUG CAA UGG GUG UGG GAG ACC A– 3'
    Met Gln Trp Val Trp Glu Thr
```

▲ **Figure 17–2.2B** In-Frame vs. Frameshift Mutations Following Insertion of Nucleotides

2.2.3 Clinical Examples

Table 17-2.2 Important Mutations in Selected Diseases

Type	Mutation	Disease
Missense	E6V	Sickle cell anemia
	E6K	HbC disease
	C282Y	Primary hemochromatosis
Nonsense	UGG → UGA Codon 17	β°-thalassemia • *Note:* > 200 mutations described for β-thalassemia
	Various	Hurler syndrome
Insertions	Triplet repeat expansions CAG	Anticipation in pedigree Huntington disease
Deletions	CFTR-ΔF508	Cystic fibrosis: • 3 base pair deletion in *CFTR* gene
	CCR5-Δ32	HIV/AIDS: • 32 base pair deletion in *CCR5* gene • Homozygous individuals are resistant to HIV
Frameshifts	Can occur in repeated sequences	Some cancers (e.g., colorectal)
	Can occur in splice sites	Some cases of Tay-Sachs, thalassemia

3 Ribosomes

- Cytoplasmic structures made of rRNA and proteins:
  - Ribonucleoproteins
  - 70S in prokaryotes
  - 80S in eukaryotes
  - Svedberg unit:
    - "S" measures the rate of sedimentation in centrifugation, not size
- Made of two subunits:
  - Large subunit:
    - 50S in prokaryotes
    - 60S in eukaryotes
    - Contains peptidyltransferase
  - Small subunit:
    - 30S in prokaryotes
    - 40S in eukaryotes

A. Prokaryotic Ribosome

- 16S rRNA (antiparallel + complementary to Shine-Dalgarno sequence)
- +21 proteins
- 30S Subunit
- 50S Subunit
  - 5S rRNA
  - 23S rRNA (Peptidyltransferase)
  - +31 proteins
- → 70S Ribosome

B. Eukaryotic Ribosome

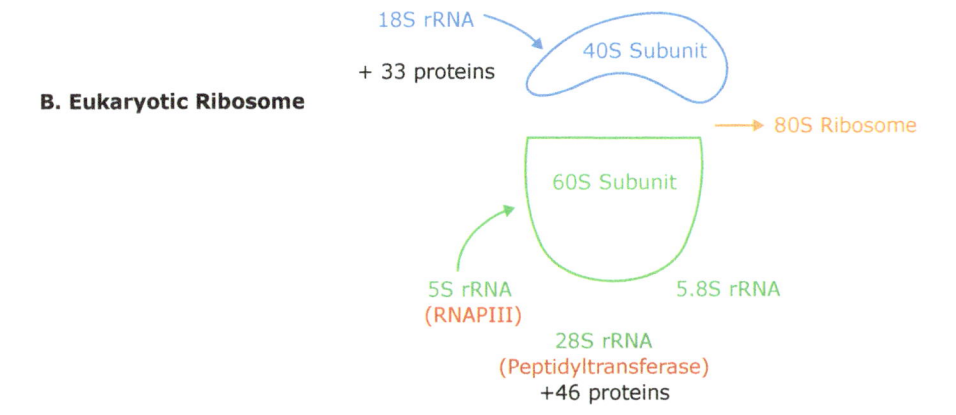

- 18S rRNA
- + 33 proteins
- 40S Subunit
- 60S Subunit
  - 5S rRNA (RNAPIII)
  - 5.8S rRNA
  - 28S rRNA (Peptidyltransferase)
  - +46 proteins
- → 80S Ribosome

▲ Figure 17-3.0 Prokaryotic and Eukaryotic Ribosomes

3.1 Binding Sites

- Ribosomes have binding sites for tRNA:
  - P-site:
    - —Peptidyl site
    - —Initiation complex formation
    - —Holds onto nascent peptide
  - A-site:
    - —Aminoacyl or acceptor site
    - —Entry of next aminoacyl-tRNA during elongation
  - E-site:
    - —Ejection site
    - —Used tRNA leaves and gets recycled

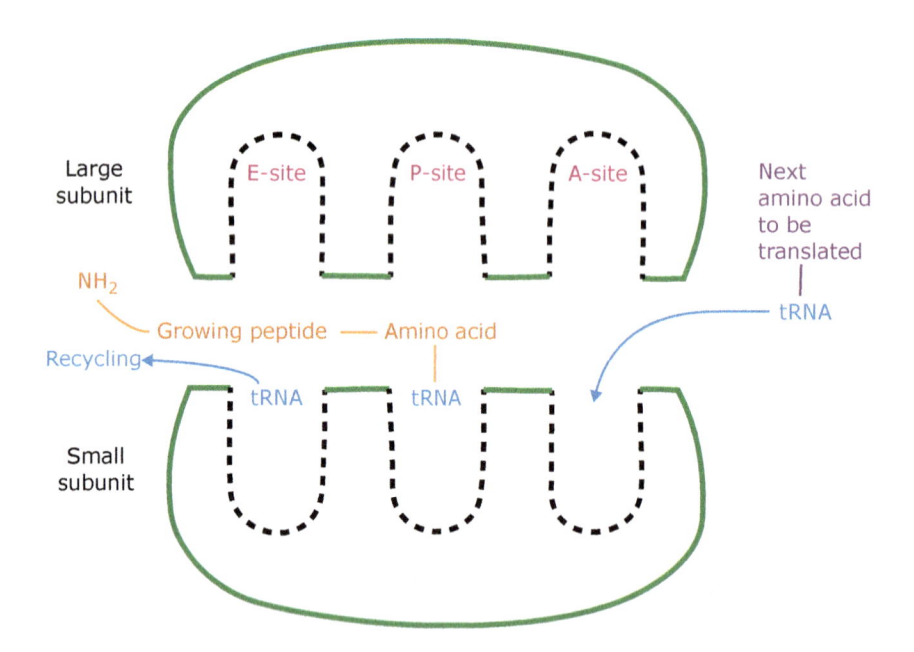

▲ Figure 17–3.1 Ribosome/tRNA Binding Sites

3.2 Clinical Relevance

3.2.1 Shiga Toxin and Verotoxin
- RNA glycosylases from *Shigella* and EHEC, respectively
- Cleave one adenine residue from 28S rRNA:
  - Inactivate protein synthesis
- Associated with hemolytic uremic syndrome:
  - B subunit binds to Gb3:
    - Cell membrane glycolipid
    - Vascular endothelium
    - Allows cellular entry
  - A subunit blocks translation:
    - Damages endothelial cell
    - Small vessel tropism:
      - GI, kidney, CNS

3.2.2 Ricin
- Toxin from *Ricinus communis*, castor oil plant
- < 2 mg pure ricin kills an adult (LD50 in μg/kg)
  - Chemical/biological warfare agent
- Ribosome-inactivating peptide:
  - RNA glycosylase:
    - Identical to Shiga toxin
- No antidote

Chapter 17 • Gene Expression: Translation

4. Transfer RNA (tRNA)

- Adaptor molecule with cloverleaf structure:
  - Anticodon arm:
    — Base pairs with mRNA codon
  - Acceptor arm:
    — Attaches respective amino acid to 3'OH end
    — Has CCA sequence
  - D Loop:
    — Has dihydrouridine
  - T ψ C loop:
    — Has ribothymidine (T)
    — Has pseudouridine (ψ)

- Attachment of amino acid to 3'OH of acceptor arm:
  - Performed by aminoacyl-tRNA synthetases:
    — Covalently attach amino acid to 3' end of CCA sequence:
      - Esterification between carboxyl group of amino acid and 2' or 3'OH of acceptor arm terminal adenosine
    — Captures two high-energy bonds from ATP:
      - tRNA is "activated" or "charged"
      - Energy later released to form a peptide bond during translation
    — Single aminoacyl-tRNA synthetase for each amino acid:
      - Stem of acceptor arm has different sequences:
        - Accommodates various shapes of 20 amino acids
      - Self-checking capabilities:
        - Ensures correct amino acid is attached to 3' end

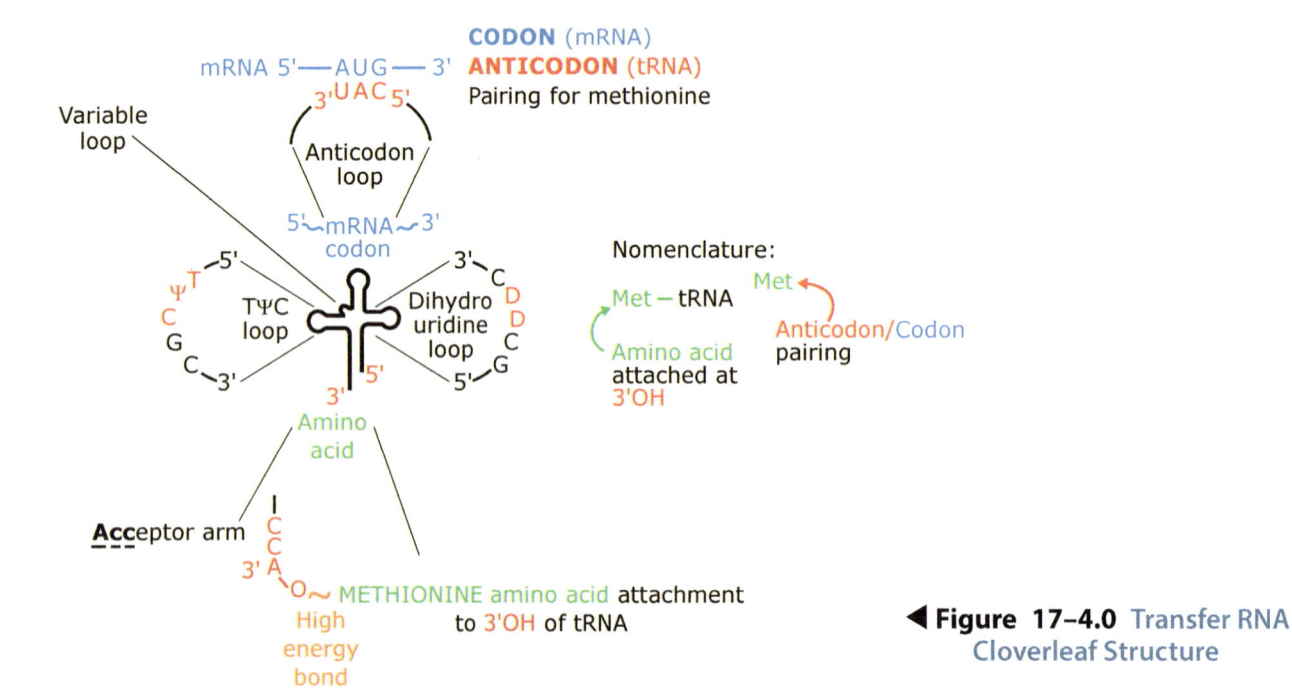

Figure 17-4.0 Transfer RNA Cloverleaf Structure

5 Translation Factors

- Proteins required to help initiation, elongation, and termination of translation
- Eukaryotic translation factors have "e" in front:
  - eEF2, for example

Table 17-5.0 — Translation Factors

Step	Cell	Factor
Initiation	Prokaryotes	IF1 through -3 IF2 is a G-protein
	Eukaryotes	eIF1 through 6 eIF2 is a G-protein
Elongation	Prokaryotes	EF-Tu EF-G EF-Ts EF-P
	Eukaryotes	eEF1 eEF2 is a G-protein
Termination	Prokaryotes	RF1 and RF2
	Eukaryotes	eRF1 recognizes stop codons

- Clinical relevance of eukaryotic translation factors:
  - ADP ribosylation of eEF2 by *Pseudomonas* and diphtheria exotoxins
    - Toxins cleave nicotinamide moiety from NAD and transfer ADP-ribosyl group onto eEF2
    - Prevent elongation of peptide
    - Necrotizing effect at bacterial colonization site

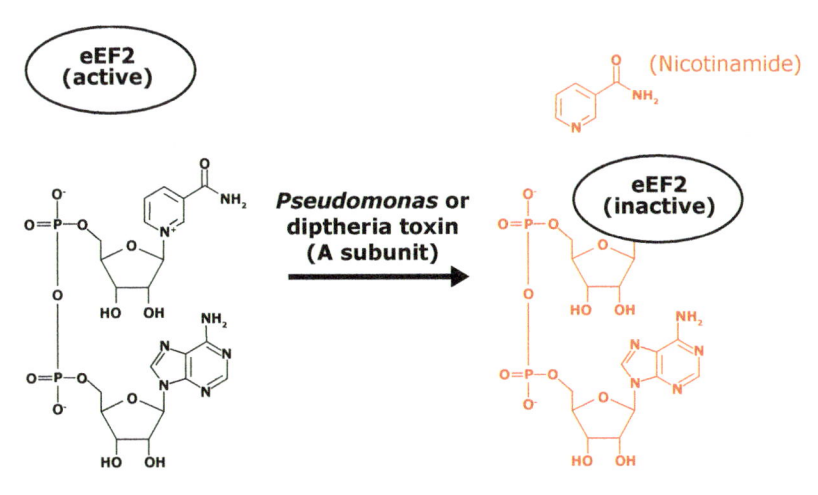

▲ Figure 17-5.0 ADP Ribosylation

6 Peptide Bond Formation

- Proteins are polymers of amino acids
- Amino acids are covalently bound by peptide bond:
  - Between carboxyl terminus of first amino acid and amino terminus of next amino acid
  - Gives two distinct ends (polarity) to proteins

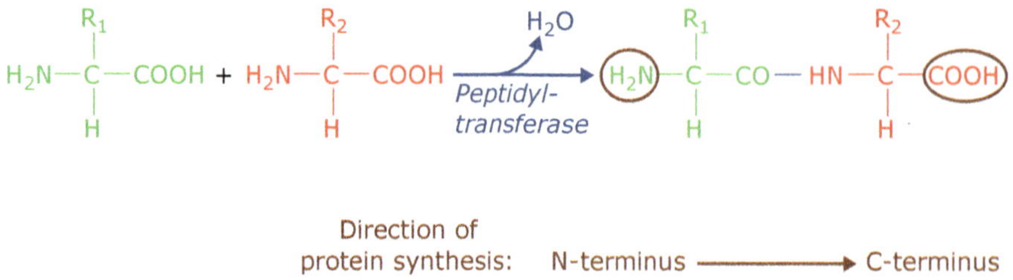

$$H_2N-\underset{H}{\underset{|}{\overset{R_1}{\overset{|}{C}}}}-COOH + H_2N-\underset{H}{\underset{|}{\overset{R_2}{\overset{|}{C}}}}-COOH \xrightarrow[\text{Peptidyl-transferase}]{H_2O} H_2N-\underset{H}{\underset{|}{\overset{R_1}{\overset{|}{C}}}}-CO-HN-\underset{H}{\underset{|}{\overset{R_2}{\overset{|}{C}}}}-COOH$$

Direction of protein synthesis: N-terminus ⟶ C-terminus

▲ Figure 17–6.0 Peptide Bond

- Catalyzed by peptidyltransferase:
  - Associated with a big subunit of ribosome
  - Ribozyme:
    —Enzymatic activity mediated by rRNA, not a protein
    —23S rRNA of prokaryotes
      - Blocked by chloramphenicol
    —28S rRNA of eukaryotes

7 Translation Process

7.1 Initiation

- Formation of initiation complex:
  - mRNA
  - Ribosome
  - Initiator tRNA:
    - Methionyl-tRNA in eukaryotes
    - Formylmethionyl-tRNA in prokaryotes
  - Initiation factors and GTP
- Only time an aminoacyl-tRNA enters the P-site
- Initiation complex formation inhibitors:
  - 30S P-site: Aminoglycosides
  - 50S P-site: Linezolid

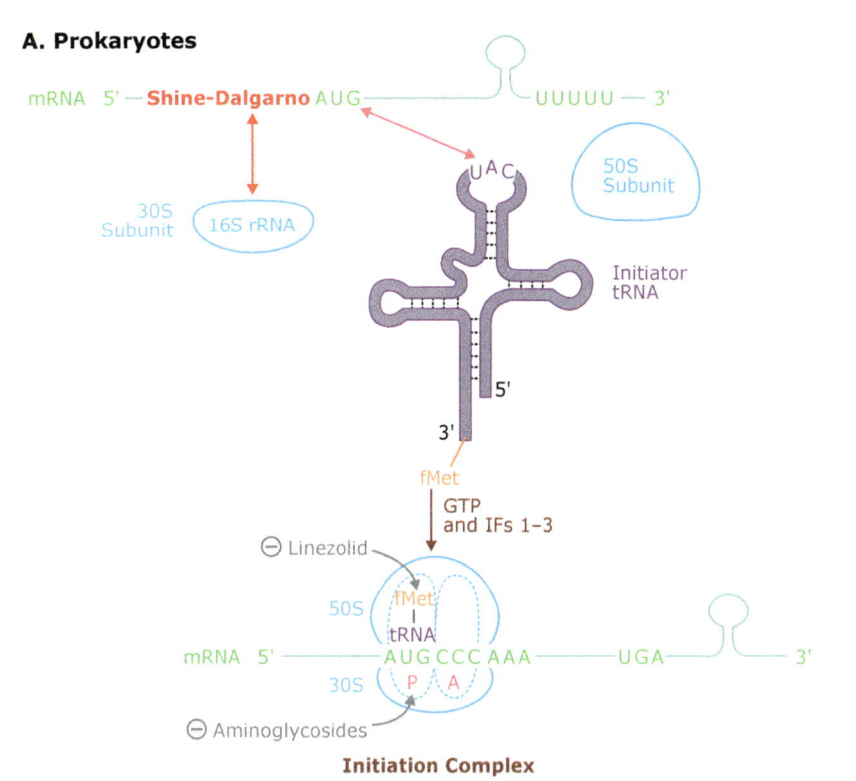

A. Prokaryotes

B. Eukaryotes

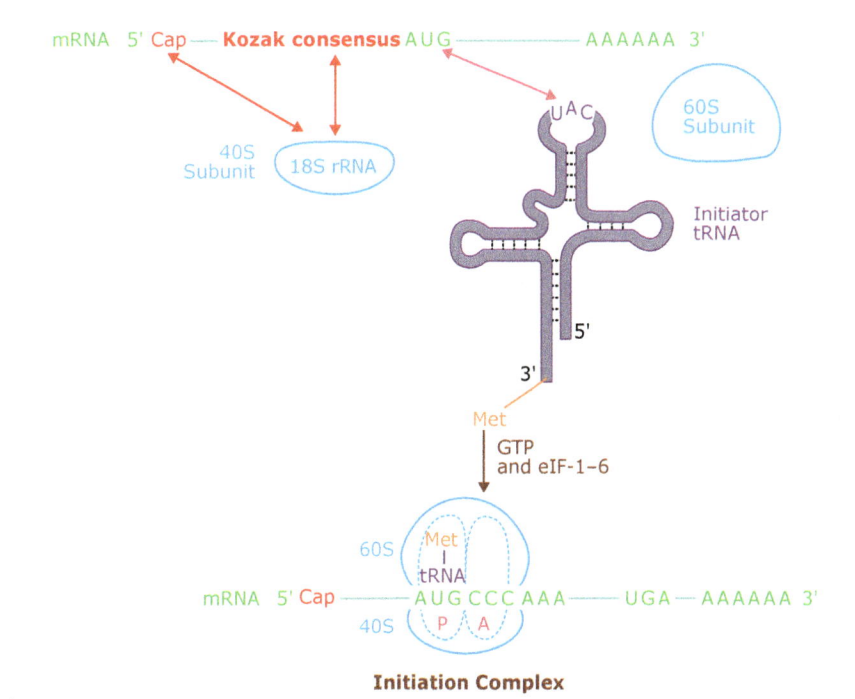

▲ Figure 17-7.1 Formation of Initiation Complex

7.2 Elongation

- Three-step cycle:
  - Aminoacyl-tRNA enters A-site
  - Peptide bond formation
  - Translocation:
    —Ribosome slides 1 codon downstream
- Requires elongation factors and energy:
  - Four high-energy bonds per amino acid added to protein
    —Two from GTP conversion to GDP
    —Two from ATP captured during tRNA activation
      - Used by peptidyltransferase
- Prokaryotic elongation is inhibited by the majority of protein synthesis inhibitor antibiotics

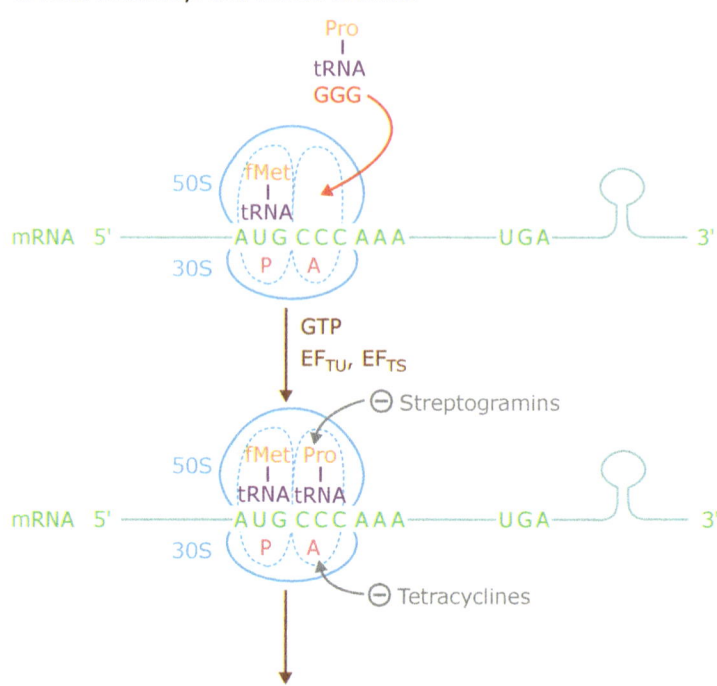

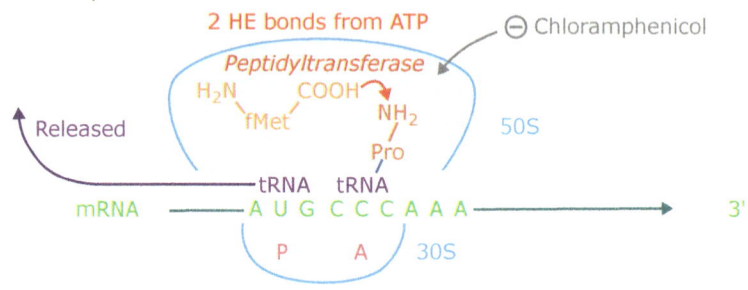

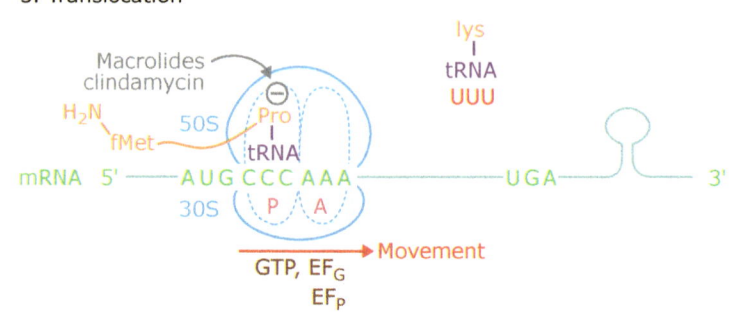

A. Prokaryotes

1. Next aminoacyl tRNA binds to A site
2. Peptide bond formation
3. Translocation

▲ Figure 17–7.2 Elongation

B. Eukaryotes

1. Next aminoacyl tRNA binds to A site

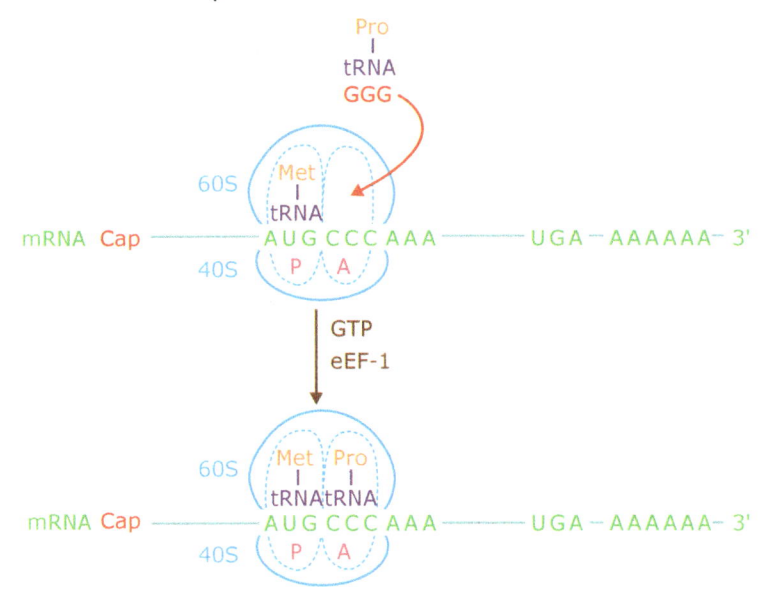

2. Peptide bond formation

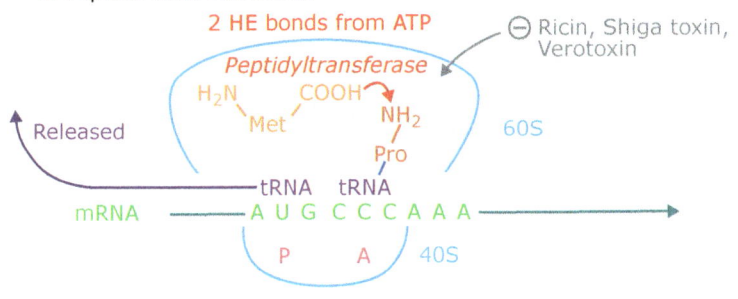

3. Translocation

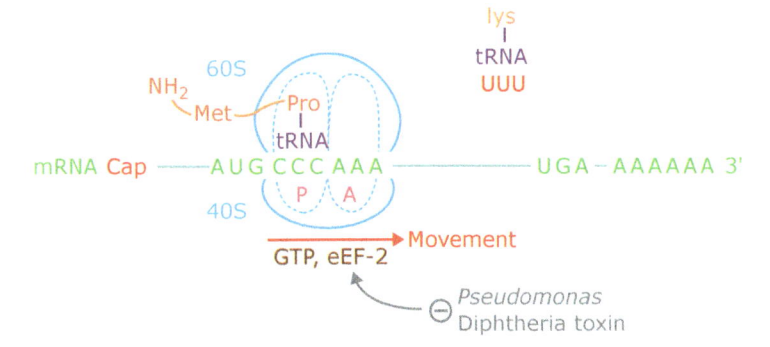

▲ Figure 17-7.2 **Elongation** *(continued)*

7.3 Termination

- Stop codon in A-site
- Energy and release factors

A. Prokaryotes

NH$_2$-fMet — Pro — Lys — aa — tRNA — STOP
mRNA 5'—AUG CCC AAA———UGA———3'
50S / 30S ribosome, P and A sites

GTP, RF$_{1-2}$ ↓

Protein release: NH$_2$—fMet ProLys———COOH

B. Eukaryotes

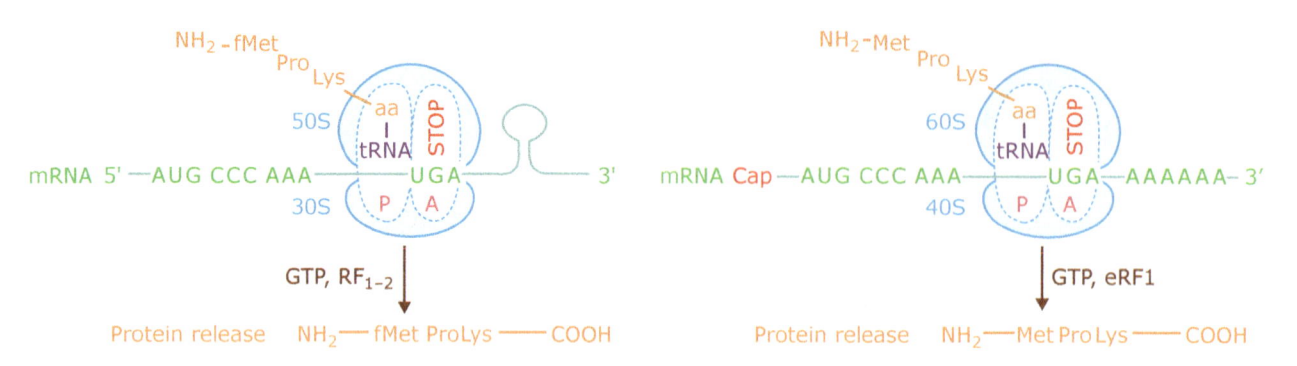

NH$_2$-Met — Pro — Lys — aa — tRNA — STOP
mRNA Cap—AUG CCC AAA———UGA—AAAAAA-3'
60S / 40S ribosome, P and A sites

GTP, eRF1 ↓

Protein release: NH$_2$—Met ProLys———COOH

▲ Figure 17–7.3 Termination

8 Protein Folding

- Proper folding is critical to function and recognition as self-protein:
  - Chaperones are proteins that assist foldings:
    —Many chaperones are heat shock proteins
  - Noncovalent interactions include:
    —H bonds
    —Ionic/electrostatic bonds
    —Hydrophobic bonds
  - Covalent interactions include disulfide bonds between Cys residues
- Four distinct levels of protein structures:
  - Primary structure:
    —Sequence of amino acid translated from mRNA
    —Held by peptide bonds
  - Secondary structure:
    —α-helices
    —β-pleated sheets
  - Tertiary structure:
    —Three-dimensional arrangement of secondary structures
    —Globular
    —Fibrillar
  - Quaternary structure:
    —Three-dimensional structure of multi-subunit proteins
- Misfolded protein and ubiquitination:
  - Misfolding can be the result of mutations:
    —Example: CFTR-ΔF508 in cystic fibrosis
  - Ubiquitin ligases attach multiple ubiquitin to misfolded peptide
  - Targeting to 26S proteasomes:
    —Multi-subunit structures found in cytoplasm
    —20S core particle is filled with proteases:
      - Digestion of misfolded protein
    —19S regulatory particle:
      - Contains ATPases
      - Opens "gate" into core particle
    —Proteasomes play a key role in adaptive immunity:
      - Viral and cancer antigens can be processed and presented onto MHCI complexes
      - Recognition by CTL targets the cell for apoptosis
    —Bortezomib is proteasome inhibitor used in multiple myeloma
      - Decreases destruction of I-κB (the "inhibitor" of NF-κB)

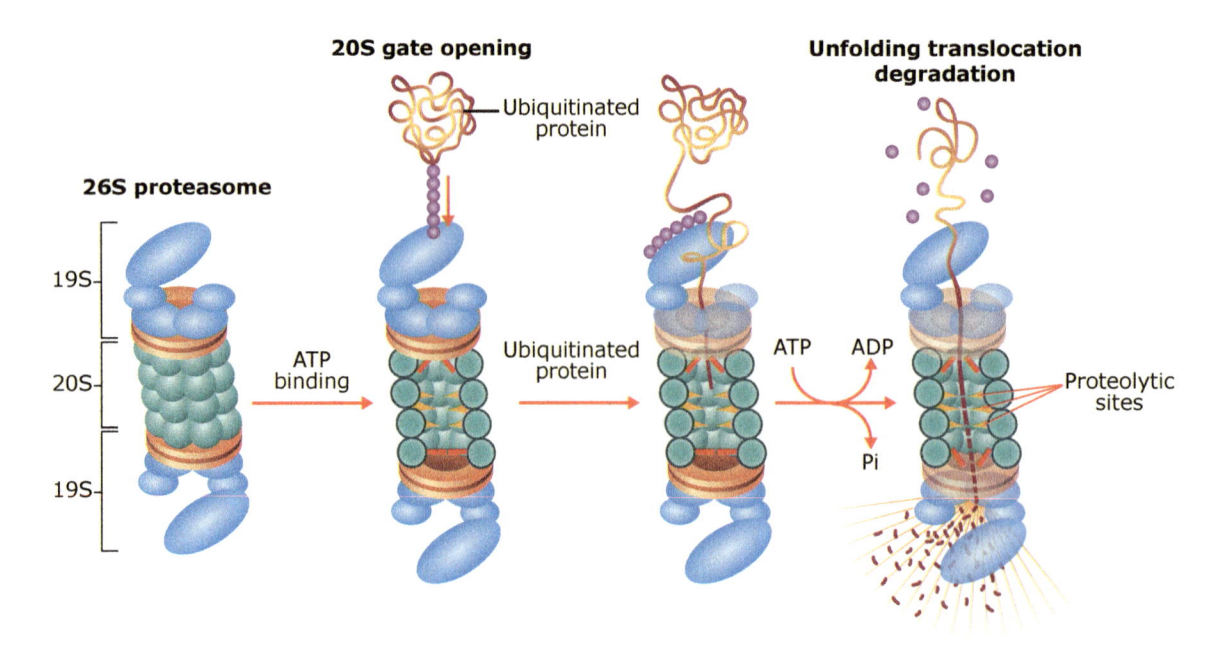

▲ Figure 17–8.0 Proteasome Digestion

- β-pleated sheets and amyloid
  - Stacks of β-pleated sheets form extracellular amyloid plaques
  - Apple-green birefringence on Congo Red
  - Causes disruption in tissue architecture
- Example: β-amyloid of Alzheimer disease

9 Protein Targeting

- Translation is cytoplasmic:
  - Cytoplasmic proteins are translated on free ribosomes
- Targeting proteins to specific organelles, membrane, or extracellular compartment requires targeting or signaling sequences

9.1 Targeting Nuclear Proteins

- Nuclear localization sequences (NLS):
  - ⊕ Charged Lys or Arg residues in short sequences
  - Importins recognize and bind to NLS:
    — "Import" protein into nucleus through channels called nuclear pore complexes

9.2 Targeting Mitochondrial Proteins

- Many mitochondrial proteins are not encoded by mitochondrial DNA
- Alternating pattern of hydrophobic and ⊕ charged amino acids:
  - Called mitochondrial targeting signal
  - Localized at N-terminus
  - 10–70 amino acid long

9.3 Targeting Peroxisome Proteins

- Requires peroxisomal targeting signals (PTS):
  - PTS 1:
    — Ser-Lys-Leu at C-terminus
  - PTS 2:
    — Less conserved
    — N-terminus

9.4 Targeting Extracellular, Plasma Membrane, or Lysosomal Proteins

- Requires N-terminal hydrophobic signal sequence:
  - 5–30 lipid-soluble amino acid residues at N-terminus
- Signal recognition particles (SRP) bind to signal sequence while ribosomes translate mRNA in cytoplasm:
  - Synthesis pauses
  - Ribosome-protein-mRNA complex is transferred to an SRP receptor:
    — SRP receptors are on the endoplasmic reticulum (ER)
    — Nascent protein is fed into ER through translocon
      - Translocon is a doughnut-shape channel
      - Made of Sec61 proteins
    — Smooth ER becomes rough ER
    — Once fed in ER, signal peptide is removed by signal peptidase
  - Translation resumes; protein is fed into RER lumen

- ER transfers protein to Golgi complex:
  - Golgi is responsible for sorting out appropriate final destination
- Important co-/posttranslational modifications occur in ER/Golgi:
  - Appropriate folding
  - Glycosylation:
    - N-linked on Asn or Arg side chains:
      - Requires dolichol-P, an intermediate of the cholesterol synthesis pathway
    - O-linked on Ser, Thr, Tyr, hydroxylysine or hydroxyproline:
      - Can occur in ER and in Golgi
    - N-linked glycosylation of Asn residues with mannose-6-phosphate in Golgi targets proteins to lysosomes
      - Done by N-acetylglucosamine-1-phosphotransferase
      - Enzyme is deficient in I cell disease
        - Lysosomes have no enzyme
          - Inclusion bodies
        - ↑ Serum lysosomal enzymes is diagnostic
        - Early death from organ failure
- In the absence of mannose-6-phosphate residues, proteins are:
  - Secreted:
    - Constitutively (no tag)
    - Clathrin-mediated
  - Placed in membrane of cell:
    - Involves GTPases called Rab proteins:
      - Key in targeting to membrane
    - SNAP and SNARE proteins:
      - Mediate vesicle fusion with membranes
      - Target of botulinum and tetanus toxins
      - Synaptosomal associated proteins
  - Returned to ER from Golgi:
    - Requires a KDEL sequence
    - KDEL stands for Lys-Asp-Glu-Leu
    - Found at C-terminus of protein

Chapter 17 • Gene Expression: Translation

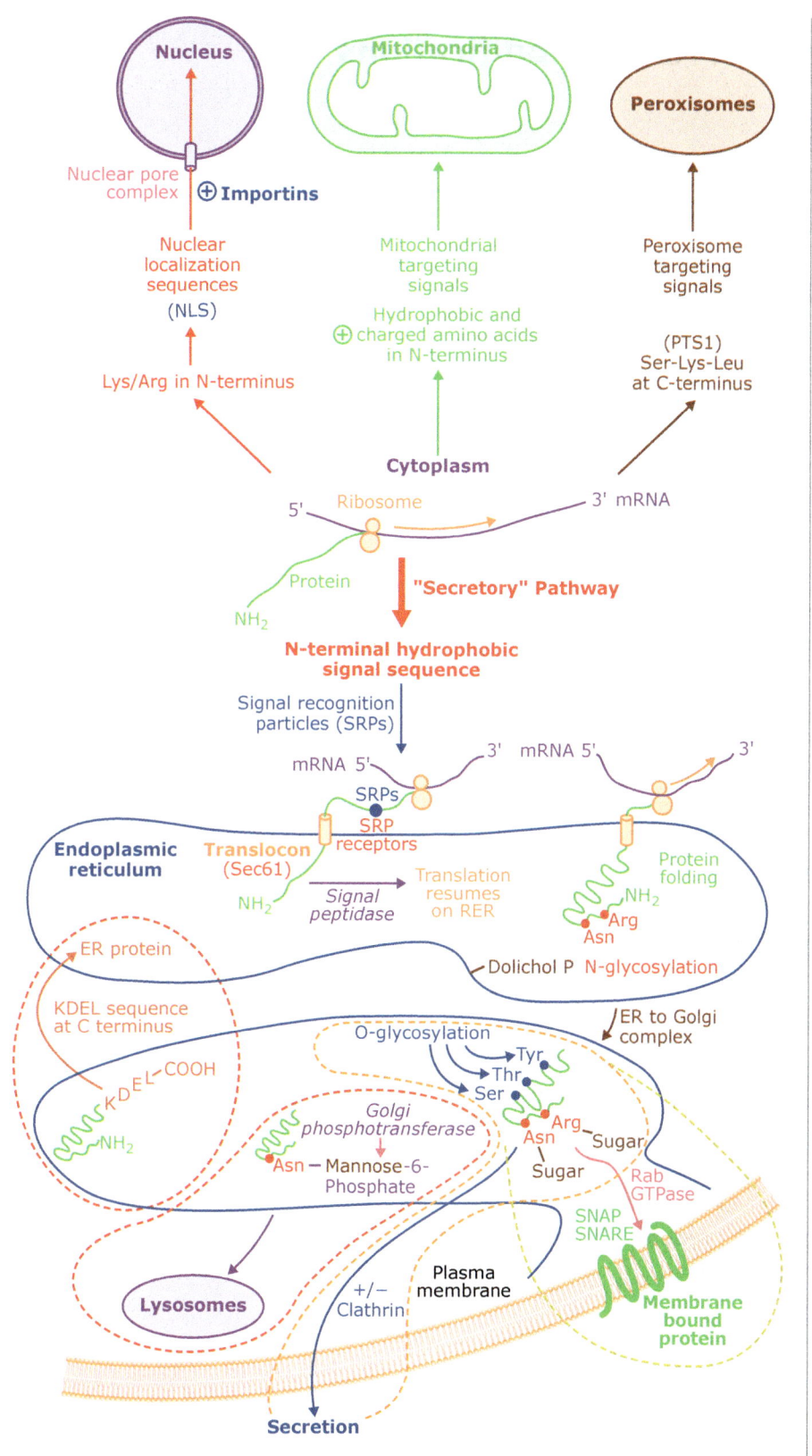

▲ **Figure 17-9.4** Targeting Proteins to Their Appropriate Locations

10. Other Important Protein Modifications

- γ-carboxylation:
  - Posttranslational:
    - Allows Ca^{2+}-binding
  - Vitamin K-dependent proteins:
    - Clotting factors II, VII, IX, and X
    - Anticoagulant proteins C and S
  - Gamma-carboxylase converts reduced vitamin K into vitamin K epoxide
    - Warfarin blocks vitamin K epoxide reductase
      - ↓ Vitamin K recycling to reduced form
- Prenylation:
  - Addition of lipid anchors to membrane proteins:
    - Transfer of cholesterol synthesis intermediates (farnesyl, geranylgeranyl) to C-terminal Cys

11. Example of Collagen

- Most abundant extracellular protein
- Collagen structure:
  - Primary structure:
    - $(Gly-X-Y)_n$
    - X and Y are often Lys or Pro
  - Secondary structure:
    - α-helix
  - Tertiary/quaternary structure:
    - Triple helix of collagen
    - Stabilized by hydroxyproline and hydroxylysine
    - Cross-linked by covalent bonds between deaminated lysines
- Collagen is an extracellular protein:
  - N-terminal hydrophobic sequence:
    - Synthesis in RER:
      - Hydroxylation of selected Lys and Pro residues
      - Lys and Pro hydroxylases require vitamin C
      - OHPro is unique to collagen
      - Glycosylation
      - Formation of triple helix
      - Secretion
  - Extracellular modification:
    - Proteolysis of secreted triple helix into tropocollagen
    - Fibril/fiber formation
      - Cross-linking of tropocollagen molecules
      - Lys deamination by lysyl oxidase
      - Requires Cu^{2+}
- Clinical relevance: Collagen disorders

Table 17-11.0 — Collagen Disorders

Disease	Collagen Type	Presentation

Osteogenesis imperfecta	Type I	• Skin/bones/tendons/cornea
		— AD type I
		  • Skeletal fragility
		  • Dentinogenesis imperfecta
		  • Hearing impairment
		  • Blue sclera
		— AR type II:
		  • Death in utero

Ehlers-Danlos type 4	Type III	• Loose connective tissue, viscera — AD/AR — Hyperextensible skin/joints — Vascular aneurysms — GI rupture — Cannot scar

Menke disease or EDS type IX	Collagens and other copper-requiring oxidases	• Copper deficiency
		— XLR
		  • Defect in ATP7A gene, copper ATPase in gut
		  • Affects lysyl oxidase
		  • Brittle, "kinky" hair
		  • Fractures
		  • Neurologic defects

Goodpasture disease	Type IV	• Type II hypersensitivity — Autoimmune • Affects renal GBM — Crescentic GN • Affects lungs — Pulmonary hemorrhage
Alport syndrome	Type IV	• Hereditary nephritis • Deafness • Eye abnormalities • 85% X-linked
Scurvy	All types	• Vitamin C deficiency • Acquired/dietary • Bleeding — Mucous membranes — Skin • Affects RER lysyl and prolyl hydroxylases

CHAPTER 18: Molecular Technologies

1 Overview

- Molecular technologies are common in laboratory practice
  - Polymerase chain reaction
  - Gel electrophoresis:
    - Southern blot: DNA
    - Northern blot: RNA
    - Western blot: Proteins
    - Southwestern blot: DNA binding proteins
    - Sequencing: Identifications of mutations
- Recombinant DNA technologies provide:
  - Probes for blots
  - Proteins used in diagnostic testing
  - Proteins used in therapeutic management
  - Gene/DNA sequence to study:
    - Identification of polymorphisms
  - Gene for gene therapy or transgenic animals
- These technologies require a good command of:
  - Restriction enzymes and palindromes
  - Hybridization of probes
  - Differences between prokaryotic and eukaryotic gene expression
  - Vectors:
    - Plasmids
    - Viruses
    - Artificial systems

USMLE® Key Concepts

For Step 1, you must be able to:

- Describe blotting techniques, restriction enzymes and palindromes, and various probes.
- Analyze and differentiate Southern, Northern, and Western blots.
- Explain PCR and recognize its need in studying polymorphisms and in sequencing DNA.

2 Restriction Enzymes and Palindromes

- Specific endonucleases originally isolated from bacteria:
  - Digest viral/phage DNA
  - Recognize and cut at palindromes ("restriction sites")
  - Commercially available (> 600!)
  - Used to cut study DNA into manageable fragments
    —Called restriction fragments
- Palindromes:
  - DNA sequences 4 to 8 base pairs long
  - When read 5' to 3', the sequences are identical on both DNA strands
- Restriction endonucleases:
  - Cut asymmetrically to yield sticky ends
  - Or cut symmetrically to yield blunt ends

Sticky Ends

EcoRI
5' GAATTC 3'
3' CTTAAG 5'

-G   AATTC-
-CTTAA and G-

BamHI
5' GGATCC 3'
3' CCTAGG 5'

-G   GATCC-
-CCTAG and G-

Blunt Ends

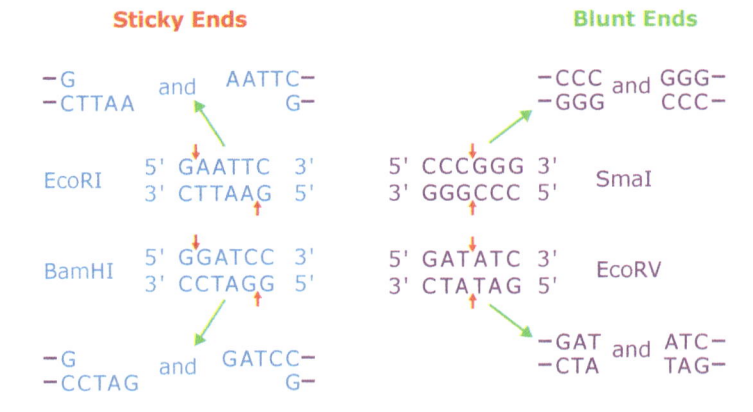

SmaI
5' CCCGGG 3'
3' GGGCCC 5'

-CCC   GGG-
-GGG and CCC-

EcoRV
5' GATATC 3'
3' CTATAG 5'

-GAT   ATC-
-CTA and TAG-

▲ Figure 18–2.0A Examples of Palindromes and Restriction Enzymes

- To recognize a palindrome based on a single strand sequence:
  - Fold sequence and base pair:

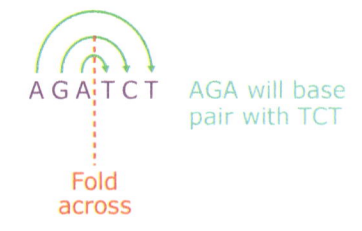

A G A T C T   AGA will base pair with TCT

Fold across

Chapter 18 • Molecular Technologies

- In recombinant DNA technology, fragments with antiparallel and complementary sticky ends can be ligated together:
  - With blunt ends, artificial sticky ends can be added

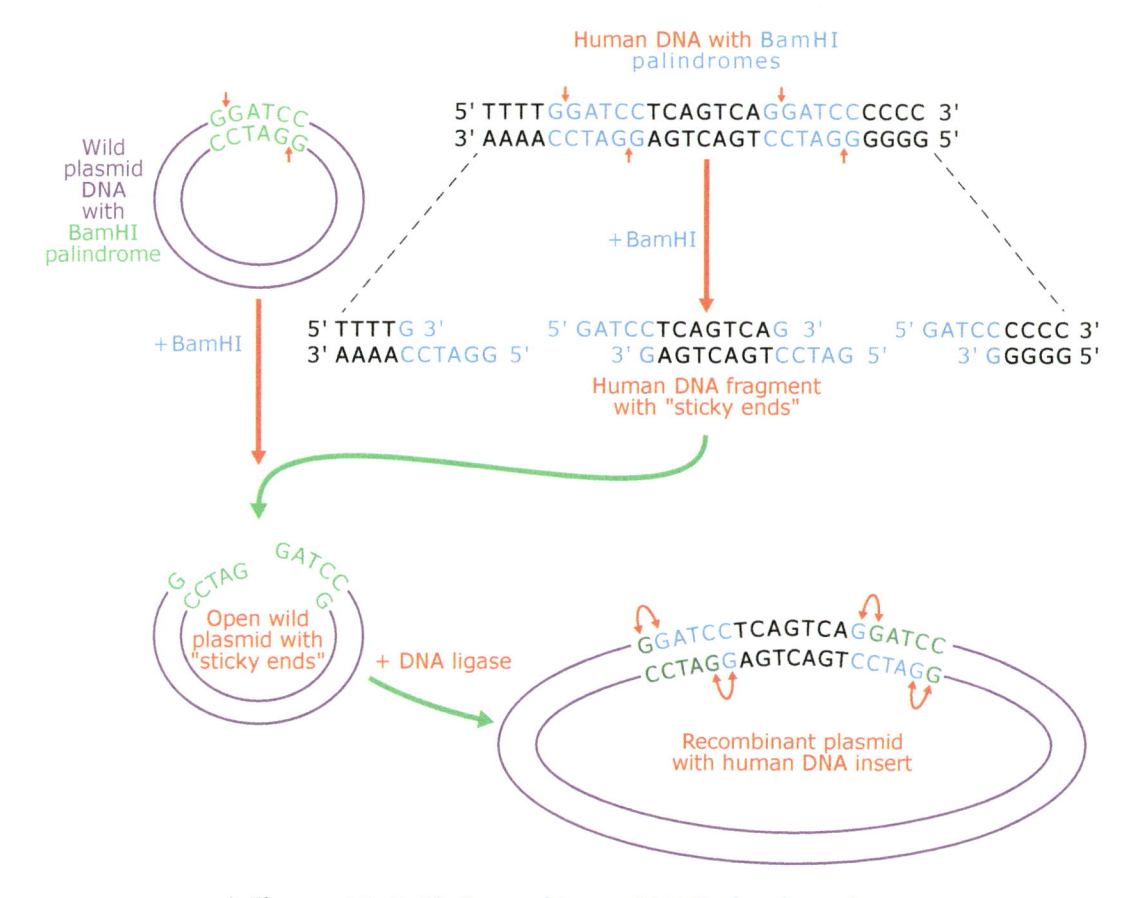

▲ Figure 18–2.0B Recombinant DNA Technology Concept

- Restriction enzyme mapping:
  - Palindromes occur in all DNA of sufficient length
  - Restriction maps are linear depiction of DNA with palindrome locations indicated
  - Restriction maps have a scale in kilobase pairs to identify restriction fragment length
  - Predict number and size of restriction fragments

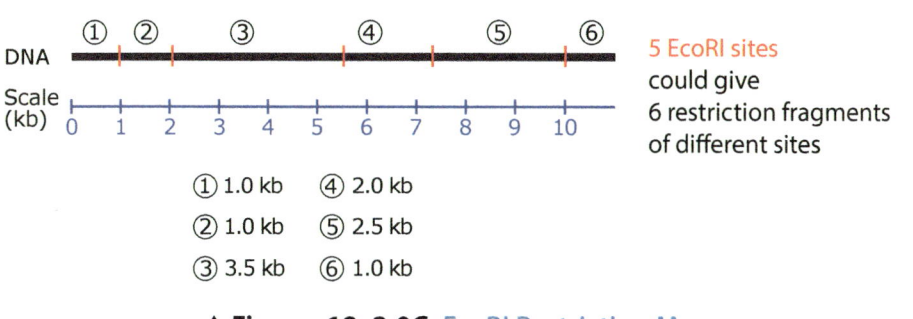

① 1.0 kb   ④ 2.0 kb
② 1.0 kb   ⑤ 2.5 kb
③ 3.5 kb   ⑥ 1.0 kb

5 EcoRI sites could give 6 restriction fragments of different sites

▲ Figure 18–2.0C EcoRI Restriction Map

3 Blotting Techniques

- Material to analyze is separated by gel electrophoresis:
  - Gel is sieve:
    - Small molecules move through easily
  - Electrophoresis moves molecules based on charges:
    - Negatively charged molecules move towards positive electrode
- Material separated on gel is blotted:
  - Transfer to a solid substrate:
    - Nitrocellulose paper, for example
    - Capillary, electrophoretic, or vacuum transfer
- Probing of material on blot:
  - Use of complementary, antiparallel DNA probes, or antibodies to proteins
  - Probes are labeled:
    - With radioactivity:
      - ^{32}P-DNA, ^{125}I-antibody
    - With biotin or digoxigenin
- Probe detection:
  - If radioactive, autoradiography (X-ray film)
  - If nonradioactive:
    - Antibodies against biotin or digoxigenin
    - Antibodies are conjugated to an enzyme
    - Enzyme substrate is metabolized to a chemiluminescent or colorful product:
      - Chemiluminescence impresses a film
      - Colorful product is direction visualized

Table 18-3.0 Blotting Techniques

Material Separated	Blot Name	Purpose
DNA	Southern	Identify gene sequence: • Mutations • Polymorphisms
RNA	Northern	Study gene expression: • Quantitation • Alternative splicing
Proteins	Western	Detect and quantitate specific proteins: • Antibodies to an infectious disease
DNA-binding proteins	Southwestern	Study gene regulation: • Transcription factors and DNA-binding sites

Chapter 18 • Molecular Technologies

Normal ASO	3'-GAGGACTCCTCTTCA-5'	
Normal β-globin chr.11	5'-CTCCTGAGGAGAAGTCTGC-3'	
Sickle β-globin	5'-CTCCTGTGGAGAAGTCTGC-3'	
SCA ASO	3'-GAGGACACCTCTTCA-5'	

- **Two short probes**
  - 15–20 nucleotides
  - Complementary and antiparallel to DNA sequence with mutation
  - DNA is first amplified by PCR
- **Used in dot/slot blot**

ASO Probes
↑
Probes
↙ ↘

Single Gene Probes
- Longer probes:
  - Complementary and antiparallel to region closely linked to gene of interest
  - Used in RFLP analysis of genetic diseases

Broadly Specific Probes
- Recognize short repeated sequences in spacer DNA
  - Short tandem repeats (STR)
- Used in forensic identity testing
- STRs are first amplified by PCR

Normal HTT gene chr. 4

5'━━━(CAG)━━━3'
         <26
   ↕ 3'━5' Single gene probe
5'━━━(CAG)━━━3'
         >40

Huntington disease

Spacer DNA from crime scene

5'━━CGCGCGCGCGCG━━3'
         6 repeats
   ↕ Probe binds to or near the repeat
5'━━CGCGCG━━3'
         3 repeats

Spacer DNA from defendant

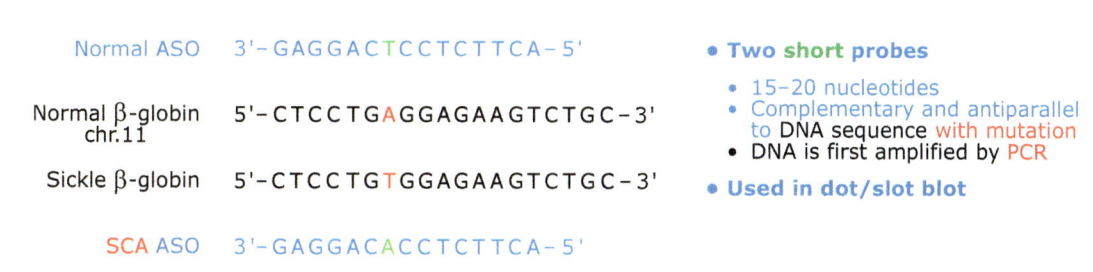

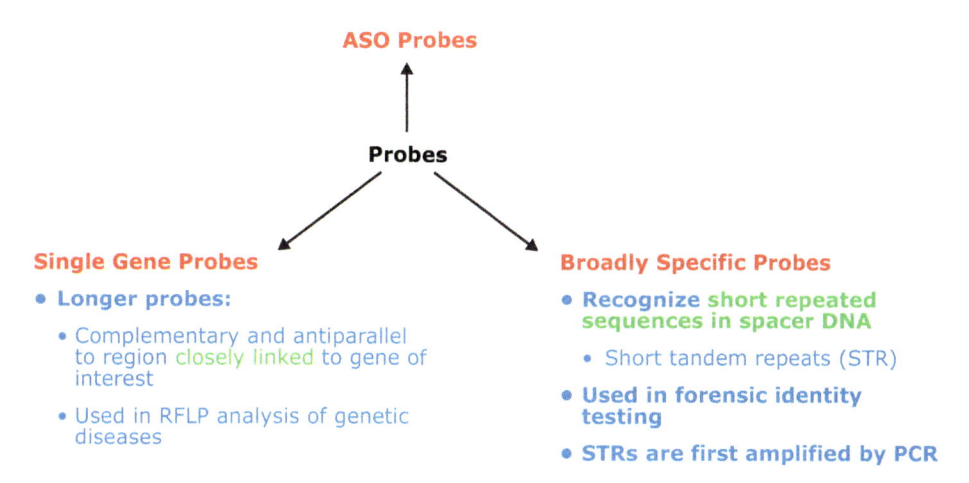

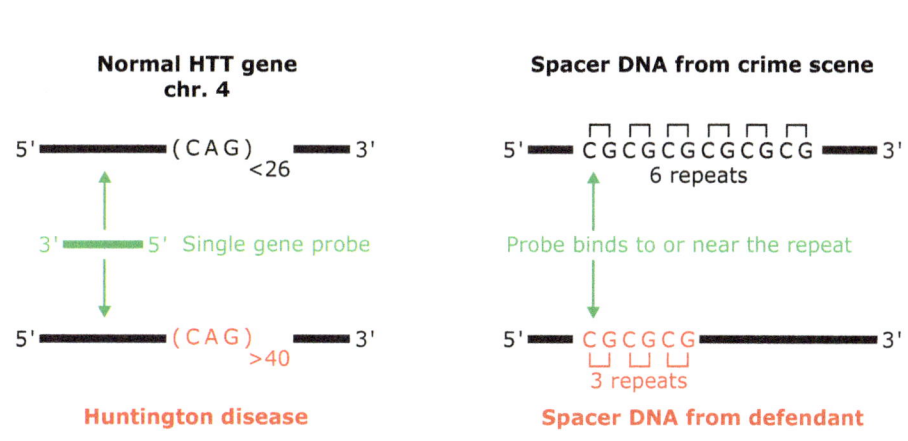

▲ **Figure 18–3.0** ss Labeled DNA or RNA Probes

4 DNA Polymorphisms

- Variations in DNA sequences between different individuals:
  - Due to inherited and acquired mutations:
    — Substitutions (point mutations)
    — Insertions or deletions
- Polymorphisms are anywhere in DNA:
  - Most likely in spacer DNA
  - Can be within genes
- Polymorphisms are used as:
  - Markers for diseases
  - Markers for genetic identity
- Restriction fragment length polymorphisms: RFLP
  - Digestion of DNA with restriction endonucleases
  - Length of restriction fragments differ between individuals:
    — Mutations affecting palindromes:
      - Affect size and number of fragments
    — Repetitive sequences:
      - The greater number of repeats, the longer the fragment

4.1 Southern Blot Analysis of RFLPs

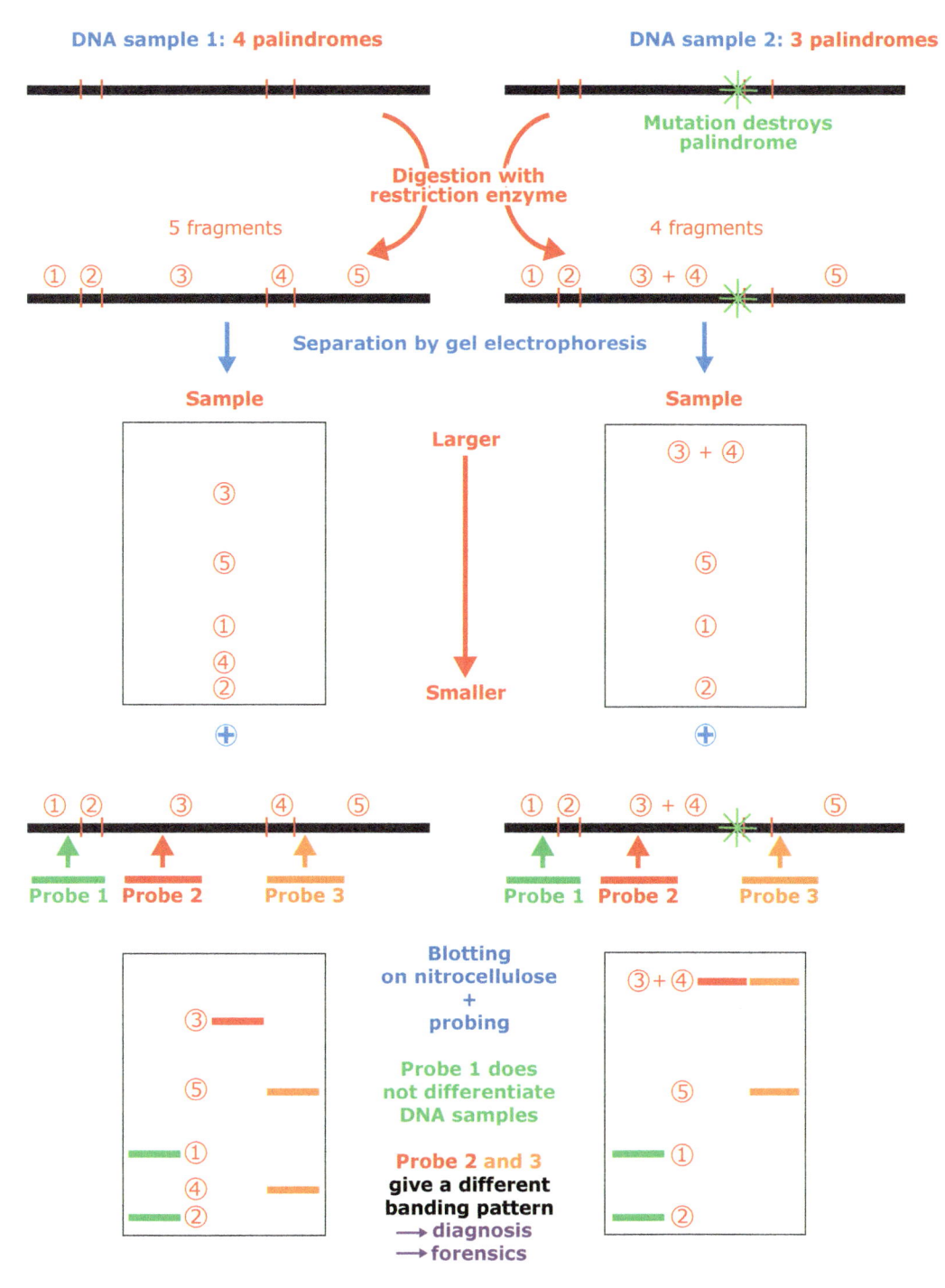

▲ Figure 18-4.1 Southern Blot Analysis of RFLPs

- Clinical Application of RFLP:
  - Mst II analysis of sickle cell anemia (SCA):
    — The point mutation in SCA destroys a palindrome for Mst II

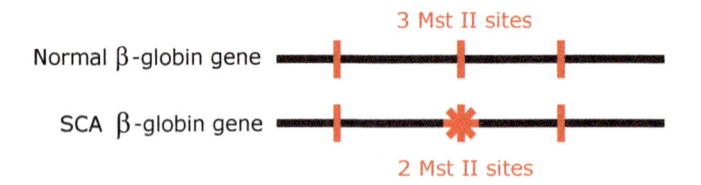

— Probing near the mutation will give different banding patterns

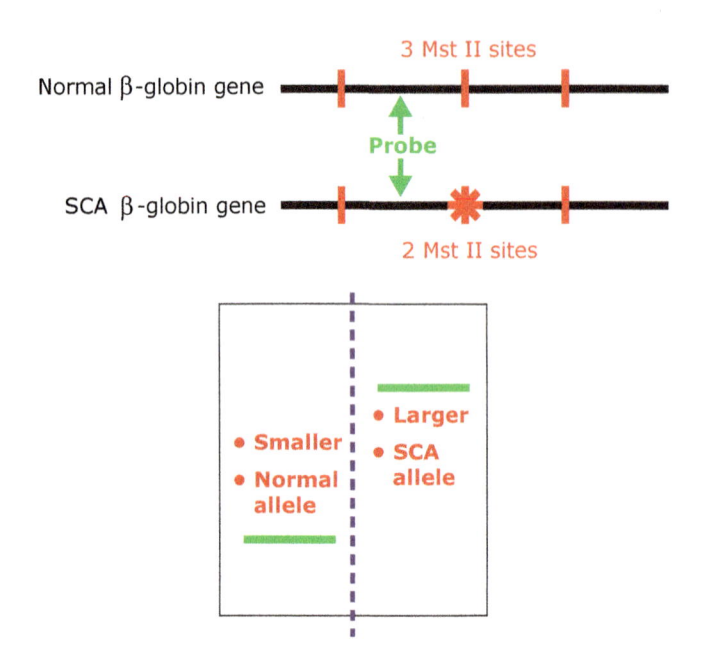

— Each individual inherits two β-globin gene alleles, giving rise to three different genotypes:
- Homozygous normal: Two small Mst II restriction fragments
- Heterozygous carrier: One small and one large Mst II fragment
- Homozygous for SCA: Two large fragments

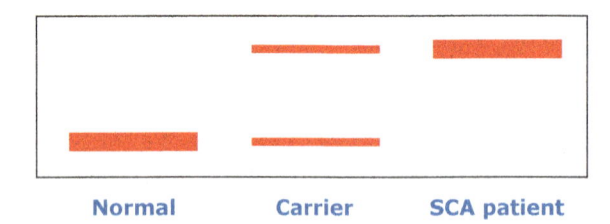

4.2 Repetitive Sequences and RFLPs

- Variable number of tandem repeats (VNTRs):
  - Short nucleotide sequence repeated in tandem multiple times:
    - Microsatellites:
      - < 5 base pairs repeats
      - Also known as short tandem repeats (STRs)
      - Include triplet repeats
    - Minisatellites:
      - Up to 60 base pair repeats
- Cutting restriction fragments containing VNTRs will give different banding patterns once probed

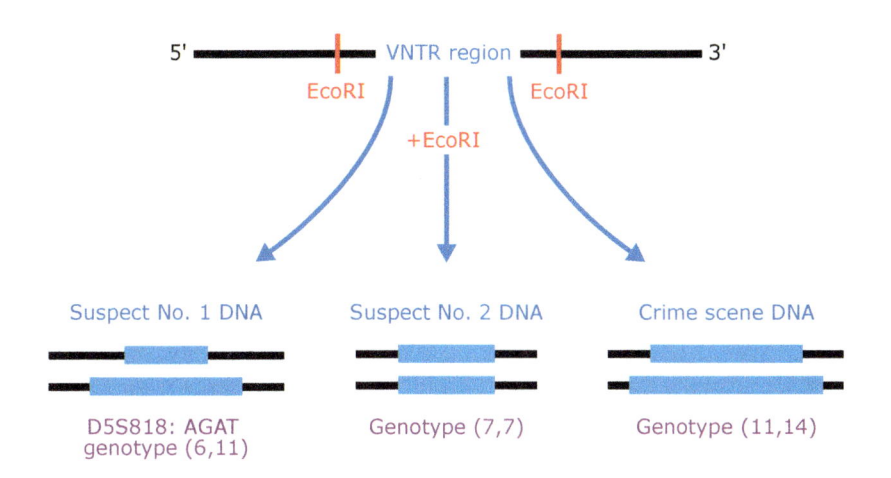

▲ Figure 18-4.2 Repetitive Sequences and RFLPs: Forensic Application

- D5S818 is one of 13 STRs analyzed by the FBI:
  - Combined DNA Information System (CODIS)
  - AGAT repeats exist 7 to 14 times in general populations
  - On chromosome 5 at 5q23.2:
    - Two separate alleles with variable number of repeats
  - Genotype frequencies of populations are statistically analyzed:
    - Sorted by ethnicities
    - Sorted by geographic location
  - The matching probability depends on the number of STR regions (loci) studied:
    - The greater the number, the less likely a match is random
    - The frequency of a set of alleles (genotype) in a population is the product of the frequency of each allele separately (product rule)
      - Example: 7 repeats in locus D5S818 occur in 1/100 people therefore genotype (7,7) would be expected in 1/100 × 1/100 (or 1 in 10,000) individuals

5 Dot/Slot Blots and ASO Probes

- No electrophoresis
- DNA sample is amplified and probed with two ASO probes as shown in Figure 18-5.0

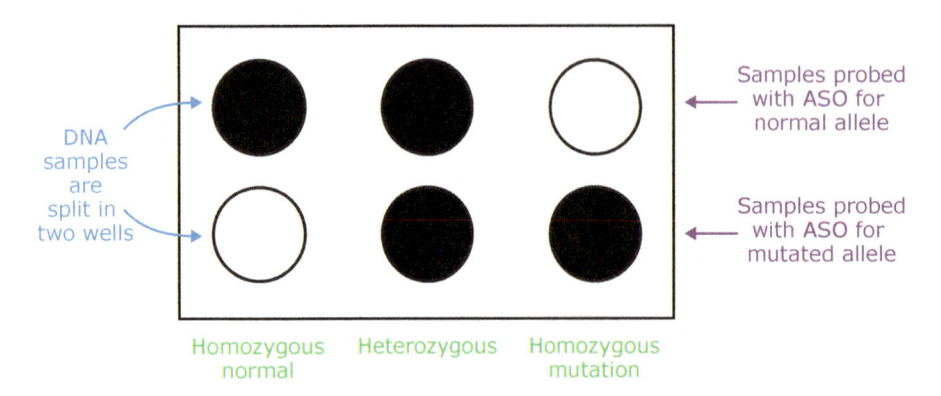

▲ Figure 18-5.0 Dot Blot Analysis

6 Northern Blots

- Used to answer questions about gene expression:
  - Investigate RNA quantity and structure:
    — The thicker a band, the more RNA is produced
    — Smaller RNA may be the result of alternative splicing
    — Larger RNA can result from expansion of repeats
- mRNAs from tissues are isolated and separated by gel electrophoresis, blotted, and probed as in Southern blots

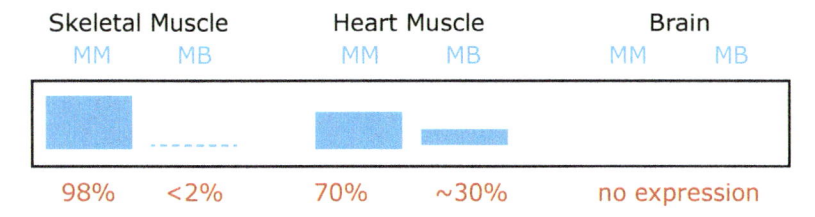

Skeletal Muscle		Heart Muscle		Brain	
MM	MB	MM	MB	MM	MB
98%	<2%	70%	~30%	no expression	

▲ Figure 18–6.0 Northern Blot of Creatine Kinase MM and MB mRNA in Various Tissues

- Array technologies: Gene expression profiling
  - Measurement of thousands of genes at the same time
    — Probes for different genes are attached to a solid surface, such as a glass slide (DNA chip) or a glass bead
    — mRNAs from tissues are reverse transcribed to cDNAs using fluorescent nucleotides
    — cDNAs are allowed to hybridize with probes on DNA chip
    — Fluorescence intensity correlates with level of expression
  - Gene expression profiling is useful to type tumors:
    — Molecular signature is critical to subtype the tumor and is used for prognosis and treatment protocol:
      - Example: ER ⊕ versus ER ⊖ breast tumors expressing ErbB2 oncogene

7 Western Blot

- Proteins are separated by gel electrophoresis and blotted
- Antibodies from patient's serum hybridize to immobilized proteins on blot
- Probes consist of radiolabeled or enzyme-linked antibodies to Fc regions of patient's immunoglobulins
- Examples include HIV, Lyme disease, HBV (infection or vaccination), etc.

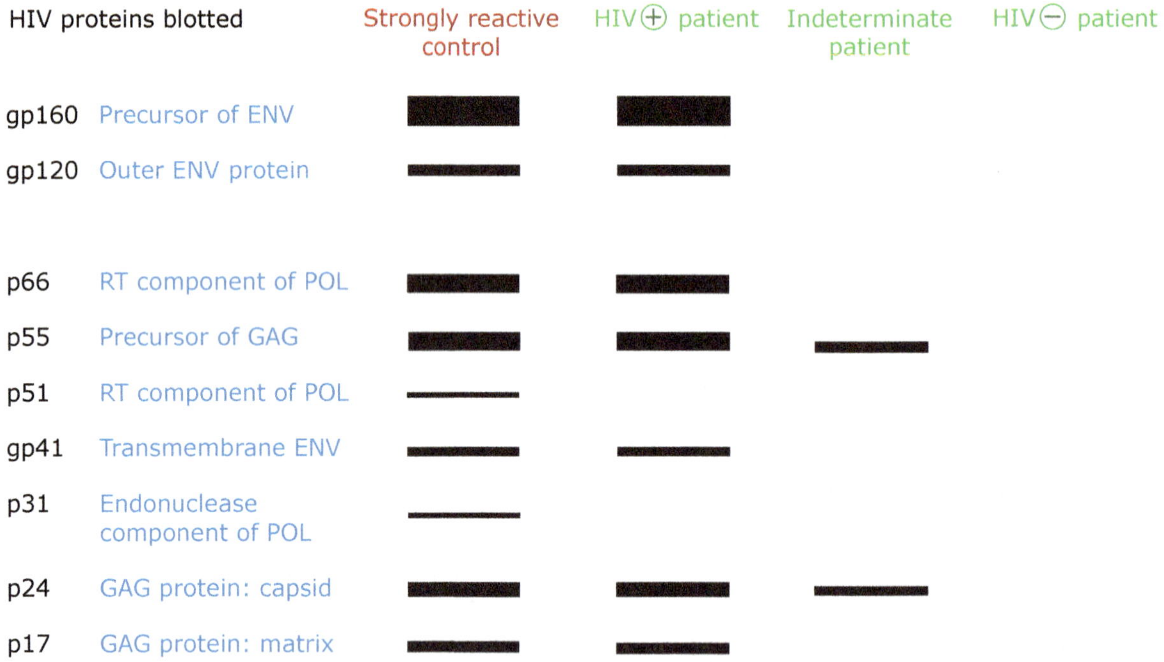

HIV proteins blotted		Strongly reactive control	HIV⊕ patient	Indeterminate patient	HIV⊖ patient
gp160	Precursor of ENV	■	■		
gp120	Outer ENV protein	■	■		
p66	RT component of POL	■	■		
p55	Precursor of GAG	■	■	■	
p51	RT component of POL	■			
gp41	Transmembrane ENV	■	■		
p31	Endonuclease component of POL	■			
p24	GAG protein: capsid	■	■	■	
p17	GAG protein: matrix	■	■		

Analysis and conclusions:

  HIV Negative: No bands present

  HIV Positive: Any two or more of the following bands— p24, gp41, and gp120/160

  Indeterminate: Any bands present, but pattern does not meet criteria for "positive"

▲ Figure 18–7.0 Western Blot and HIV Testing

8 Polymerase Chain Reaction

- In vitro replication
- Rapid production of large amounts of specific DNA sequences
- Requires very small sample to start with:
  - Single strand of hair, single blood drop
- PCR requires four components:
  - Target dsDNA must be present
  - Two specific primers in excess:
    - Both templates of DNA will be copied
    - Each primer binds to 3' flanking sequences of DNA of interest
    - Critical component of PCR
    - 20–30 nucleotides-long
  - Excess nucleotides for new DNA synthesis (dNTPs)
  - Heat-stable DNA polymerase:
    - Taq polymerase, isolated from *Thermus aquaticus*, a bacteria living in hot springs
- PCR is a three-step process:
  - Denaturation:
    - Heating to 95° C separates DNA strands
    - Takes 20–60 seconds
  - Annealing:
    - Cooling to 50°–70° C allows primers to bind 3' flanking sequences
    - Most critical step for specificity
    - Takes 20–90 seconds
  - Extension:
    - Taq polymerase copies templates
    - Occurs at 70° C
    - Takes 10–60 seconds

Chapter 18 • Molecular Technologies

- Repeating this process 20 to 40 cycles results in millions of copies of target DNA:
  - PCR products can be blotted and probed
  - PCR products can be sequenced

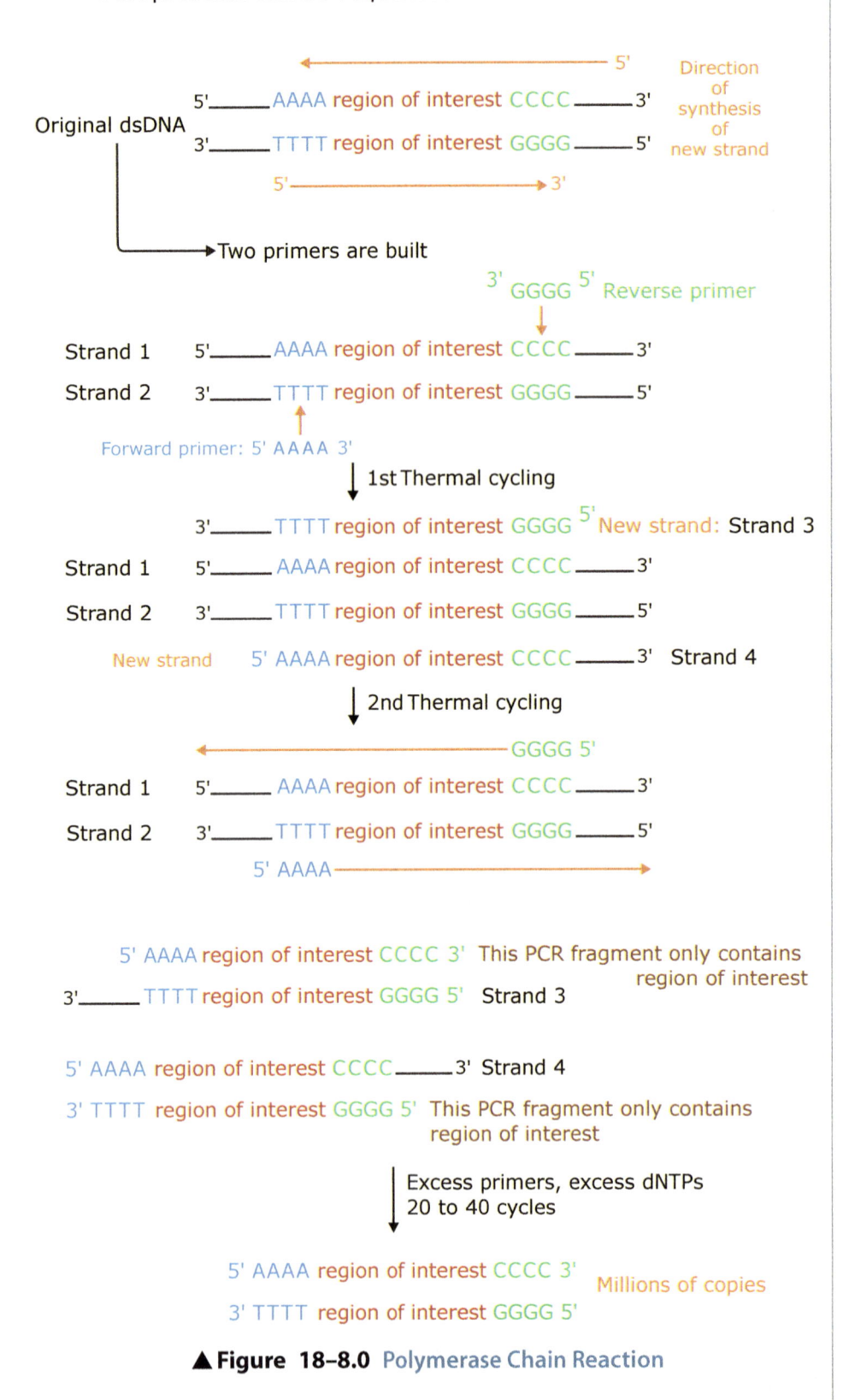

Original dsDNA

5'_____AAAA region of interest CCCC_____3'
3'_____TTTT region of interest GGGG_____5'

Direction of synthesis of new strand

→ Two primers are built

Reverse primer: 3' GGGG 5'

Strand 1   5'_____AAAA region of interest CCCC_____3'
Strand 2   3'_____TTTT region of interest GGGG_____5'

Forward primer: 5' AAAA 3'

↓ 1st Thermal cycling

3'_____TTTT region of interest GGGG 5'   New strand: Strand 3
Strand 1   5'_____AAAA region of interest CCCC_____3'
Strand 2   3'_____TTTT region of interest GGGG_____5'
New strand   5' AAAA region of interest CCCC_____3'   Strand 4

↓ 2nd Thermal cycling

←———————— GGGG 5'
Strand 1   5'_____AAAA region of interest CCCC_____3'
Strand 2   3'_____TTTT region of interest GGGG_____5'
5' AAAA ————————→

5' AAAA region of interest CCCC 3'   This PCR fragment only contains region of interest
3'_____TTTT region of interest GGGG 5'   Strand 3

5' AAAA region of interest CCCC_____3'   Strand 4
3' TTTT region of interest GGGG 5'   This PCR fragment only contains region of interest

↓ Excess primers, excess dNTPs
20 to 40 cycles

5' AAAA region of interest CCCC 3'   Millions of copies
3' TTTT region of interest GGGG 5'

▲ **Figure 18-8.0 Polymerase Chain Reaction**

Chapter 18 • Molecular Technologies

8.1 PCR in HIV Diagnosis

- Amplification of HIV cDNA is required for diagnosis when ELISA and Western blot are not relevant:
  - Infant of HIV ⊕ mother:
    —Has mother's IgGs
    —Would have ⊕ Elisa and Western blot whether infected or not
  - Immunosuppressed patients
  - High risk of exposure, but too early to test for antibodies:
    —Rape victim
    —IVDU
    —Needle stick

Infected CD4 ⊕ Cell

HIV diploid (+) ssRNA

Fusion/Entry
- gp120/gp41
- CD4/CCR5
- CD4/CXCR4

(+) ssRNA →[HIV reverse transcriptase]→ cDNA →[DNA polymerase]→ ds cDNA

Human ds 5'_____ HIV ds _____ 3'
DNA   3'_____ cDNA _____ 5'

Integrase

⇩

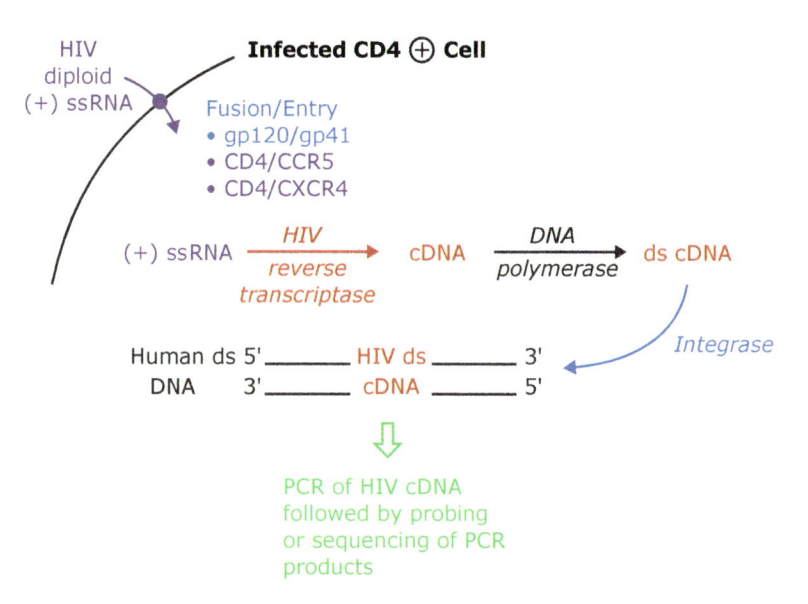

PCR of HIV cDNA followed by probing or sequencing of PCR products

▲ Figure 18-8.1 PCR for HIV Provirus (cDNA)

8.2 HIV Viral Load: RT-PCR

- Reemergence of viremia shortly precedes AIDS-defining diseases
- Viral load can be quantitated using reverse transcriptase PCR
- Viral load is not for diagnosis, but for monitoring
- Use of Tth polymerase:
  - *Thermus thermophilus* DNA polymerase has reverse transcriptase activity
- RT-PCR is used to detect other RNA viruses:
  - Coronaviridae responsible for SARS, for example

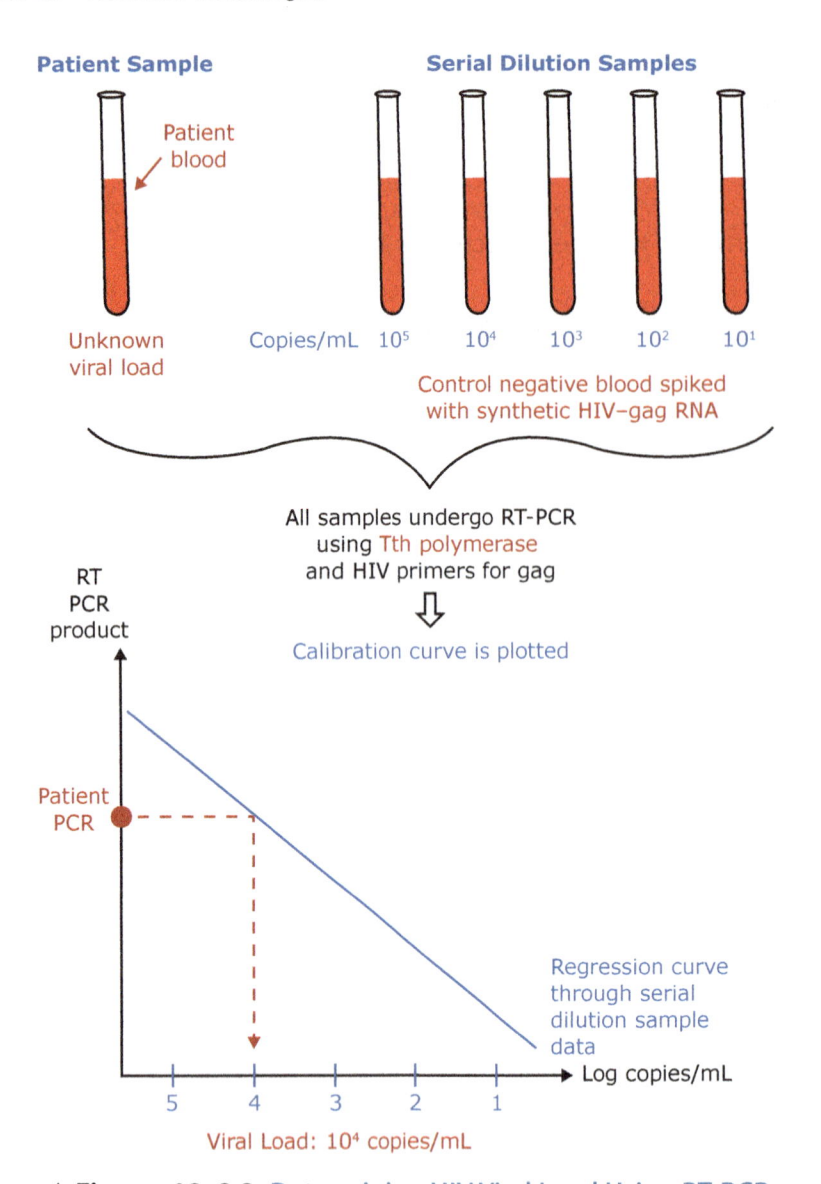

▲ Figure 18-8.2 Determining HIV Viral Load Using RT-PCR

8.3. PCR in Direct Mutation Testing

- Mutations affect small DNA regions or can be single nucleotide substitutions
- PCR is used to amplify the DNA region of interest
- Fragments can be blotted and probed or sequenced

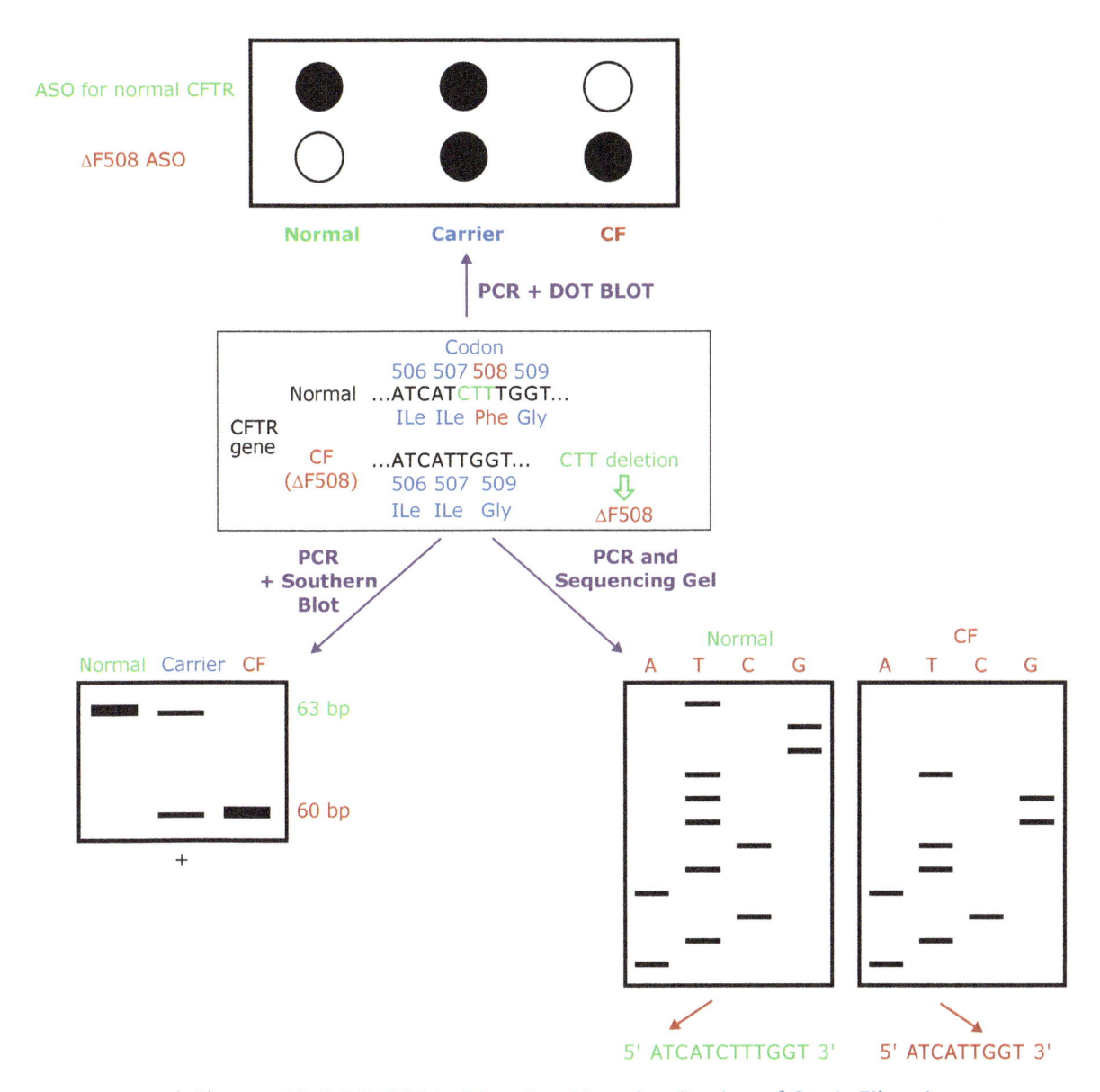

▲ Figure 18-8.3A PCR in Direction Mutation Testing of Cystic Fibrosis

Chapter 18 • Molecular Technologies — Biochemistry

- **Sequencing DNA:**
  - DNA sample to be sequenced is amplified in four different test tubes
  - Each test tube contains a dideoxyribonucleoside triphosphate
    — ddNTPs lack a 3'OH
    — Cause chain termination:
      - Similar to zidovudine or didanosine in replication (Chapter 15)
    — PCR product ends with dideoxynucleotide
  - Gel is read from bottom to top:
    — Smallest PCR fragment is 1 nucleotide long:
      - DNA polymerase took a ddNTP first
    — Sequence read is antiparallel and complementary to original template

PCR strand 5' A————————→ 3'
            3' TAGTAGAAACCA 5'
            Template DNA to sequence
          + Excess primers, dNTPs, DNA pol

+ddATP   +ddTTP   +ddCTP   +ddGTP
   A   T   C   G

— All PCR fragments end with —

5' A   5' AT   5' ATC   5' ATCATCTTTG
5' ATCA   5' ATCAT   5' ATCATC   5' ATCATCTTTGG
                  5' ATCATCT
                  5' ATCATCTT
                  5' ATCATCTTT
                  5' ATCATCTTTGGT 3'

Read gel from bottom up

5' PCR product

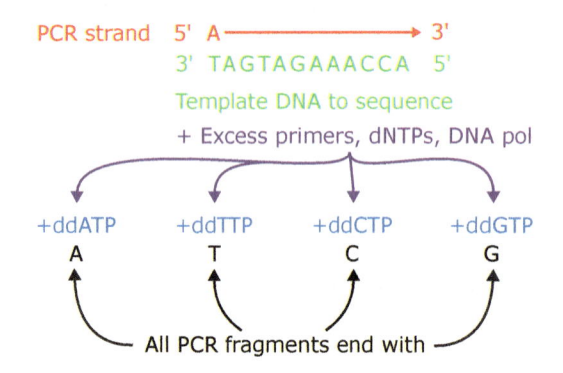

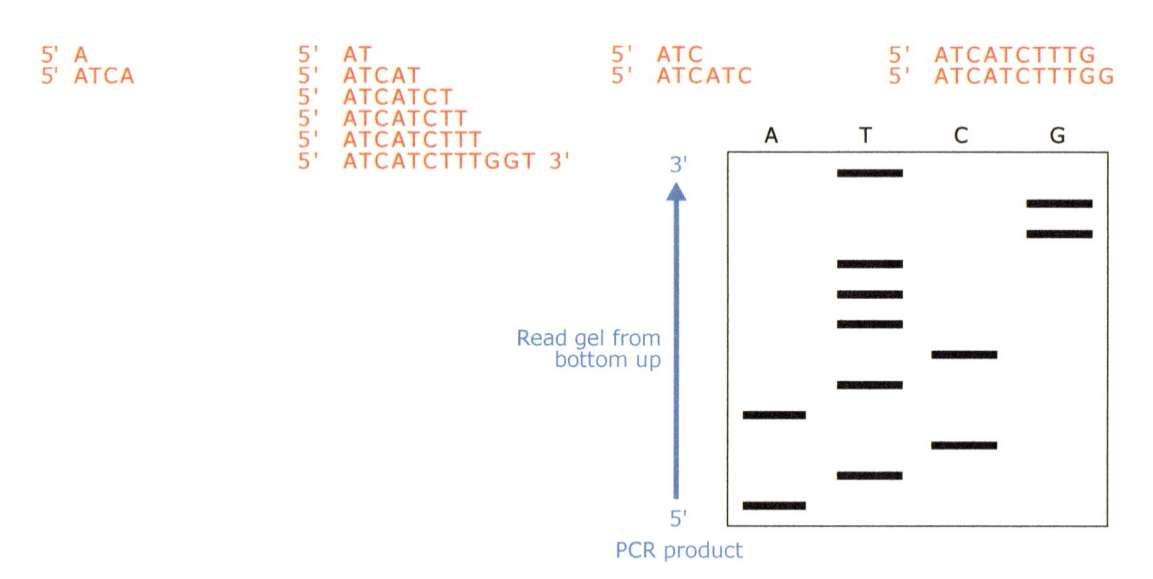

▲ **Figure 18-8.3B** Dideoxy Chain Termination Sequencing (Sanger Method)

CHAPTER 19 — Recombinant DNA Technology

1 Overview

- Cloning is a technique for amplifying DNA sequences
- Cloning differs from PCR:
  - The segment of DNA is inserted in a vector
  - The vector infects a host cell
  - The host cell replicates or expresses the inserted human DNA
  - The copied DNA or protein expressed is isolated, purified
- Applications include:
  - Production of therapeutic proteins
  - Gene therapy
  - Transgenic animals

USMLE® Key Concepts

For Step 1, you must be able to:
- Describe cloning techniques.
- Differentiate uses of genomic versus expression libraries.
- Understand the roles and requirements of vectors.
- Describe applications of recombinant DNA technologies.

2 Sources of Human DNA

- Two sources:
  - Genomic DNA:
    - Any nucleated cell
    - Genome is cut by restriction endonucleases into manageable fragment sizes
    - All DNA is cloned:
      - Spacer DNA with promoters, enhancers, silencers
      - Genes with UTRs, exons, and introns
    - Sequence of interest may be fragmented
  - mRNAs from tissues expressing genes of interest:
    - mRNAs are reverse transcribed to cDNA
    - No need for fragmentation
    - Only UTRs and exons are cloned
    - Ideal approach for the therapeutic protein expression

3 Vectors and Cloning Strategy

- cDNAs from mRNAs or restriction fragments from genomic DNA are inserted into vectors to produce recombinant vectors
- All vectors must have:
  - ORI to allow replication in host cell
  - Palindromes to allow insertion of human DNA
  - Modes of selection:
    - Antibiotic resistance genes:
      - Host cells with recombinant vectors are plated on differential media
    - Reporter genes:
      - Some vectors contain genes encoding for a specific enzyme or fluorescent protein, conferring unique characteristics to transformed cells
- If the goal of cloning is expression, the vector must also have:
  - Transcription start sequence, such as a TATA box
  - Transcription termination signal, such as a GC-rich hairpin loop sequence for prokaryote transcription
  - Ribosome binding sequence, such as a Shine-Dalgarno sequence for prokaryote translation
- Types of vectors vary with host cell chosen for cloning:
  - Plasmids or phages are used for bacteria:
    - Plasmids are extrachromosomal dsDNA that can infect bacteria
    - Phages are bacteria viruses
    - Host cells with plasmids are called transformed cells
    - Host cells with phages are called transduced or transfected cells
  - Retroviruses, adenoviruses, and liposomes are used for eukaryotic cells
- A collection of host cells with recombinant human genome fragments is called a genomic library
- A collection of host cells with recombinant human cDNAs from mRNAs is called a cDNA or expression library

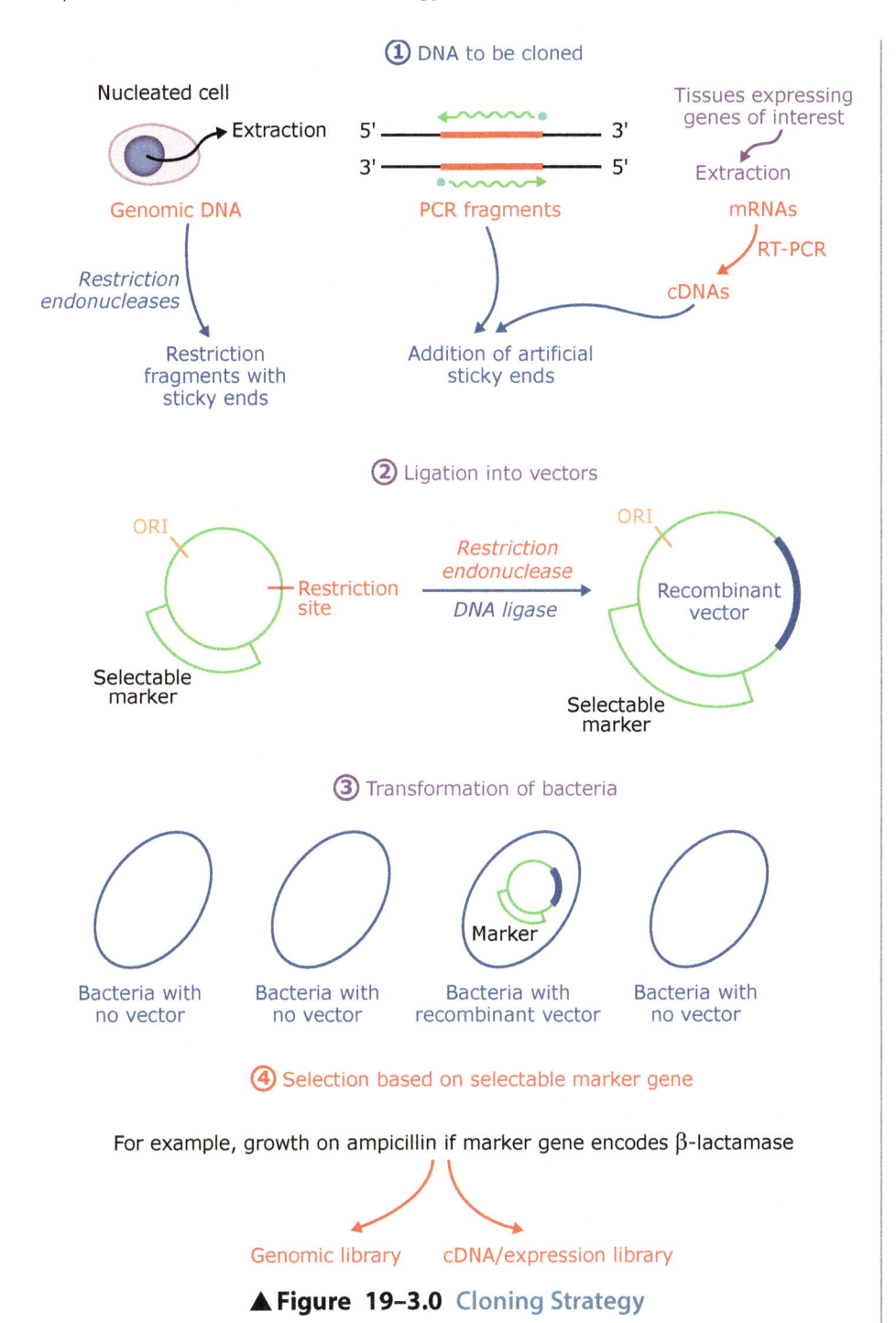

Chapter 19 • Recombinant DNA Technology

① DNA to be cloned

Nucleated cell → Extraction → **Genomic DNA**

PCR fragments

Tissues expressing genes of interest → Extraction → **mRNAs** → RT-PCR → **cDNAs**

Genomic DNA → *Restriction endonucleases* → **Restriction fragments with sticky ends**

PCR fragments and cDNAs → **Addition of artificial sticky ends**

② Ligation into vectors

Vector with ORI, Restriction site, Selectable marker → *Restriction endonuclease, DNA ligase* → **Recombinant vector** (with ORI, Selectable marker)

③ Transformation of bacteria

- Bacteria with no vector
- Bacteria with no vector
- Bacteria with recombinant vector (Marker)
- Bacteria with no vector

④ Selection based on selectable marker gene

For example, growth on ampicillin if marker gene encodes β-lactamase

→ Genomic library
→ cDNA/expression library

▲ **Figure 19–3.0** Cloning Strategy

4 Cloning Applications

4.1 Production of Recombinant Proteins

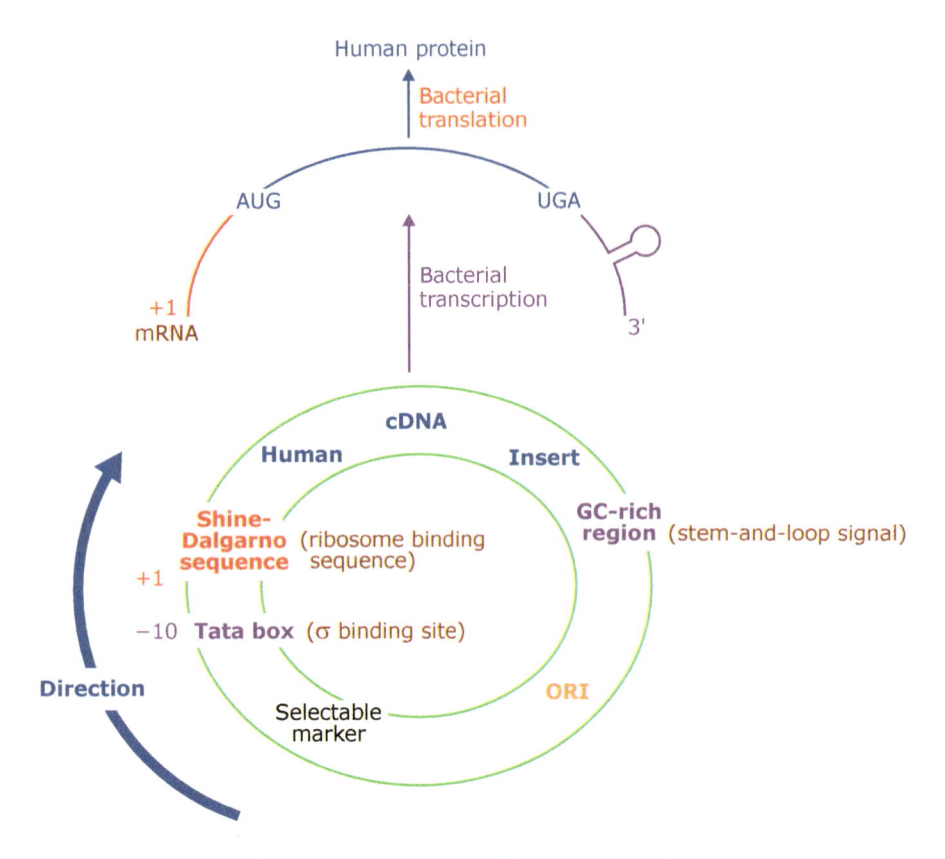

Figure 19-4.1 Use of Expression Vectors

4.2 Gene Therapy

- Goal is to introduce healthy genes into somatic cells:
  - Germ cells, such as gametes, are not used in human gene therapy
  - Hundreds of clinical trials are underway in the U.S.
- Healthy gene product is expressed:
  - Correcting a genetic deficiency:
    — Replacing factor VIII in hemophilia, for example
  - Interfering with other proteins expressed in that tissue:
    — Making an antibody against an infectious agent or an oncogenic protein
- Introduction of gene is achieved with viral vectors or direct injection of naked DNA or liposomal preparations of DNA

Table 19-4.2 **Viral Vectors in Human Gene Therapy**

Virus	Advantages	Disadvantages
Retroviruses	• Reverse transcriptase • Integrase	• Only infect replicating cells • Integration is random
Lentiviruses	• Subclass of retrovirus • Can infect nondividing cells	• Integration is random
Adenoviruses	• Can infect nondividing cells	• Does not integrate in genome • Many humans have existing antibodies (common cold)

- Random integration can occur next to promoters of oncogenes:
  - Can result in tumor genesis
- Lack of integration requires repeated administration:
  - Host immune response develops against viral vector
- Viral vectors are genetically engineered to be replication-defective:
  - Re-administration as cells die
  - Re-administration results in resistance from host through immune response
- Viral vectors can be modified to target a specific cell type:
  - Called pseudotyping
  - Addition of envelope glycoproteins from other viruses to alter tropism
- Gene therapy can be done in vivo or ex vivo:
  - Ex vivo: Infection is done in cell cultures in vitro; successfully infected cells are reinjected into the patient

4.3 Transgenic Animals

- Introduction of defective gene into animal genome creates a transgenic animal
- Deletion of gene creates a knockout animal
- Gives more realistic animal model of human disease
- Original technique: Fertilized ovum microinjection
  - Microinjection of defective gene into pronucleus of fertilized mouse oocyte
  - Reimplantation of genetically engineered embryo into female mouse
  - Litter of transgenic animals
  - Defective gene coexists with animal's own copy of gene:
    — Issue with recessive traits

- **Stem cell transgenesis:**
  - Insertion or knockout in blastocysts of a selected mouse strain
  - Merging of engineered blastocysts with those of another strain:
    — Produces a chimera
  - Chimeras are inbred for as many as 20 generations:
    — Resulting population comprises homozygous and heterozygous individuals
    — Allows for study of dominant and recessive traits

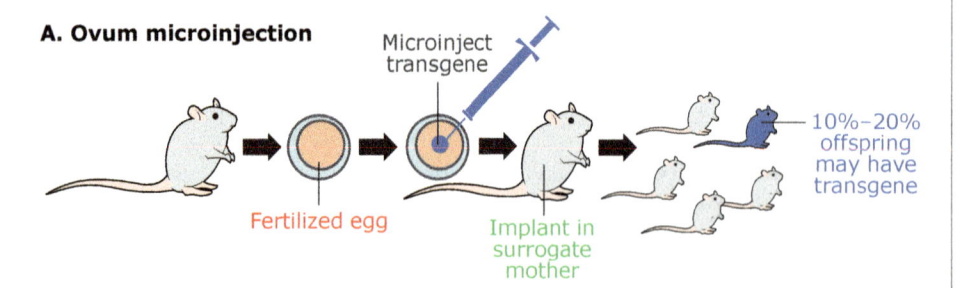

A. Ovum microinjection

B. Chimera production

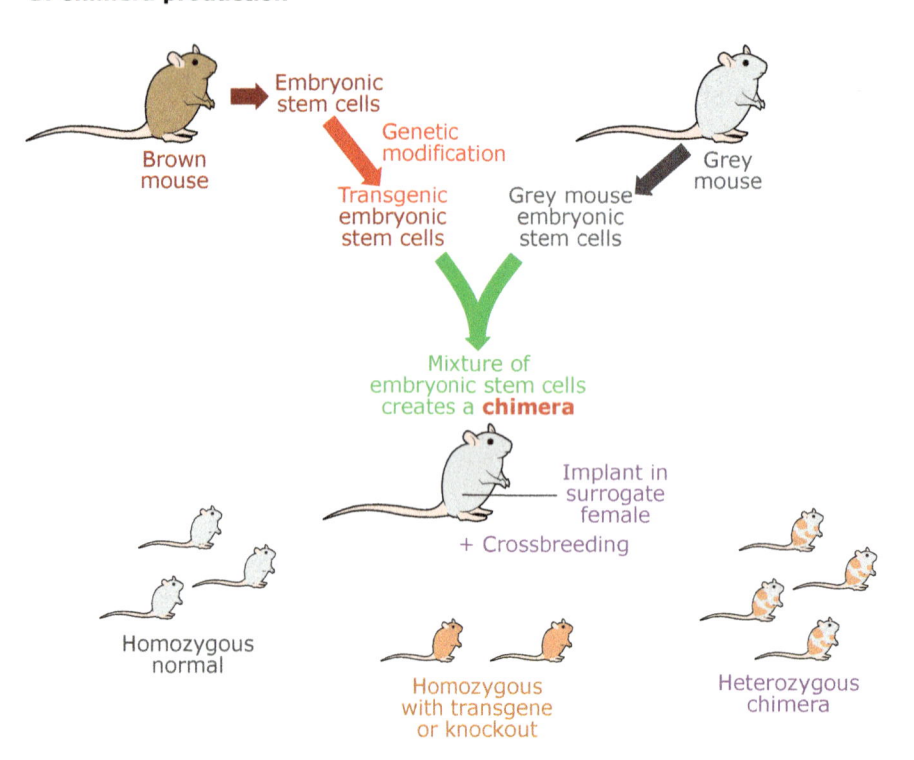

▲ Figure 19–4.3 Transgenic Animals

Genetics

CHAPTER 1: Mendelian Inheritance

1 Overview

1.1 The Human Genome

- The human genome contains the genetic information required for differentiation of all cells, including the code for all proteins synthesized by cells and the instructions to control the expression of these proteins during development.
- The genome is 3×10^9 base pairs in length, spread over 23 chromosomes—analogous to an encyclopedia split into 23 volumes of different sizes.
- Each chromosome consists of a single double helix of DNA.
- Every nucleated somatic cell has two copies of each chromosome.
- Within the genome, genes code for the amino acid sequence of proteins (see *Biochemistry*, Chapter 17):
  - The genome contains ~23,000 genes with coding portions (exons).
  - The position of a gene on the DNA sequence is its locus (meaning its place)—the terms gene and locus are often used interchangeably.
  - A significant number of genes do not encode proteins, but are transcribed to RNA and function only in translation (rRNA, tRNA) or in the regulation of gene expression (miRNA, XIST, etc.).
- Makeup of genome:
  - Coding portions (exons) constitute ~1.5%.
  - Conserved non-coding sequences (mostly to insure the proper expression of genes during development) account for 3.5%.
  - Repeat sequences, pseudogenes ("nature's failed experiments"), and genetic material for which the possible function has yet to be determined make up the remainder (~95%).

USMLE® Key Concepts

For Step 1, you must be able to:
- Describe the role of genes in human development.
- Identify the mode of inheritance from a pedigree.
- Recall the mode of inheritance for the most frequently encountered mendelian disorders.
- Identify exceptions to the mendelian rules of inheritance.

1.2 Language of Mendelian Inheritance

Table 1-1.2	Basic Mendelian Terminology
Term	Definition
Phenotype	Characteristics, such as eye color, height, or disease state (e.g., cystic fibrosis)
Gene	Portion of DNA sequence encoding protein or functional transcript
Allele	Form of a gene inherited from one parent (e.g., the alleles for brown and blue eyes are different forms of the same gene)—each parent passes one allele of each gene to each of their offspring
Homozygote	Individual who has inherited the same allele from each parent
Heterozygote	Individual who has inherited a different form of the gene from each parent
Dominant	The phenotype seen in a heterozygous individual
Recessive	The phenotype hidden in a heterozygous individual but revealed among the offspring of a heterozygous couple

1.3 Mendel's Law of Segregation

- If each parent is homozygous for different alleles of the same gene, their offspring will all be heterozygous and will exhibit the dominant phenotype (Figure 1–1.3A).
- The chance that a heterozygous individual will pass on a given allele at each mating is 50% (Figure 1–1.3B).
- The segregation of alleles is often illustrated using a Punnett square (Figure 1–1.3C).

> **Important Concept**
>
> The alleles of different genes are passed to the next generation independently—we now know this does not apply if the genes are on the same chromosome.

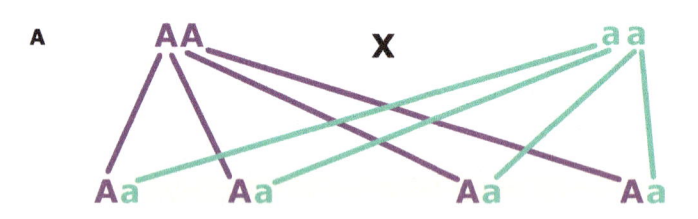

▲ Figure 1–1.3A Segregation of Alleles: Homozygous Parents

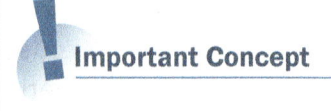

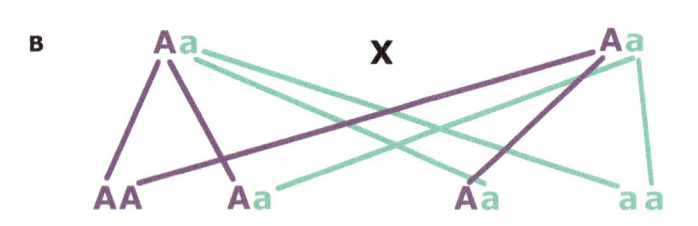

▲ Figure 1–1.3B Segregation of Alleles: Heterozygous Parents

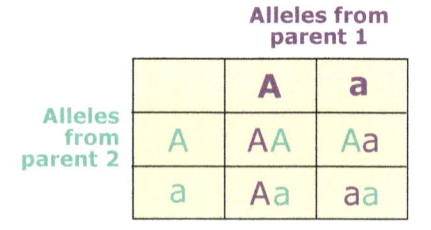

▲ Figure 1–1.3C Segregation of Alleles: Punnett Square

2 Patterns of Mendelian Inheritance

- Phenotypes that result from the variation in a single gene (including single gene disorders, such as cystic fibrosis, Marfan syndrome, hemophilia A) are said to exhibit mendelian inheritance and can be either:
  - Dominant or recessive
  - Autosomal or X-linked
- Inheritance patterns can be determined from the pedigree or family tree (Figure 1–2.0).
- Some phenotypes may display dominant or recessive inheritance across different families when due to mutations in different genes, but within any one family the inheritance of the phenotype will always be consistent (e.g., congenital deafness can exhibit autosomal dominant or recessive inheritance depending on the mutated gene).
  - If an individual heterozygous for a mutation is affected, the phenotype is dominant.
  - If an individual heterozygous for a mutation is not affected, the phenotype is recessive.

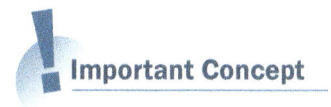

Important Concept

The terms dominant and recessive only should be used to describe the phenotype and not a gene or allele.

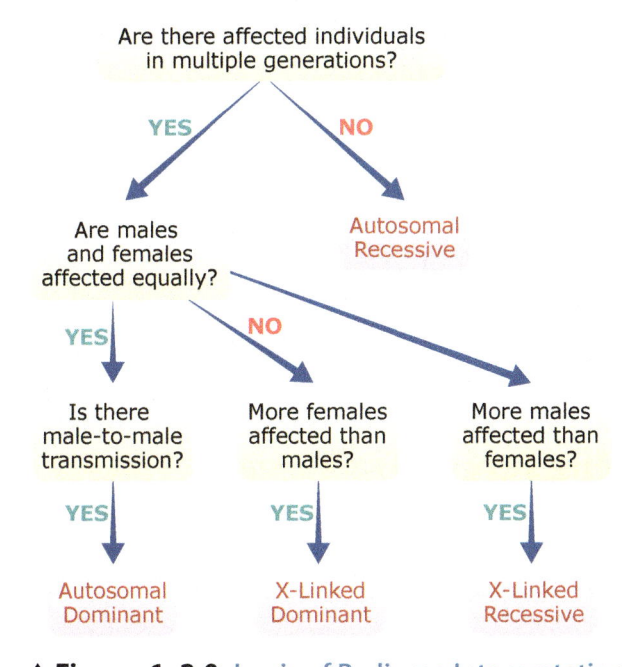

▲ Figure 1–2.0 Logic of Pedigree Interpretation

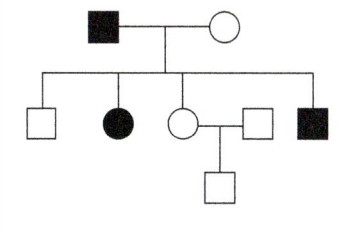

▲ Figure 1–2.1A Autosomal Dominant Pedigree

2.1 Autosomal Dominant Inheritance

- Phenotype will be present in successive generations.
- Phenotype will be present equally in males and females.
- Only autosomal dominant phenotypes will exhibit father-to-son transmission (Figure 1–2.1A).
- Affected individuals have a 50% chance of passing the phenotype to each child (Figure 1–2.1B).

	Alleles from affected parent	
	A	a
Alleles from unaffected parent a	Aa	aa
a	Aa	aa

▲ Figure 1–2.1B Punnett Square for Autosomal Dominant Inheritance

2.2 Autosomal Recessive

- Pedigrees exhibiting autosomal recessive inheritance will typically have affected males and females in a single generation with unaffected parents (Figure 1-2.2A).
- Recessive phenotypes are commonly revealed in consanguineous families, in which the parents are second cousins (or closer).

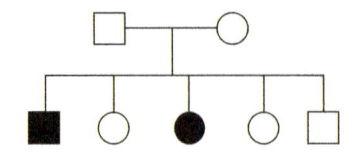

▲ Figure 1-2.2A
Autosomal Recessive
Pedigree

- When both parents are heterozygous for mutations in the same gene, each has a 50% chance of passing on the mutant allele and therefore each child has a 25% chance of being affected (Figure 1-2.2B).
- Consideration of the Punnett square indicates that the unaffected sibling of an individual with an autosomal recessive phenotype has a two thirds (66%) chance of being a carrier, not a 50% chance.
  - The Punnett square shows the situation at conception for each child of a carrier couple.
    — Once a child can be seen to be unaffected, one of the four possibilities has been eliminated, and in two of the remaining three possibilities, the children would be carriers.

	Alleles from carrier parent	
	A	a
Alleles from carrier parent A	AA	Aa
a	Aa	aa

▲ Figure 1-2.2B Punnett Square for Autosomal Recessive Inheritance

2.3 X-Linked Recessive

- Because females have two X chromosomes and males have only one, mutations in genes located on the X chromosome may show their effects only in males (Figure 1–2.3A).
- Because males receive their X chromosome from their mother, the mothers of affected males must be heterozygous (obligate carriers).

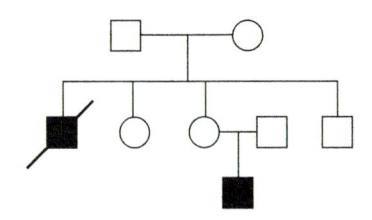

▲ **Figure 1–2.3A** X-Linked Recessive Pedigree

- The unaffected females who "link" affected males in an X-linked recessive pedigree are obligate carriers.
- Because carrier females are heterozygous, they will pass the mutation to half of their children so each daughter has a 50% chance of being a carrier and each son has a 50% chance of being affected (Figure 1–2.3B).
- All daughters of affected males will be carriers.

	Alleles from carrier mother	
	X	X^m
Alleles from normal father — X	XX	$X^m X$
Alleles from normal father — Y	XY	$X^m Y$

▲ **Figure 1–2.3B** Punnett Square for X-Linked Recessive Inheritance

- In a population with approximately equal numbers of males and females, only one third of all X chromosomes are in males in contrast to half of autosomes. Thus, one third of all X-linked mutations are in males.
  - Because most of the X-linked phenotypes are genetic lethal (affected individuals die before passing on the mutation), it follows that one third of X-linked mutations would be lost in each generation.
  - Because X-linked phenotypes have not disappeared, geneticists hypothesized (and subsequently proved) that there must be a high mutation rate for the X chromosome.
  - From the above, it becomes clear that, in the absence of family history, one third of affected males are the result of a new mutation and only two thirds of mothers of affected males are heterozygous.

Looking Ahead

X-inactivation is discussed in Chapter 4.

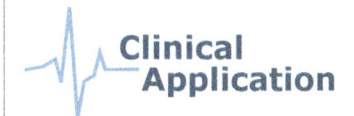

Clinical Application

In autosomal recessive pedigrees, the *unaffected* sibling of an affected individual has a two thirds chance of being a carrier.

In X-linked recessive pedigrees, in the *absence of a family history*, the mother of an affected boy has a two thirds chance of being a carrier.

2.4 X-Linked Dominant

- X-linked dominant phenotypes are usually dramatically more severe in males than in females and may often show male lethality (Figure 1–2.4).
- Heterozygous females will pass the mutant allele to half their children, so half their children will be affected as seen for autosomal dominant inheritance.
- All daughters and none of the sons of an affected male will be affected because males only pass the Y chromosome to their sons.

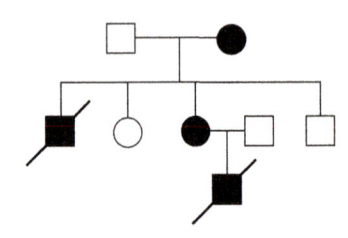

▲ Figure 1–2.4 X-Linked Dominant Pedigree

2.5 Exceptions

- The majority of single gene disorders demonstrate one of the patterns of inheritance discussed above.
- In real-life situations, a given family may not show all of the characteristics to allow absolute identification of the pattern of inheritance, so it is essential to know the mode of inheritance for the most commonly encountered mendelian disorders (Table 1–2.5).

Table 1-2.5 — Mendelian Disorders

	Autosomal	X-Linked
Dominant	• Achondroplasia • Acute intermittent porphyria (AIP) • Familial hypercholesterolemia (FH) • Huntington disease (HD) • Marfan syndrome (MFS) • Myotonic dystrophy (DM1) • Neurofibromatosis (NF1) • Osteogenesis imperfecta (OI) • Polycystic kidney disease (PCKD)	• Fragile X syndrome • Pyruvate dehydrogenase deficiency • Rett syndrome • Vitamin D-resistant rickets
Recessive	• Cystic fibrosis (CF) • Glycogen storage diseases • Hemoglobinopathies • Maple syrup urine disease (MSUD) • Phenylketonuria • Tay-Sachs disease and most other metabolic disorders	• Duchenne and Becker muscular dystrophies (DMD and BMD) • Glucose–6–phosphate dehydrogenase (G6PD) deficiency • Hemophilia A and B • Lesch-Nyhan syndrome • Menkes syndrome • Ornithine transcarbamoylase (OTC) deficiency

2.5.1 New Mutation and Mosaicism

- When a new mutation occurs during gametogenesis in either parent and is passed to a child, then the child will be heterozygous for the mutation and may exhibit an autosomal dominant phenotype.
- Typically, a single affected individual will be observed and neither parent will exhibit the phenotype or have the mutation in his or her somatic cells.
- Occasionally, the mutation arises early in gametogenesis, such that the parent may produce multiple gametes with the mutation and have more than one child who is heterozygous (and hence affected). This type of inheritance is known as germline mosaicism.

2.5.2 Pseudodominance

- If a mutation (or mutations) resulting in a recessive phenotype is very common in a population, then a homozygous individual is fairly likely to have children with somebody who is heterozygous for the same mutation.
- Because the homozygote can only pass on the mutant allele, and the heterozygote will pass it on 50% of the time, half the children will be affected and the pedigree will appear dominant when the phenotype is actually recessive.
- Examples include blue eyes or the O blood group in European populations and sickle cell disease in West African populations.

2.5.3 Mitochondrial Inheritance

- Because essentially all mitochondria are passed in the egg from the mother and none in the sperm, mutations in the mitochondrial genome (encoding some components of the oxidative phosphorylation complexes and mitochondrial-specific translation machinery) will only be passed from the mother and never from the father (Figure 1–2.5A).
- The proportion of affected children depends on the concept of heteroplasmy—the proportion of mitochondria in the egg carrying the mutation.
- The severity of the phenotype also varies with the proportion of mitochondria with the mutation (Figure 1–2.5B).

2.5.4 Reduced Penetrance

- Genes and their products must act in a coordinated fashion for normal differentiation and development to proceed—thus variation at a second gene may exacerbate or ameliorate the effect of a mutation.

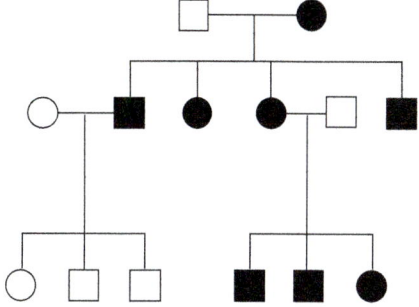

▲ **Figure 1–2.5A** Mitochondrial Inheritance Pedigree

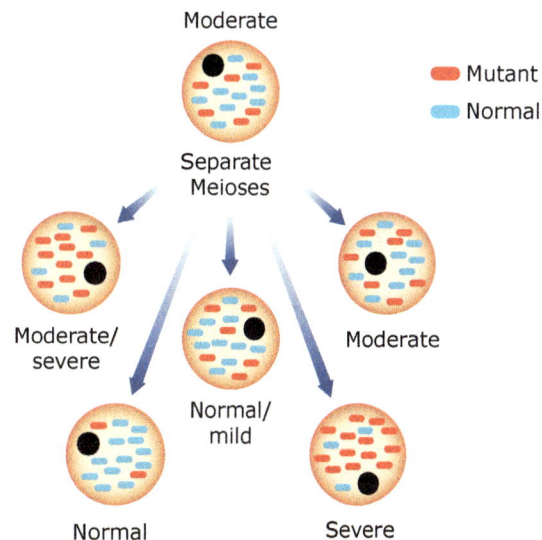

Different ratios of normal to mutant mitochondria affect severity of phenotype.

▲ **Figure 1–2.5B** Heteroplasmy of Mitochondrial Mutations

Chapter 1 • Mendelian Inheritance — Genetics

- A mutation that results in a phenotype in some individuals and not in others is said to exhibit reduced penetrance (Figure 1–2.5C).
- The unaffected individuals (arrowed in the pedigree) must be heterozygous for the mutation causing this autosomal dominant phenotype because they each have an affected parent and child.
- Penetrance is quantified as the number of individuals exhibiting the phenotype out of those who have the mutation ($7/9$ or 78% in this example) and is additive across families.
- Reduced penetrance is a crucial concept underlying multifactorial disorders (Chapter 7), but the majority of single gene disorders exhibit 100% penetrance.

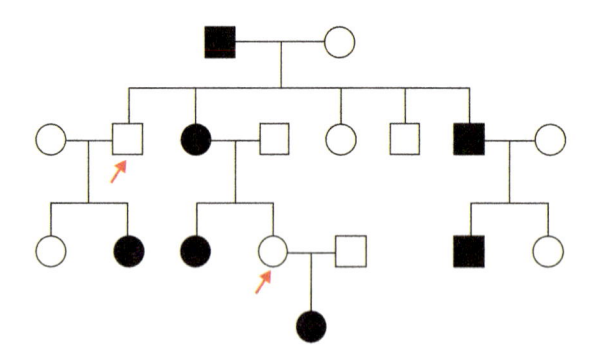

▲ Figure 1–2.5C Reduced Penetrance in an Autosomal Dominant Pedigree

2.5.5 Variable Expressivity

- Variation in other genes can also affect the range and severity of signs and symptoms for phenotypes showing 100% penetrance, which is often seen for phenotypes that exhibit pleiotropy—effects in multiple tissues that result from a single mutation.
- A hypothetical example for a Marfan syndrome pedigree is shown in Figure 1–2.5D.
- All affected individuals are heterozygous for the same mutation in the *FBN1* gene, but likely have different variants in other genes that change the probability of the different signs and symptoms.

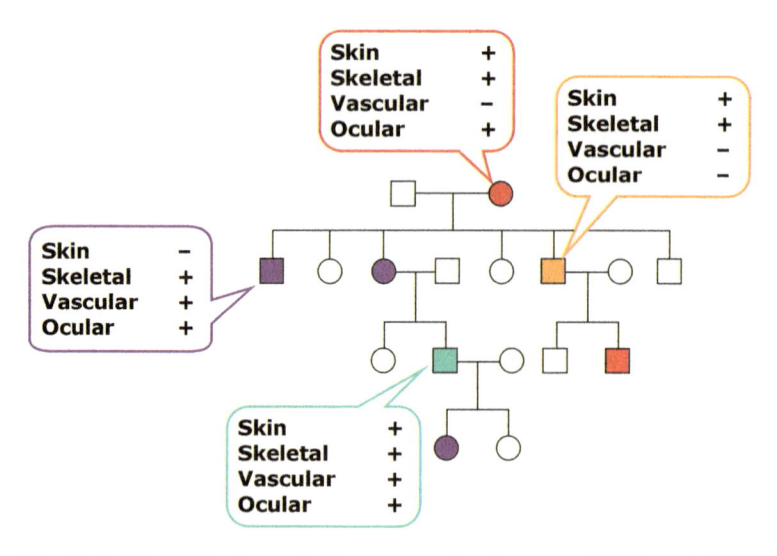

Skin	+
Skeletal	+
Vascular	−
Ocular	+

Skin	+
Skeletal	+
Vascular	−
Ocular	−

Skin	−
Skeletal	+
Vascular	+
Ocular	+

Skin	+
Skeletal	+
Vascular	+
Ocular	+

All affected individuals are heterozygous for the same *FBN1* mutation, but exhibit different aspects of the pleiotropic phenotype.

▲ Figure 1–2.5D Variable Expressivity in Marfan Syndrome

CHAPTER 2 — Chromosomes

1 Overview

- Chromosomes are essentially vehicles carrying (genetic) information from one (cell) generation to the next.
- Any disruption of the transmission process can result in an imbalance of information affecting cellular differentiation and development.
- Abnormalities of chromosomes are found in > 50% of first-trimester miscarriages and are responsible for multiple congenital anomalies in ~0.5% of newborns.

USMLE® Key Concepts

For Step 1, you must be able to:
- Differentiate between mitosis, meiosis I, and meiosis II.
- Explain how nondisjunction results in trisomies.
- Identify the common autosomal and sex chromosome aneuploidy syndromes.
- Explain the consequences of reciprocal and robertsonian translocations.

2 Mitosis

- The process of mitosis maintains the balance of information between diploid somatic cells.
- After the replication of DNA in the S phase of the cell cycle, the nuclear envelope dissolves, and the chromosomes condense (prophase) and are attached to spindles via the centromere (metaphase).
- Immediately after replication, each double helix of DNA is called a chromatid (i.e., each chromosome is composed of two chromatids).
- The spindles contract, pulling the chromosomes to opposite sides of the cell (anaphase) prior to cell division (cytokinesis) and restoration of the nuclear envelope (Figure 2–2.0).
- Because the chromatids are identical, and because one from each chromosome is passed to each daughter cell, the two daughter cells are genetically identical to each other.
- Defects in mitosis, in which both chromatids pass to one daughter cell, result in mosaic individuals who have different cell populations with 45, 46, or 47 chromosomes.
  - These rare cases of mitotic nondisjunction (abnormal segregation) are responsible for mosaic cases of Down syndrome.
  - Errors in mitosis can also occur in the development of cancer cells.

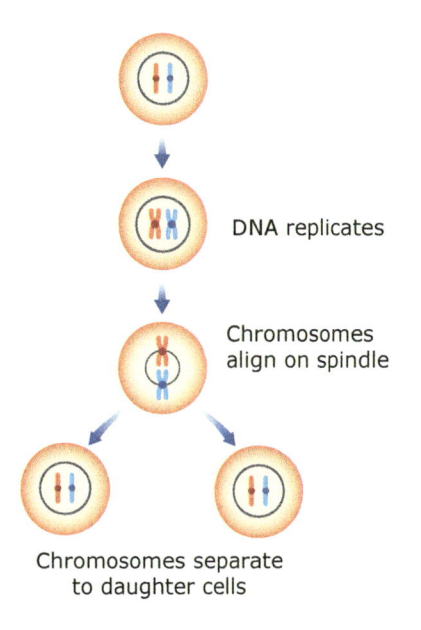

▲ Figure 2–2.0 Mitosis

Chapter 2 • Chromosomes — Genetics

3 Meiosis

- Reduction from the diploid to haploid state in gamete production utilizes a distinct process, called meiosis, which is divided into two phases: meiosis I and meiosis II (Figure 2-3.0).
- After replication in S phase, the chromosomes again condense (prophase) but, in contrast to mitosis, the homologous chromosomes align and recombination (crossing-over) takes place between two of the four chromatids.
- Strand exchange involves the cleavage of both strands in each DNA double helix and subsequent repair.
- There is at least one recombination event for each chromosome pair per meiosis (with more events on longer chromosomes).
- The exchange of homologous sequence between chromosomes is an important source of variation in eukaryotes as the alleles of genes are shuffled between maternal and paternal chromosomes.

Connection to Biochemistry

For a detailed discussion of replication, see *Biochemistry*, Chapter 15.

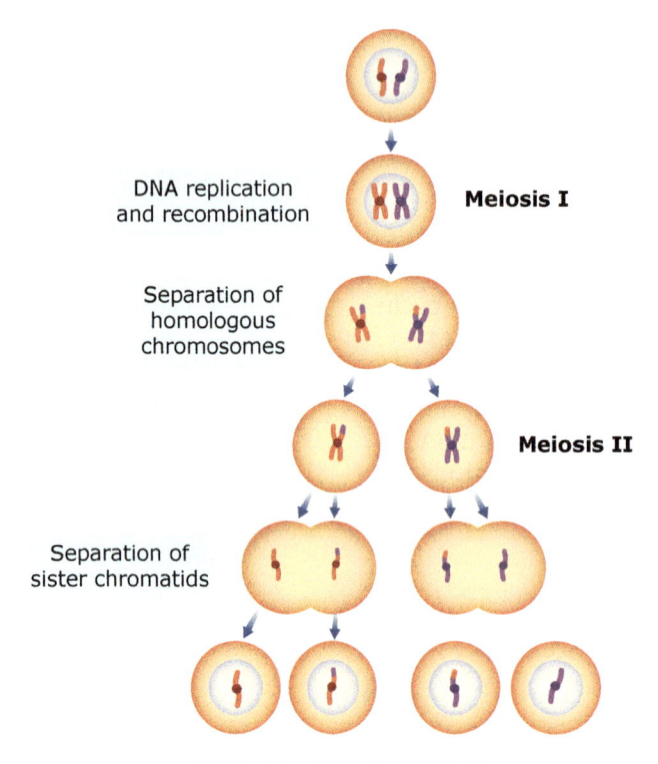

▲ Figure 2-3.0 Meiosis

- The homologous pairs of chromosomes attach to spindle fibers in metaphase I and are separated during anaphase.
- At this stage, each daughter cell has 23 chromosomes (one from each pair) comprising two chromatids.
- Both cells now move to meiosis II, which is broadly similar to mitosis in that the chromatids are separated so that from the initial diploid cell, four haploid gametes have been produced.
- Each gamete contains one copy of each chromosome, but the DNA is not identical due to the shuffling of alleles via recombination in prophase I and the random assortment of maternal and paternal chromosomes in metaphase I.

Connection to Anatomy

See *Anatomy* for a discussion of meiosis in the context of spermatogenesis and oogenesis.

Chapter 2 • Chromosomes

- The complexities of meiosis I result in the process taking much longer than mitosis:
  - ~60 days in spermatogenesis
  - ~10–50 years in oogenesis
- In females, meiosis begins early in embryonic life but is stalled in prophase I until the onset of puberty and then only one cell per month continues through the process.
- In males, the only homology between the X and Y chromosomes is at the ends of the chromosomes (called the pseudoautosomal region because males and females have two copies of all the sequence in this area, unlike the remainder of the X and the Y), and they often appear to be touching just at the ends rather than at positions along the length of the chromosome.

> **Important Concept**
>
> After the first meiotic division in females, there is one secondary oocyte and one polar body. Meiosis II only proceeds in the oocyte to yield the mature oocyte and a second polar body. Thus, each meiosis in females yields only one mature haploid gamete.

4 Karyotype

- A **karyotype** is a microscopic visualization of chromosomes.
- Karyotypes are created by the following steps:
  - Cells that are capable of division (e.g., white blood cells, amniocytes) are collected and cultured.
  - Subsequent addition of colchicine to the culture media prevents spindle formation so that mitosis is halted in metaphase when the chromosomes are condensed.
  - Lysis of the cells and staining of the chromosomes with Giemsa results in characteristic banding patterns (Figure 2–4.0).
  - Each chromosome stains differently because of the different distribution of genes on each.

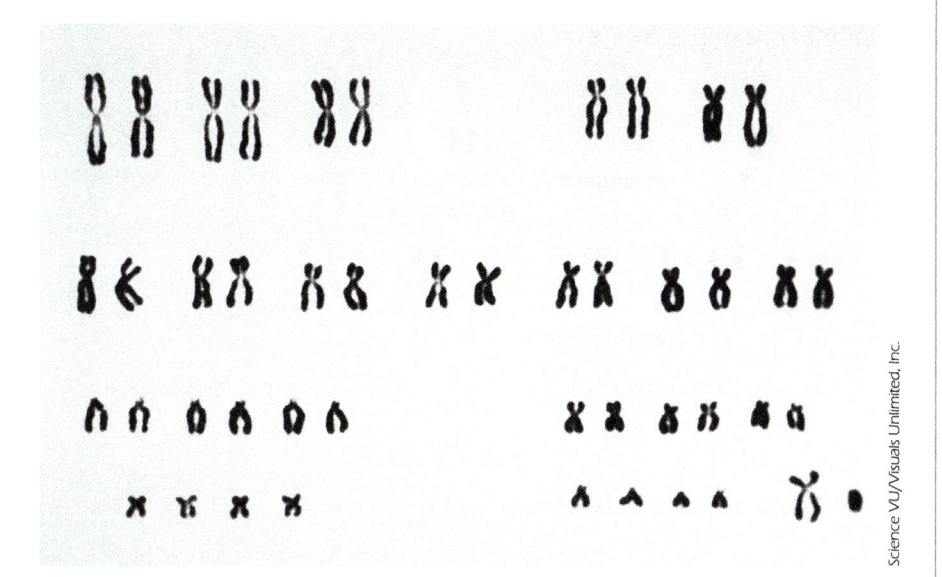

▲ Figure 2–4.0 Normal Male Karyotype

5 Nomenclature

- Chromosomes are described morphologically depending on the position of the centromere:
  - Metacentric (middle)
  - Submetacentric (to one side)
  - Acrocentric (at the end)
- The centromere is between the two arms of the chromosome—one short, one long:
  - The short arm is "p"
  - The long arm is "q"
- The bands on each arm are numbered away from the centromere and bands are divided into various levels of sub-bands depending on the microscopic resolution.
- Thus, a deletion on the long arm of chromosome 22 would be abbreviated as 46XX,del(22)(q11)—meaning, "female, deletion (on chromosome 22) (long arm, first band, first sub-band)."

6 Nondisjunction

- Failure of the chromosomes to segregate properly (nondisjunction) in meiosis results in aneuploidy.
- Theoretically, nondisjunction could occur in either meiosis I or meiosis II, resulting in disomic or nullisomic gametes and trisomic or monosomic conceptus (Figure 2–6.0), but it has been shown that the majority of autosomal nondisjunction occurs in maternal meiosis I (> 85%).
- The majority (> 80%) of aneuploid conceptus abort spontaneously.

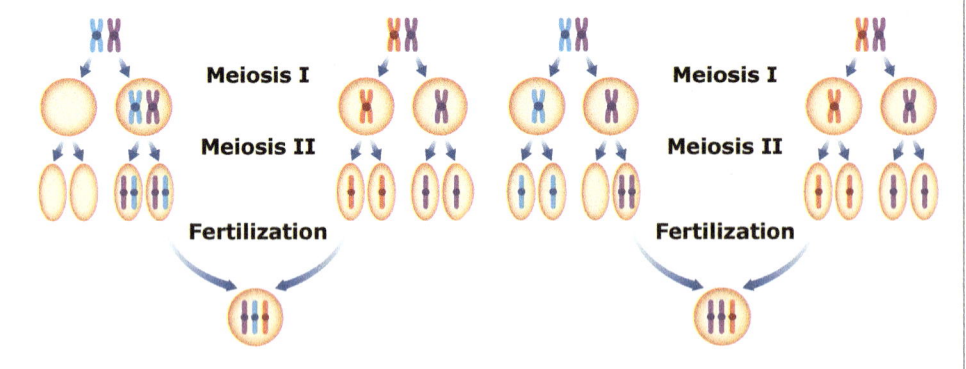

▲ **Figure 2-6.0** Nondisjunction in Meiosis I *(left)* and Meiosis II *(right)*

6.1 Autosomal Trisomies

- Only three autosomal trisomies survive gestation:
  - Chromosome 13 (Patau syndrome)
  - Chromosome 18 (Edwards syndrome)
  - Chromosome 21 (Down syndrome)
- Trisomies are associated with increased maternal age at conception (Figure 2–6.1A)—an observation at least partly due to the duration of prophase I in females.
- Prenatal screening tests have been instituted to identify the majority of trisomic fetuses by 13 weeks' gestation.
- The First Trimester Integrated Screening for Trisomies (FIRST) test is now standard of care and identifies > 80% of Down syndrome pregnancies irrespective of maternal age by measuring maternal chorionic gonadotropin levels and nuchal translucency.

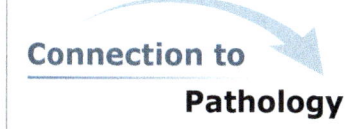

Connection to Pathology

Other aspects of prenatal testing are discussed in *Pathology*.

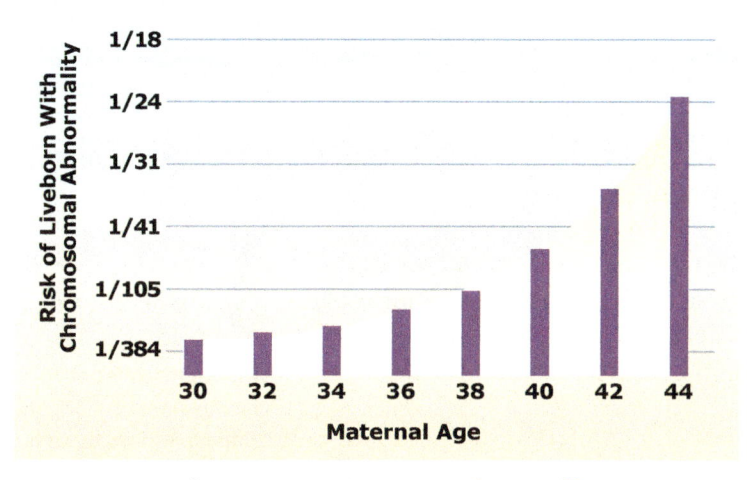

▲ Figure 2–6.1A Maternal Age Effect

6.1.1 Trisomy 21

- Down syndrome (see Figure 2–6.1B) is the most common autosomal trisomy, affecting 1:700 live births.
- Described as "the most complicated genetic insult compatible with human survival" (Reeves).
- **Etiology:**
  - ~95% are complete trisomies
  - ~4% are robertsonian translocations
  - ~1% are mosaic due to mitotic nondisjunction
    - Severity of presentation increases in proportion to the number of trisomic cells

- **Clinical features:**
  - **Neonatal:**
    - Hypotonia
    - Excess nuchal skin
    - Epicanthal folds
    - Upward slanting palpebral fissures
    - Single palmar (simian) creases
    - Congenital heart disease (40%)
    - Anal and/or duodenal atresia
    - Hirschsprung disease
    - Short stature
    - Brachycephaly
  - **Childhood:**
    - Intellectual disability
    - 10x–20x increased risk of acute lymphocytic leukemia (ALL) and acute myelocytic leukemia (AML; especially megakaryoblastic).
  - **Adulthood:**
    - After ~40 years of age, neuropathologic changes comparable to those seen in Alzheimer disease develop in almost all Down syndrome patients.
    - Advances in care have raised the median life span to 60 years.
- Management of Down syndrome patients has progressed markedly in recent years.
  - These patients can function well in group homes and other supervised environments.

▲ Figure 2–6.1B Down Syndrome

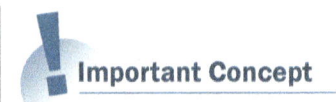

6.1.2 Trisomy 18
- Edwards syndrome affects approximately 1:3,000 live births.
- Presentation (neonatal):
  - Multiple central nervous system and cardiac abnormalities
  - Microcephaly
  - Prominent occiput
  - Micrognathia
  - Low-set ears and short neck
  - Overlapping fingers
  - Renal malformations
  - Limited hip abduction
  - Rocker-bottom feet
- Median survival is about 14 days with < 10% surviving 1 year.

6.1.3 Trisomy 13
- Patau syndrome affects approximately 1:5,000 live births.
- Presentation (neonatal):
  - Microcephaly
  - Cardiac abnormalities
  - Genitourinary and renal abnormalities
  - Polydactyly
  - Cleft lip and palate
- Mean survival is ~7 days.

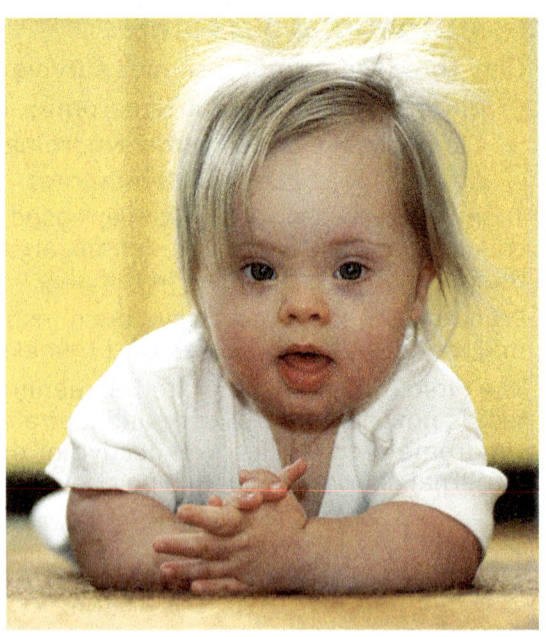

> **Important Concept**
>
> Why are trisomies of chromosomes 13, 18, and 21 the only ones to survive gestation? These chromosomes have the fewest number of genes and result in less *imbalance* than trisomy for any other autosome. Monosomic embryos miscarry earlier than trisomic embryos and fetuses, implying that nature is more tolerant of excess genetic information than insufficient information.

6.2 Aneuploidy of the Sex Chromosomes

- Aneuploidy of the sex chromosomes results in distinct phenotypes (Figures 2-6.2A and 2-6.2B).
- Klinefelter syndrome (47,XXY karyotype) is seen in ~1:500 males
  - Cases present with hypogonadism and female secondary sex characteristics, including gynecomastia and hair distribution.
  - May also show mild intellectual disability, which is also seen in individuals with 47,XXX or 47,XYY karyotypes.

▲ Figure 2-6.2A Klinefelter Syndrome

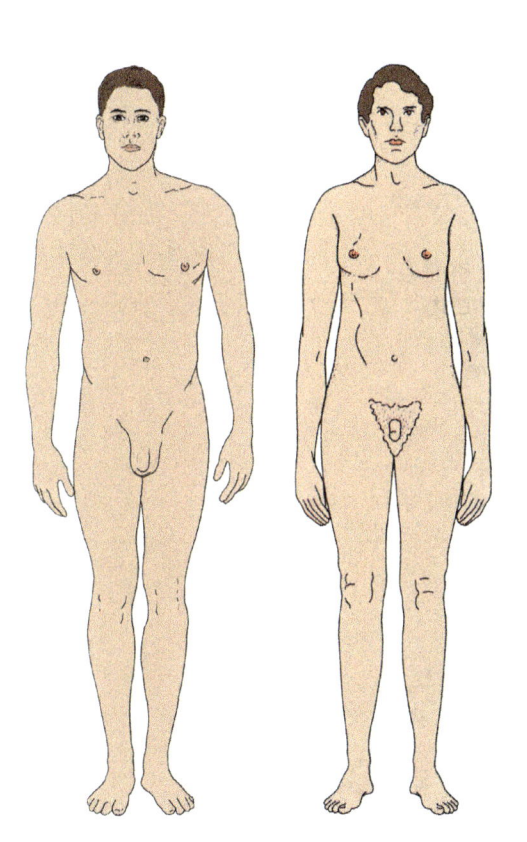

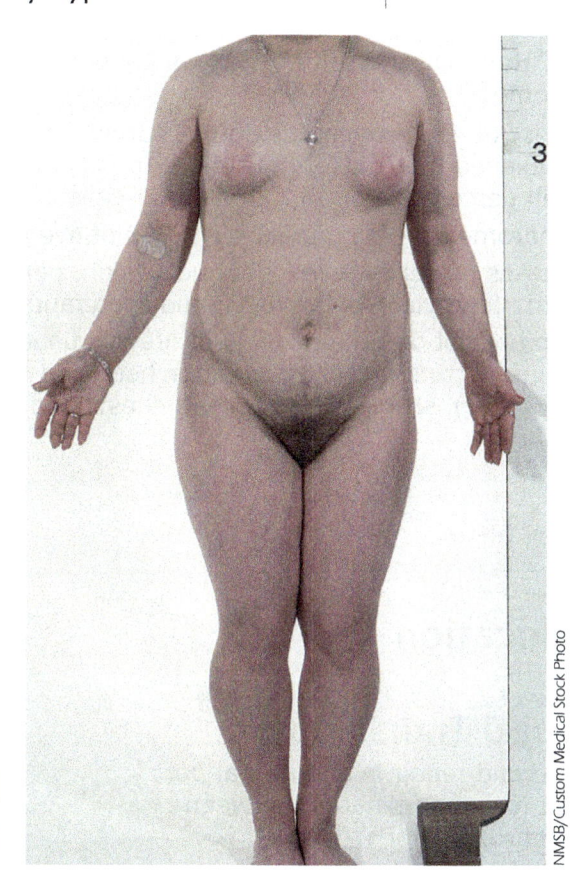

▲ Figure 2-6.2B Turner Syndrome

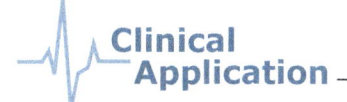

Clinical Application

Nondisjunction of Sex Chromosomes

Analysis of the potential consequences of nondisjunction of the sex chromosomes (see Table 2-6.2 on next page) reinforces understanding of differences between meiosis I and II. Because segregation of homologous chromosomes takes place in meiosis I (and the X and Y chromosomes act as homologues during meiosis), nondisjunction in paternal meiosis I can only result in 47,XXY in the offspring. Conversely, 47,XYY has to be the result of paternal meiosis II nondisjunction because the outcome requires the presence of two Y chromosomes in a single sperm.

Table 2-6.2 Nondisjunction of Sex Chromosomes

Nondisjunction During	Possible Outcomes	Impossible Outcomes
Maternal meiosis I	XXX or XXY	XYY
Maternal meiosis II	XXX or XXY	XYY
Paternal meiosis I	XXY	XYY or XXX
Paternal meiosis II	XYY or XXX	XXY

- Monosomy of the X chromosome (45,X) is known as Turner syndrome:
  - The majority of 45,X conceptus do not survive to term, and it is believed that those that do are mosaic, possessing some small percentage of 46,XX or 46,XY cells.
  - Turner syndrome cases comprise ~1:2,000 of live female births.
  - Newborn cases present with excess nuchal skin, peripheral lymphedema (especially of the feet), and coarctation of the aorta.
  - Those who are not diagnosed early in life will usually present with mild intellectual disability, amenorrhea (and no other signs of puberty), short stature, broad chest, and multiple pigmented nevi.

7 Translocation

7.1 Reciprocal Translocation

- DNA cleavage and repair is an integral part of prophase I for recombination between homologous chromosomes.
- If two pairs of chromosomes are undergoing recombination in close proximity at the same time, exchange may take place between nonhomologous chromosomes, resulting in the reciprocal translocation of genetic information.
  - A typical description might be 46,XY,t(4:16)(q13:q12), meaning "46 chromosomes, male, translocation (between chromosomes 4 and 16), (breakpoints on long arm band 1 sub-band 3 and long arm band 1 sub-band 2, respectively)."
- The continued alignment of homologous sequences results in the formation of a tetravalent (or cruciform) structure in the following metaphase (Figure 2-7.1).

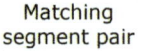

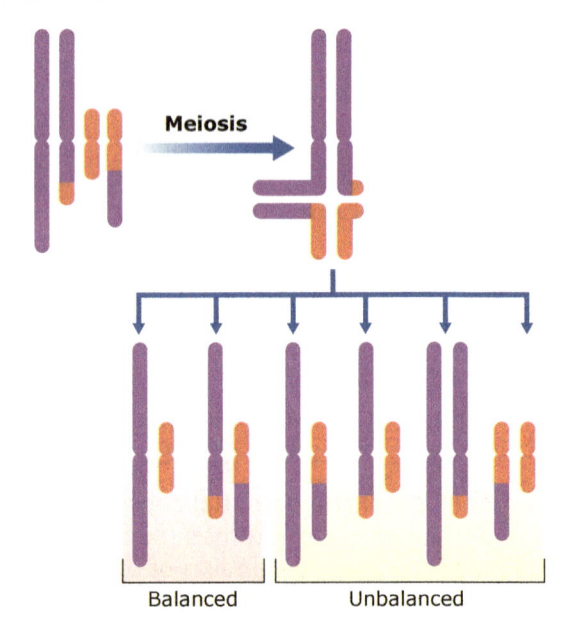

▲ Figure 2–7.1 Reciprocal Translocation

- Depending on the orientation of the tetravalent to the spindle, the chromosomes may segregate in one of three ways:
  - Only one of these (alternate segregation) results in balanced gametes with the genetic material in either the normal or reciprocal conformation.
  - The other outcomes (adjacent segregation) result in unbalanced chromosomal complements with partial disomy and partial nullisomy resulting in partial trisomy or monosomy if fertilized.
- The severity of the resulting phenotype depends on how many genes are trisomic or monosomic and their roles in development, ranging from early miscarriage to term birth with multiple congenital anomalies.
- If the chromosomal breakpoint is within, or close to, a gene, then any phenotype resulting from heterozygous loss of function of that gene will be observed in a balanced translocation carrier.

7.2 Robertsonian Translocation

- Reciprocal translocation involving the short arms of two nonhomologous acrocentric chromosomes is called a robertsonian translocation
- In this type of translocation, the material from the short arms is lost, but this is inconsequential because it codes for rRNA and there are multiples copies of these genes elsewhere in the genome.
  - Thus, a balanced carrier of a robertsonian translocation will have only 45 chromosomes but two copies of all protein-coding genes.
  - Once again, how the chromosomes segregate at meiosis will determine the outcome (Figure 2–7.2).

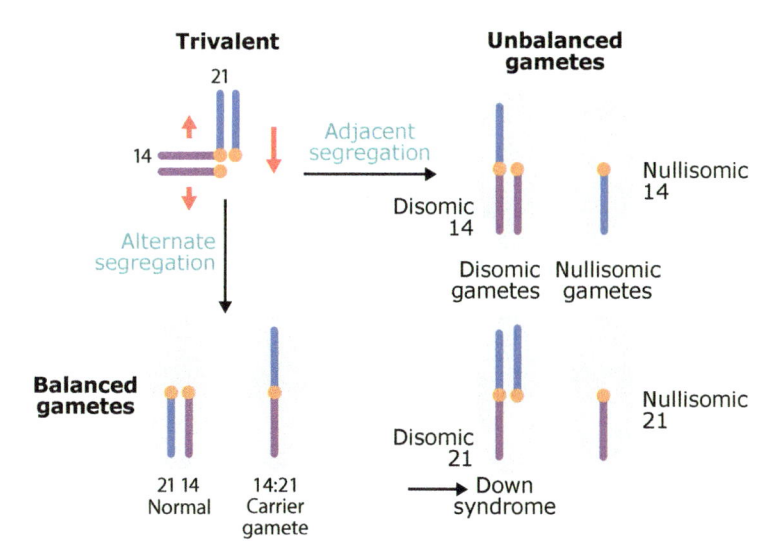

▲ Figure 2–7.2 Robertsonian Translocation

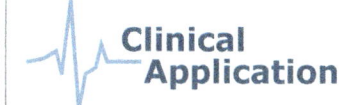

Clinical Application

Approximately 4% of cases of Down syndrome are the result of a robertsonian translocation involving chromosome 21. In a minority of these cases, one of the parents is a carrier of the translocation and is at risk of having further Down syndrome children. It is essential to obtain a karyotype in all cases of Down syndrome so that appropriate counseling can be offered.

Important Concept

Because ~50% of all protein-coding genes are expressed in the brain at some point in development, changes in copy number for more than one or two genes will almost invariably result in some effect on brain development. Thus, almost all children with unbalanced translocations or inversions show some degree of intellectual disability.

8 Inversions and Deletions

- If two breaks occur on the same chromosome, different outcomes are possible depending on the location of the breaks:
  - Two breaks on the same chromosomal arm result in either an interstitial deletion or a paracentric inversion.
  - One break on each arm can result in either a ring chromosome or a pericentric inversion.
- Ring chromosomes are usually seen in a mosaic state, as they do not segregate faithfully at mitosis.
- Interstitial deletions will result in a phenotype determined by the number and nature of deleted genes.
- Pericentric and paracentric inversions segregate differently in meiosis (Figure 2–8.0) and result in chromosomes that are:
  - Partially deleted
  - Partially duplicated
  - Normal and inverted (pericentric)
  - Normal, inverted, dicentric, and acentric (paracentric)

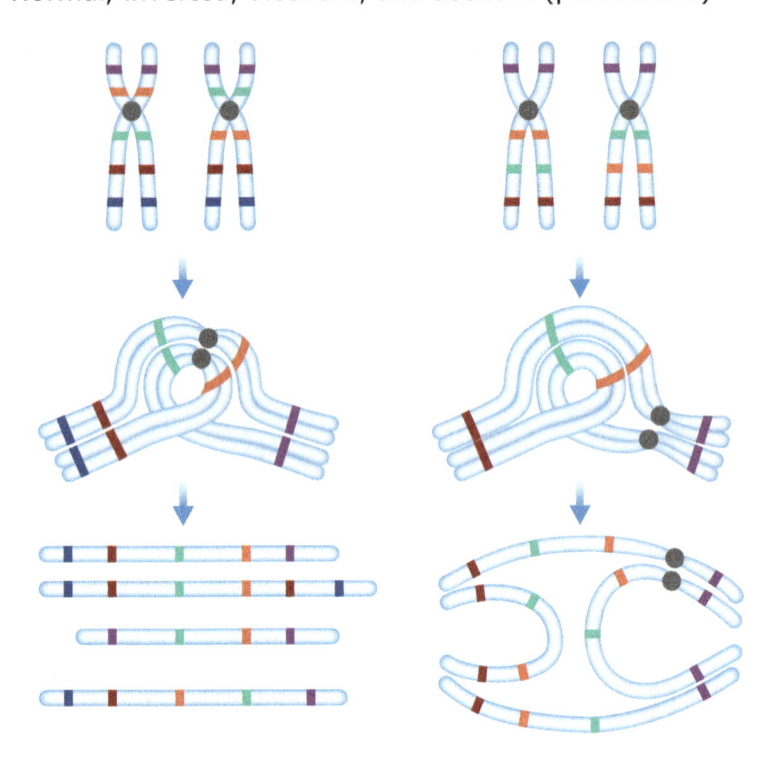

▲ Figure 2–8.0 Pericentric *(left)* and Paracentric *(right)* Inversions

CHAPTER 3 Mutations and Disease

1 Overview

- Any change in DNA sequence that affects the ability to express a gene, or affects the stability or function of its product, can potentially result in disease (Table 3-1.0).

Table 3-1.0 Consequences of DNA Mutation

Change in DNA	Possible Consequence	Disorder (Gene)
Single nucleotide substitution	Silent	Third nucleotide of codon
	Missense	• Achondroplasia (p.G380R in *FGFR*) • Sickle cell disease (p.E6V in *HBB*)
	Nonsense	Cystic fibrosis (p.G542X in *CFTR*)
	Splice	Cystic fibrosis (c.621+1G>T in *CFTR*)
Insertion/deletion	Frameshift	Tay-Sachs disease (c.1274_1277dupTATC in *HEXA*)
	Repeat expansion	• Fragile X syndrome • Huntington disease
Unequal cross-over	Deletion	• Williams-Beuren syndrome (WBS, Williams syndrome) • 22q11 deletion syndrome • α-thalassemia • Angelman syndrome • Prader-Willi syndrome
	Duplication	Williams-Beuren region duplication syndrome
	Gene conversion	Congenital adrenal hyperplasia (*CYP21B*)

USMLE® Key Concepts

For Step 1, you must be able to:

- Differentiate gain of function and loss of function mutations.
- Describe the residual activity of mutations.
- Explain the expansion and contraction of repeat sequences.

Connection to Biochemistry

Mutations are discussed in *Biochemistry*, Chapter 17.

Chapter 3 • Mutations and Disease

1.1 Types of Mutations

- Based on their effect on the structure of the genetic sequence, mutations can be generally classified into the following categories:
    - **Single-nucleotide substitutions (point mutations):**
        - Most prevalent mutations
        - Humans differ from each other at about 1 base per 1,000 (single nucleotide polymorphisms or SNPs), but only a fraction of these 6 million variants predispose to, much less cause, disease
    - **Insertion/deletion (indel) mutations:** Tend to arise in regions of repetitive sequence.
    - **Unequal crossover:** Larger (often megabase) deletions and duplications that arise as a consequence of misalignment between repeat sequences during meiosis.
- Whether a mutation results in a recessive or dominant phenotype is a feature of the gene and its product; however, the type of mutation observed may be predictive:
    - Mutations in genes encoding enzymes and transporters tend to result in recessive phenotypes (e.g., PKU, CF; exception—most porphyria).
    - Mutations in genes encoding transcription factors, signaling molecules, and structural proteins tend to result in dominant phenotypes (e.g., Waardenburg syndrome, Marfan syndrome, osteogenesis imperfecta).
    - Recessive phenotypes are almost invariably due to loss of function mutations—that is, any change that prevents synthesis of gene product or its function (nonsense, frameshift, many splice mutations, deletions and some missense mutations).
    - Dominant phenotypes may be due to loss or gain of function depending on the gene and the mutation.

Connection to Pathology

- Mutations in oncogenes are always gain of function.
- Mutations in tumor suppressor genes are always loss of function.

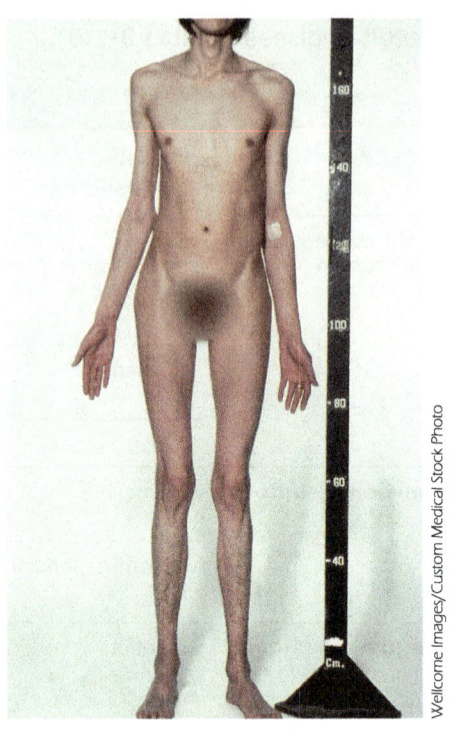

Classic musculoskeletal presentation of Marfan syndrome with long limbs (dolichostenomelia) and digits (arachnodactyly). Marfan syndrome results from heterozygous loss of function mutation in the fibrillin 1 gene (*FBN1*).

▲ Figure 3–1.1A Marfan Syndrome

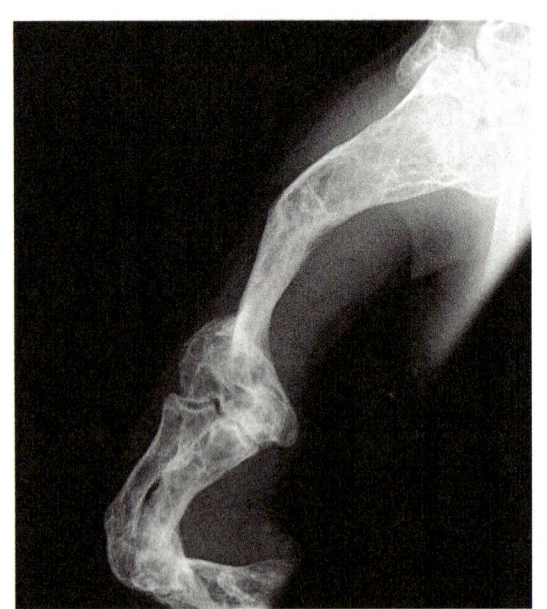

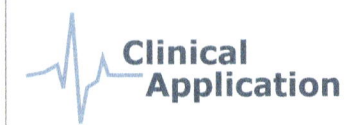

Bone deformity in OI type III due to multiple in utero fractures.

▲ Figure 3–1.1B Osteogenesis Imperfecta

Clinical Application

Achondroplasia is one of a series of skeletal dysplasias that result from missense mutations in fibroblast growth factor receptor 3 (*FGFR3*).

1.2 Dominant Phenotypes
- Dominant phenotypes result from one of three mutational mechanisms: haploinsufficiency, gain of function, and dominant-negative.

1.2.1 Haploinsufficiency
- "Half is not enough."
- Most common type of mutational mechanism for dominant phenotype.
- Means by which loss of function mutations result in a dominant phenotype.
- If a null mutation is seen in a case of a dominant phenotype, then any missense mutation causing the same phenotype must be loss of function.

1.2.2 Gain of Function
- Mutations tend to be specific and different mutations in the same gene may result in different phenotypes (e.g., *FGFR3*).
  - With *FGFR3* different mutations result in degrees of constitutive activation of the receptor and thus affect bone growth to different extents.
- Mutant protein must be made so mutations are most often missense and never null.

1.2.3 Dominant-Negative
- Represent a special class wherein the mutant gene product interferes with the function of the normal gene from the other allele, resulting in a greater effect than if mutant product had not been synthesized at all.
- Mutant protein must be made so mutations are most often missense and never null.
- Collagen mutations in osteogenesis imperfecta (OI) are a classic example.

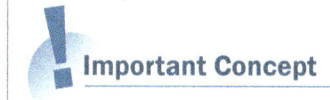

> **Important Concept**
>
> Mutations preventing synthesis of gene product are said to be null mutations.

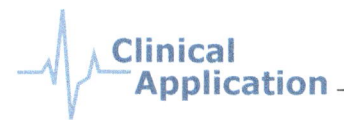

Clinical Application

Osteogenesis Imperfecta (OI)
- OI type I (mild) is the result of heterozygosity for a null mutation, which results in production of only 50% of normal type I collagen.
- More severe forms—OI type II (lethal) and OI type III (deforming)—result from heterozygosity for missense mutations, which replace glycine residues in the helical region of the collagen molecules.
- Mutant gene product interacts with gene product from the normal allele, which results in the production of only 25% of normal collagen and a more severe phenotype.
- Thus, OI type I is the result of haploinsufficiency, and types II and III are the result of dominant-negative mutations in either of the type I collagen genes—*COL1A1* or *COL1A2*.

Figure 3-1.2 Mutation Mechanism Algorithm

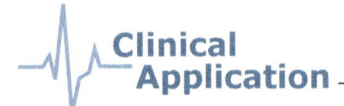

```
                    Mode of inheritance?
                   /                    \
              Recessive              Dominant
                 |                       |
         Loss of function        Null alleles observed?
           mutations              /              \
                                Yes              No
                                 |                |
                        Haploinsufficiency   Do different missense
                                             mutations yield
                                             distinct phenotypes?
                                              /            \
                                             No            Yes
                                             |              |
                                     Dominant-negative  Gain of function
```

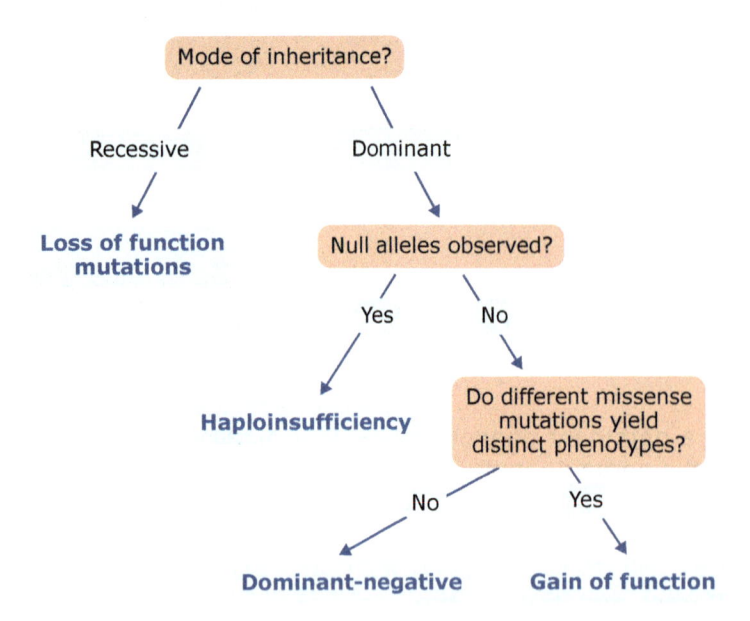

Consideration of the mode of inheritance and the nature of mutations observed allows determination of the underlying mechanism.

Important Concept

Nonsense mutations introducing termination codons prior to the last exon result in significant degradation of mutant transcript via a process called nonsense-mediated mRNA (messenger ribonucleic acid) decay, and thus DO NOT yield truncated polypeptides. This limits the number of examples of dominant-negative mutation.

Clinical Application

Determination of mutational mechanism may be important in the choice of therapeutic intervention—does an absent protein need to be replaced or should the function of a mutant protein be controlled?

2 Residual Activity

- Different mutations in a single gene may have different effects on the resulting phenotype, depending on how much gene product is synthesized and/or how much function is retained:
  - Recessive phenotypes may be less severe when one or both mutations retain some function/activity (e.g., mild hemophilia A is associated with missense mutations; severe hemophilia is due to an intragenic inversion or other null mutation).

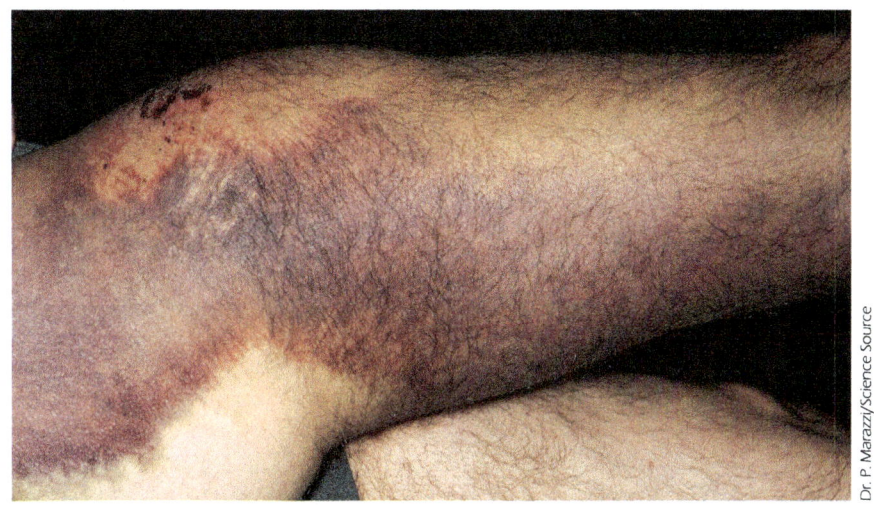

Severe hematoma following minimal trauma in a patient with hemophilia.

▲ Figure 3-2.0 Hemophilia

- Different missense mutations may have different effects depending on the location and nature of the substitution (e.g., substitution in the active site of an enzyme will have a greater effect than one elsewhere, and substitution with a more similar amino acid will have less of an effect).
- The effects of both alleles must be considered to estimate the severity of a recessive phenotype. Because heterozygotes are clinically unaffected, a combination of alleles providing close to 50% function will likely result in a milder phenotype than seen for alleles providing 30% function.

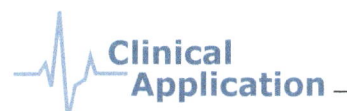

Clinical Application

Most cases of both Duchenne and Becker muscular dystrophy (DMD and BMD) are the result of deletion of multiple consecutive exons in the dystrophin gene. BMD is milder because the total loss of coding sequence is a multiple of three nucleotides in length, thus retaining the reading frame and allowing synthesis of a truncated protein with residual function.

! Important Concept

An individual with a recessive phenotype, who inherited different mutant alleles from each parent, is said to be a compound heterozygote. These individuals represent the majority of recessive phenotypes. Examples such as sickle cell disease, where all affected individuals are homozygous for the same mutation, are an exception. Most single gene disorders thus exhibit allelic heterogeneity—different mutations of the same gene that result in the same phenotype. If the same phenotype can result from mutations in different genes (e.g. deafness, spherocytosis), the mutation is said to exhibit locus heterogeneity.

Promoter/Enhancer Mutations

- Mutation of the proximal promoter drastically reduces the amount of transcript (e.g., TATA-box mutation in β-thalassemia).
- Enhancer mutations exert tissue-type or cell-type specific effects due to the tissue-specific nature of enhancer function.
- Single-nucleotide substitutions may increase or reduce the efficiency of transcription factor binding.
- Chromosomal rearrangements such as translocations or inversions may separate an enhancer from its target gene, thus affecting expression in some cells and not in others.

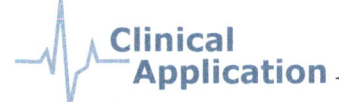

Clinical Application

One of the mutations for blue eye color is in an enhancer of the *OCA2* gene, which affects pigment deposition only in the eye and not in hair or skin.

Connection to Biochemistry

The roles of proximal promoter elements and enhancers are discussed in *Biochemistry*, Chapter 16.

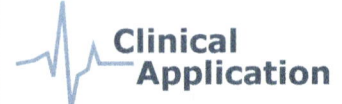

Clinical Application

Heterozygosity for mutation in an enhancer for the *SHH* (sonic hedgehog) gene is seen in some cases of polydactyly, whereas a mutation in the coding region causes holoprosencephaly.

4 Contiguous Gene Syndromes

- Changes in DNA that affect multiple genes are often the cause of complicated phenotypes.
- Mutations can occur at the chromosomal level (e.g., translocations and inversions) or via the process of unequal cross-over during meiosis.
- Where a gene, or group of genes, is flanked by direct repeat sequence, it is possible that the nonhomologous repeats could align during meiosis, resulting in chromosomes deleted or duplicated for the region (Figure 3–4.0):
  - Should one of these chromosomes be in the gamete forming a zygote, then the zygote will have one or three copies of the gene(s) between the repeats.
  - The resulting phenotype will be determined by which genes are duplicated or deleted.

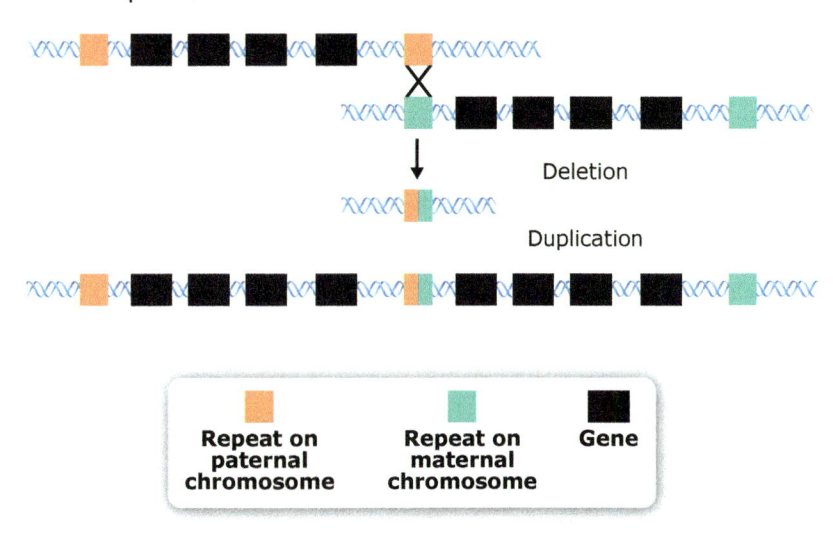

▲ Figure 3–4.0 Alignment of Nonhomologous Repeats

- The presence of repeat sequences flanking groups of genes means that these events can recur much more often than a random translocation or inversion.
- The resulting phenotypes are recognized as particular syndromes (see Table 3-1.0 on page 3–1).

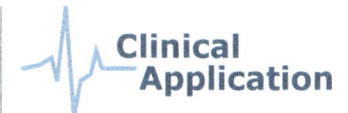

Clinical Application

- The tandem duplication of the α-globin genes on chromosome 16 results in many α-thalassemia alleles being the result of gene deletion events.
- Misalignment between a functional gene and a neighboring pseudogene can result in deletion or gene conversion, in which DNA repair interrupts recombination and mutant sequence is copied from the pseudogene into the functional gene, preventing synthesis of normal product. This unusual phenomenon is seen in congenital adrenal hyperplasia and spinal muscular atrophy.

Chapter 3 • Mutations and Disease

5 Dynamic Mutations and Anticipation

- Once a mutation has occurred in DNA, it tends to be stable over many generations.
- An important exception is encountered with the expansion or contraction of simple repeat sequences.
- Expansion or contraction can occur over successive generations, in which case the mutation is said to be a *dynamic mutation*.
  - If the expanding or contracting repeat is within or close to a gene, then any effect on gene function may change with the size of the repeat.
  - Consequently, the severity of any resulting phenotype may change.
- The observation that a phenotype can become more severe in successive generations (with symptoms becoming apparent at an earlier age) is termed *anticipation* (Figure 3–5.0A)— a phenomenon that is now known to be due to the expansion of repeat sequences within particular genes (Table 3-5.0).

Table 3-5.0	Phenotypes for Expansion of Repeat Sequences					
Phenotype	Friedreich Ataxia	Fragile X Syndrome	FXTAS[2]	Huntington Disease	Myotonic Dystrophy
Inheritance	AR	XD	X-linked	AD	AD
Gene product	Frataxin	FMRP[1]	FMRP	Huntingtin	DMPK[3]
Position of repeat	Intron	5' UTR[4]	5' UTR	Exon 1	3' UTR
Repeat	GAA	CGG	CGG	CAG	CTG
Normal range	5–33	5–54	5–54	≤35	5–34
Pathogenic range	66–~1700	>200	55–200	≥36	>50
Germline expansion	Maternal?	Maternal	Maternal	Paternal	Maternal
Mechanism	Loss of function	Loss of function	Gain of function (RNA)	Gain of function (protein)	Gain of function (RNA)

[1] Fragile X mental retardation protein
[2] Fragile X tremor-ataxia syndrome
[3] Dystrophia myotonica-protein kinase
[4] Untranslated region

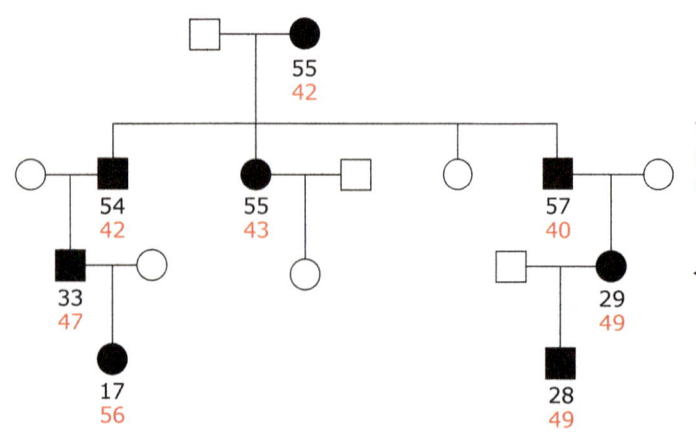

The age of onset in each affected person is in black; the number of CAG repeat units (repeated trinucleotide sequence) in the mutant allele is in red.

◀ **Figure 3–5.0A** Anticipation in a Pedigree Segregating Huntington Disease

- The following features of dynamic mutation phenotypes should be noted:
  - Because Friedreich ataxia shows recessive inheritance anticipation is not observed.
  - When the CGG repeat in the *FMR1* gene exceeds 200 units, it becomes hypermethylated, which prevents transcription.
  - The FMR1 premutation (55–200 repeats) stabilizes mutant transcripts, but limits translation, resulting in the late-onset FXTAS phenotype in normal transmitting males (NTM; Figure 3–5.0B).
  - CAG expansion occurs in the paternal germline; others occur in the maternal germline.
  - Expansion in the 3' UTR of DMPK transcripts results in formation of a stem-loop structure that attracts RNA binding proteins preventing them from splicing, and otherwise regulating, other transcripts.

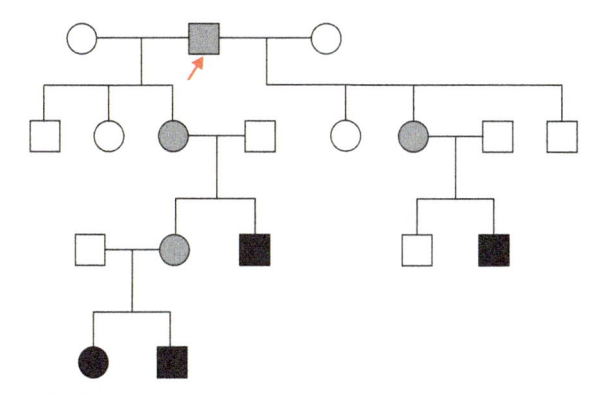

Individuals with Fragile X syndrome are shown by black symbols and will have > 200 CGG repeats. Individuals who MUST have a premutation (55–200 repeats are cross-hatched. Note that despite the mutation being X-linked, the common ancestor (indicated by arrow is male.

▲ **Figure 3–5.0B** Fragile X Syndrome Pedigree

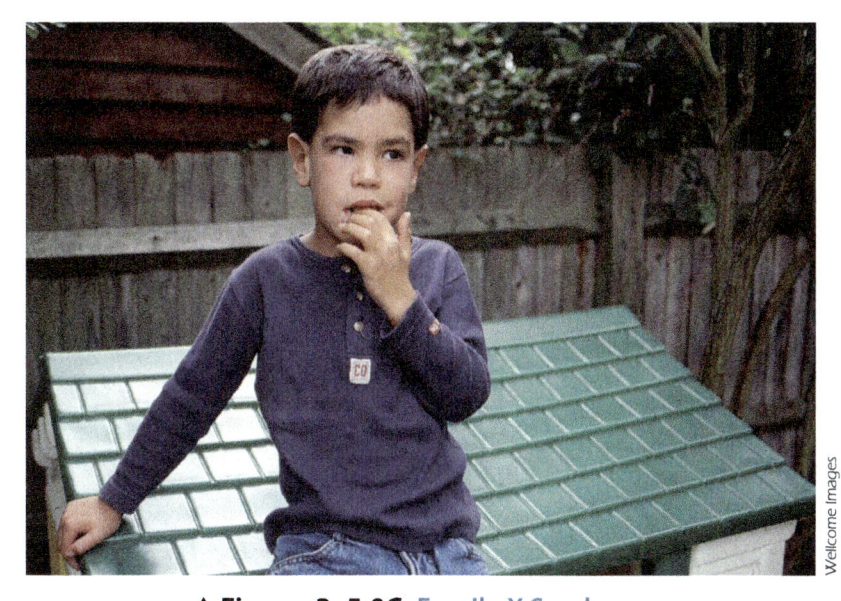

▲ **Figure 3–5.0C** Fragile X Syndrome

CHAPTER 4: X-Inactivation and Epigenetics

1 Overview

- The mechanism(s) by which gene expression is regulated can be as important as DNA sequence in determining the outcome of developmental processes.
- Geneticists originally coined the term epigenetics to describe matters outside of conventional genetics, but the term is now taken to mean changes to DNA that DO NOT change the genetic sequence, but affect gene expression.
- Epigenetic effects are mediated primarily via methylation.
- The role of epigenetics in the etiology of disease is becoming progressively clearer, but the two main examples remain X-inactivation (to accomplish dosage compensation) and parent of origin effects (because a minority of autosomal genes must only be expressed from one allele).

USMLE® Key Concepts

For Step 1, you must be able to:

- Describe random X-inactivation.
- Explain the consequences of selection after X-inactivation in heterozygotes.
- Describe the basis of parent of origin effects.
- Explain the mechanism and consequences of uniparental disomy.

Looking Back

DNA methylation is described in *Biochemistry*, Chapter 3.

2. Dosage Compensation

- Because the products of ~900 genes on the X chromosome have to interact with those encoded by autosomal genes, and most cellular processes are identical in males and females, there must be a means of adjusting for the presence of two X chromosomes in females and one in males.
- Dosage compensation is accomplished by inactivation of one of the two X chromosomes.
- X-inactivation is RANDOM. Either the maternal or paternal X chromosome is randomly inactivated at the late blastocyst stage in female development.
- The pattern of inactivation is clonal. Once inactivation occurs, all daughter cells will show the same pattern of inactivation (Figure 4–2.0). The inactivated X is imprinted and the imprint is passed from one cell generation to the next via methylation.

Important Concept

There is no 5-methyl-dCTP in the cell to be incorporated during replication. The pattern of methylation is maintained through successive cell generations by a DNA methylase, which recognizes 5-methylcytosine on the template strand and methylates the corresponding cytosine on the newly synthesized strand. Recall that methylation occurs at CpG dinucleotides.

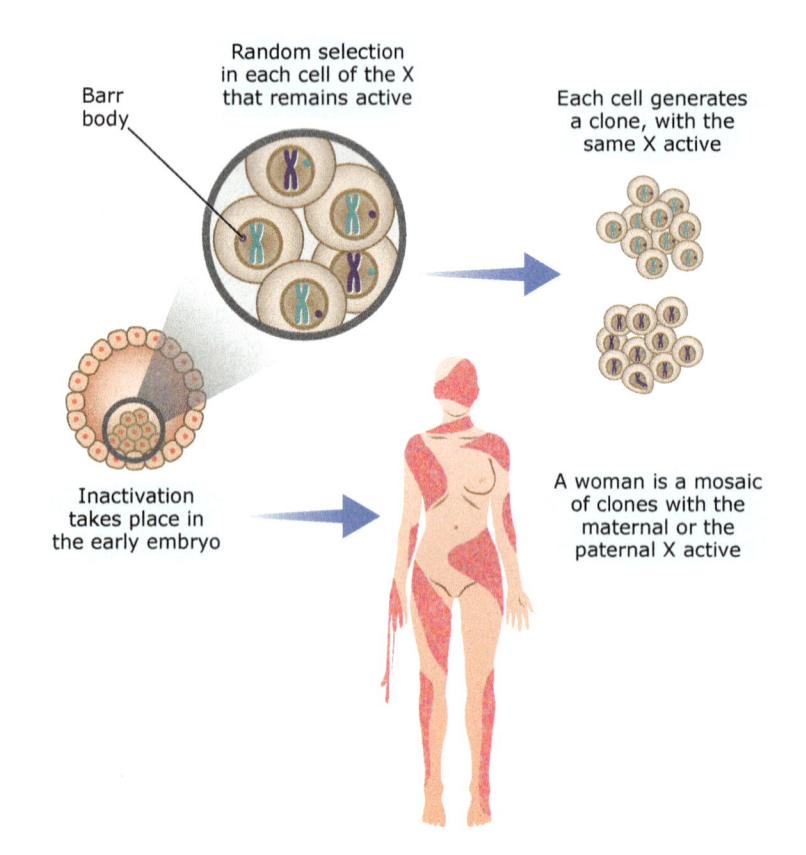

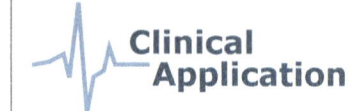

▲ **Figure 4–2.0** Random X Inactivation Results in Mosaic Females

- All females are mosaic with two distinct cell populations—one with the paternal X inactivated, the other with the maternal X inactivated.
- The pseudoautosomal region (PAR) at the tip of the short arm escapes inactivation because the genes in this region are also present on the Y chromosome and all humans have two copies. All other genes on the Y chromosome are involved in male sexual differentiation and spermatogenesis.

Clinical Application

- Deamination of 5-methylcytosine results in C → T transition mutations.
- CpG dinucleotides represent mutation hotspots in the genome.
- Many recurrent point mutations are at CpG dinucleotides (e.g., p.G380R in *FGFR3* is spontaneous in ~80% of achondroplasia cases).

Mechanism of X Inactivation

- During oogenesis, the previously inactive X is reactivated so that all eggs have one active X. In spermatogenesis, the X is temporarily inactivated and then reactivated. Thus, in a female zygote, both X chromosomes are active.
- At the late blastocyst stage, the *XIST* gene is transcribed from both X chromosomes to yield an mRNA (messenger ribonucleic acid) that remains in the nucleus and does not code for protein.
- One of the two X chromosomes becomes coated with XIST transcript and is methylated. It then undergoes histone deacetylation and thus becomes heterochromatin, which is the inactive X (X_i).
- On the other X chromosome, an autosomal-encoded protein (believed to be synthesized at levels to bind only one X chromosome) blocks the spread of XIST. This chromosome is the active X (X_a). This model explains the number of Barr bodies (X_i) in human cells—one fewer than the number of X chromosomes no matter how many X chromosomes are present.

"Nonrandom" or "Skewed" Inactivation

- X inactivation is always random. Variation around an expected mean of 50:50 paternal:maternal inactivation, to as much as 30:70 or 70:30, is normal.
- Deviation outside of the normal range is the result of selection against cells with a mutant allele on X_a.
- Examples of selection and the relevant explanation are provided in Table 4-4.0.

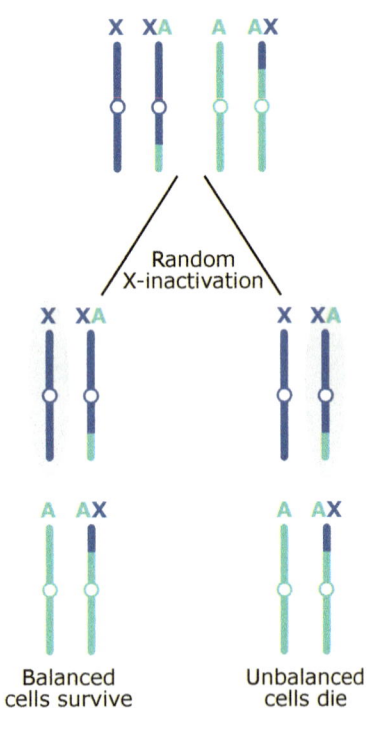

Random X-inactivation gives two populations of cells. Cells with the non-translocated X inactivated have balanced gene expression and have a selective advantage for proliferation during embryogenesis.

▲ Figure 4–4.0 X-Autosome Translocation

Table 4-4.0	"Nonrandom" Inactivation	
Example	Observation in Adult Cells	Explanation
X-autosome translocation	The non-translocated X is ALWAYS inactivated.	Imbalance of X and autosomal genes occurs in cells where the translocated X is inactive (Figure 4–4.0).
α-thalassemia with mental retardation, X-linked (ATRX)	> 90% of cells have mutation on X_i.	Selection against cells with mutation on X_a during development since gene product is required for normal genome-wide expression.
X-linked severe combined immune deficiency (X-SCID)	Almost all white blood cells have mutation on X_i. 50:50 in other cells.	Selection against cells with mutation on X_a during development since gene product required for differentiation. No selection occurs in cells where gene is not expressed.
Hemophilia	Mutation on X_i in ~50% of cells.	Presence/absence of gene product has no bearing on cell survival.

5 Parent of Origin Effects

- Over 100 autosomal genes are expressed from only one, not both, alleles in one or more cell types. The allele that is not expressed is methylated and is said to be imprinted.
- These genes are not distributed randomly in the genome, so their expression is coordinately regulated.
- All imprints are removed during gametogenesis and a new imprint specific to that germline (maternal or paternal) is applied (Figure 4–5.0A).

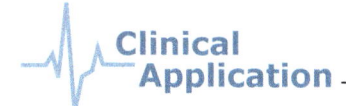

Clinical Application

Methylation and Disease

- Methylation across the genome increases during development as the cells become more specialized and express a smaller subset of genes.
- Aberrations in methylation result in abnormal gene expression and hence disease.
- Inappropriate methylation of an allele would have the same effect as a loss of function mutation.
- A loss of methylation would result in over-expression and be the equivalent of a gain of function mutation.
- Changes in methylation are important markers in tumor progression. Loss of methylation of oncogenes and excessive methylation of tumor suppressor genes both favor rapid cell growth and division.

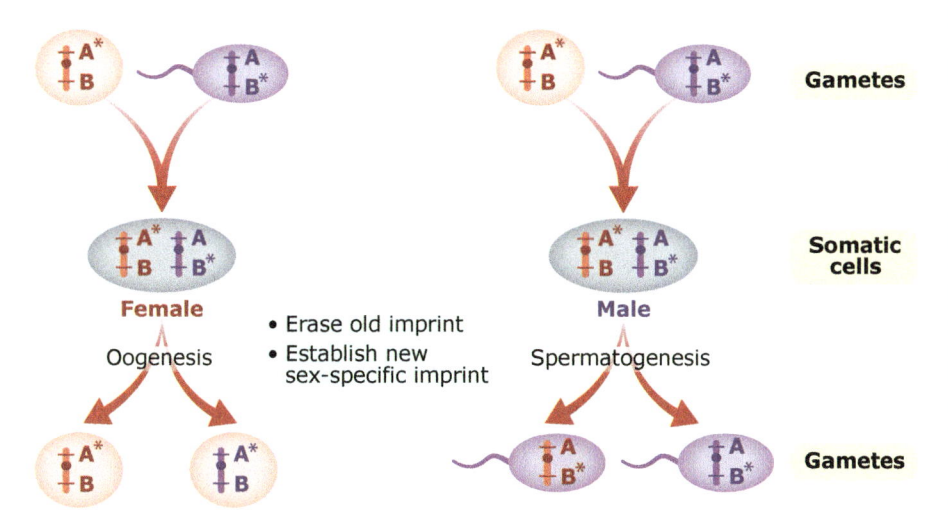

Parent of origin imprints are reapplied each time a chromosome passes through gametogenesis. Imprinted alleles are marked with an asterisk (*).

▲ Figure 4–5.0A Parent of Origin Imprints and Gametogenesis

Chapter 4 • X-Inactivation and Epigenetics

- Mutations in imprinted genes lead to parent of origin effects. If, by chance, a particular chromosome happens to pass through the same germline for multiple generations (e.g., from mother to daughter to granddaughter), a mutation in a maternally imprinted gene on that chromosome would remain hidden since the normal paternal allele would be expressed (Figures 4–5.0B and 4–5.0C).
- The phenotype is only seen when the mutation is on the allele that should be expressed—regardless of whether the parent passing on the mutation was affected. At the DNA sequence level, all affected individuals are heterozygous.

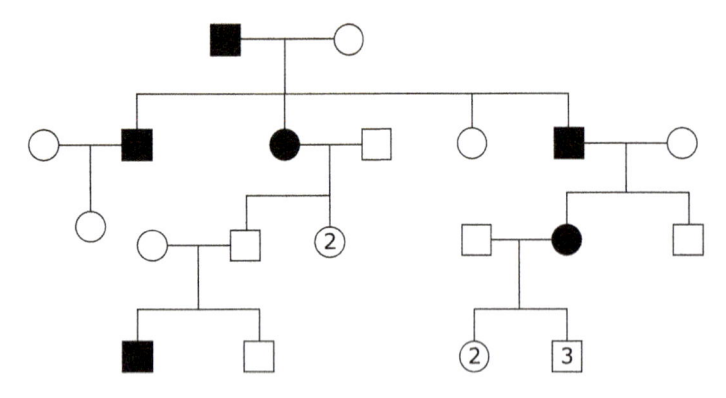

▲ **Figure 4–5.0B** Pedigree for Mutation in Maternally Imprinted, Paternally Expressed Gene

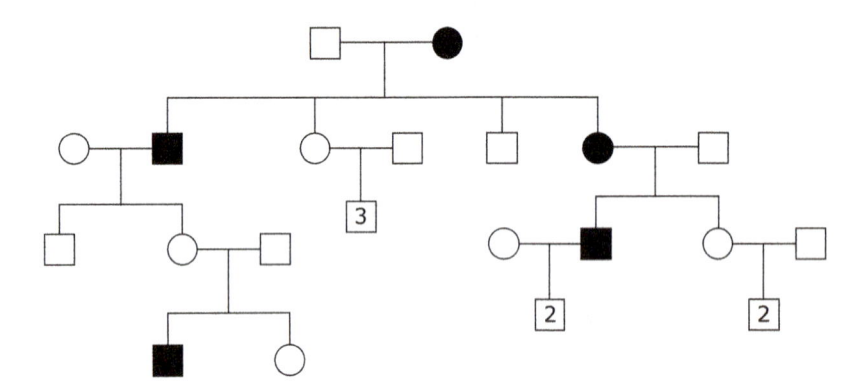

▲ **Figure 4–5.0C** Pedigree for Mutation in Paternally Imprinted, Maternally Expressed Gene

6 Uniparental Disomy

- The rare finding of both copies of an autosome being from the same parent is referred to as uniparental disomy (UPD).
- If any genes on a UPD chromosome are subject to imprinting, then UPD will result in the same phenotype as the mutation of that gene on the opposite chromosome. Maternal UPD is the functional equivalent of a paternal mutation; paternal UPD is the equivalent of a maternal mutation.
- Most cases of UPD arise via a process termed trisomy rescue (Figure 4–6.0A). Nondisjunction in gametogenesis results in a disomic gamete and trisomic zygote. At an early mitotic division, one of the extra chromosomes is lost. The daughter cell with 46 chromosomes has a selective advantage over those with 45 or 47, and its descendants come to dominate the embryo.
  - There is a two thirds chance that the chromosome that is lost will be the "extra" one from the disomic gamete and there will be no evidence that anything abnormal had occurred.
  - In one third of cases, the chromosome from the normal gamete will be lost and the embryo will have UPD.

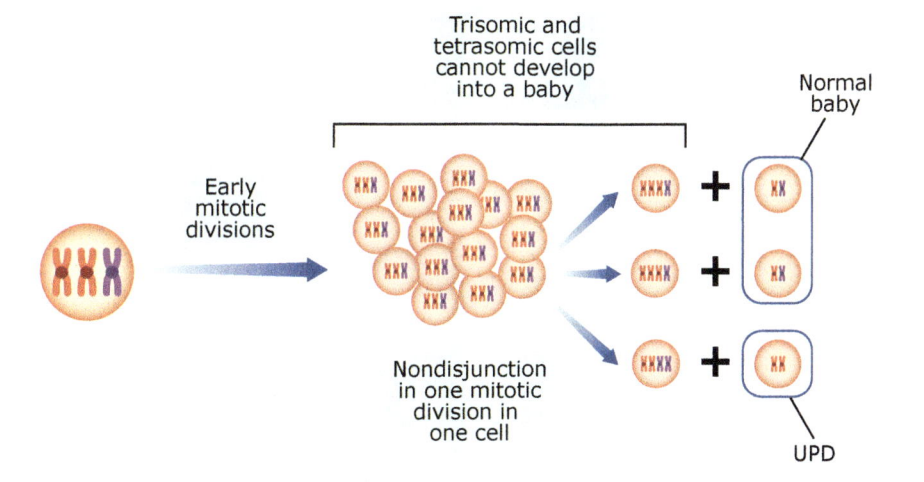

▲ Figure 4–6.0A Uniparental Disomy Follows From Trisomy Rescue

- When UPD follows from nondisjunction in meiosis I, it is termed heterodisomy (because the chromosomes are a homologous pair and are not identical).
- UPD following from nondisjunction in meiosis II is termed isodisomy because the chromosomes are identical. Because an individual with isodisomy is homozygous for all alleles on the chromosome, the individual may show a recessive phenotype for which the parent was a heterozygous carrier.
- If no genes on a UPD chromosome are methylated, there may be no clinical consequences.

Connection to Pathology

UPD for the entire genome results in the development of hydatidiform moles (46 paternal chromosomes) or ovarian teratomas (46 maternal chromosomes).

Looking Back

The different consequences of nondisjunction in meiosis I versus meiosis II, and what would follow for UPD, are discussed in Chapter 2.

Clinical Application

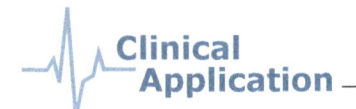

Prader–Willi Syndrome and Angelman Syndrome

- Because maternally and paternally expressed genes are grouped, different phenotypes may arise from mutation in a given region, depending on whether the mutation is on the maternal or paternal chromosome.
- The genes diagrammed in Figure 4–6.0B are located in a region of chromosome 15 that is sometimes deleted because it is flanked by repeat sequences which may misalign at meiosis (see Chapter 3).
- Some genes are expressed only from the paternal chromosome and others only from the maternal chromosome:
  - Deletion of this region from the paternal chromosome results in Prader-Willi syndrome (PWS).
  - Deletion of the region from the maternal chromosome results in Angelman syndrome (AS).

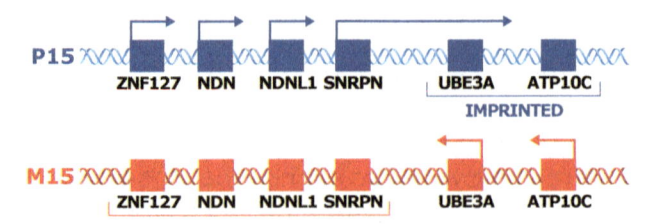

▲ Figure 4–6.0B Gene Cluster on Chromosome 15 Deleted in PWS and AS

- Infants with PWS are hypotonic. Later development is characterized by hyperphagia, obesity, and intellectual disability.
- Children with AS exhibit delayed developmental milestones, frequent laughter, ataxia, seizures, and severe intellectual disability with almost absent speech.
- Approximately 70% of cases of both PWS and AS are the result of *de novo* deletions on chromosome 15—confirmed by FISH analysis (Figure 4–6.0E).
- Over 25% of cases of PWS are due to maternal UPD.
  - Maternal UPD is the functional equivalent of a paternal deletion (no expression of the SNRPN cluster genes).
- ~3% of PWS and AS cases are due to imprinting errors.
- 5%–10% of AS cases are due to mutation of the maternal UBE3A gene.

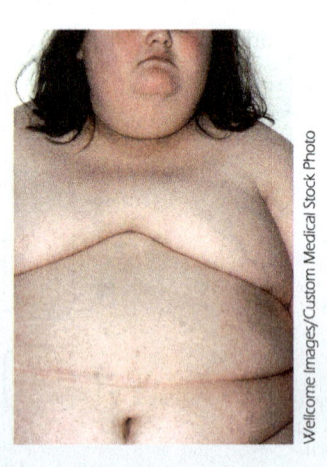

▲ Figure 4–6.0C Prader-Willi Syndrome

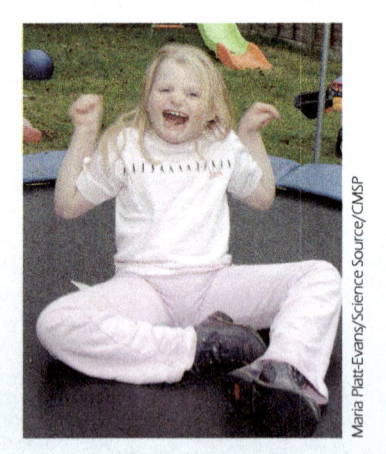

▲ Figure 4–6.0D Angelman Syndrome

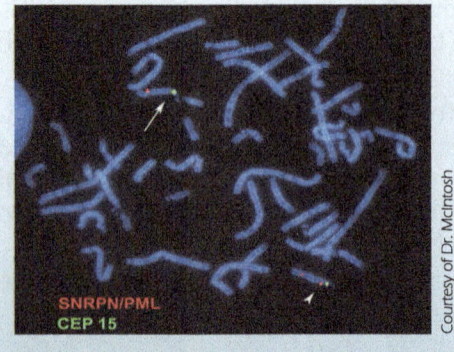

▲ Figure 4–6.0E FISH Showing Deletion on Chromosome 15 (*long arrow*) Versus Normal (*arrowhead*)

CHAPTER 5 — Genetic Testing and Gene Identification

1 Overview

- Analysis of DNA allows for:
  - Confirmation of diagnosis or discrimination between differential diagnoses.
  - Prediction of affected status including prenatal diagnosis using DNA from chorionic villus biopsy.
  - Identification of disease genes.
- Diagnosis may be direct or indirect:
  - Direct diagnosis—precise identification of the DNA mutation causing disease.
  - Indirect diagnosis—tracking of a mutant allele in a family using linkage without knowing the identity of the mutation.

> **USMLE® Key Concepts**
>
> For Step 1, you must be able to:
> - Interpret DNA sequencing and genotyping data.
> - Explain the methods used to identify disease genes.

2 Direct Testing

- **DNA sequencing:** Specifically identifies single nucleotide changes in DNA. In a heterozygote, DNA from both alleles is sequenced simultaneously and so the difference between the two alleles will result in two fragments of the same size in different reactions (Sanger method) or with different terminating dideoxy nucleotides (Figure 5–2.0A).

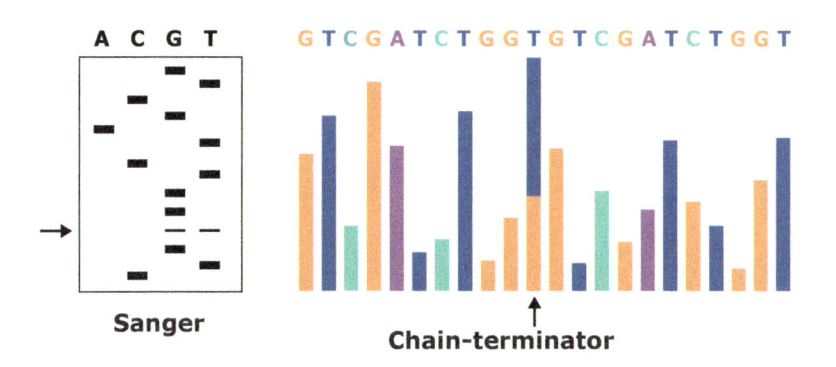

▲ Figure 5–2.0A Heterozygous Point Mutation: Sanger Method *(left)* and Chain-Terminator Sequencing *(right)*

> **Connection to Biochemistry**
>
> Molecular techniques, such as PCR and sequencing, are discussed in *Biochemistry*, Chapter 18.

- **Allele-specific oligonucleotides (ASOs):** Can be used to screen individuals for mutations that are common in a population:
  - The region in which the mutation is known to be (usually a particular exon) is amplified by polymerase chain reaction (PCR) and the product is hybridized separately with oligonucleotide probes specific for the mutant and normal alleles.
  - The specificity of DNA base-pairing allows discrimination between perfectly and imperfectly matched strands (Figure 5–2.0B).

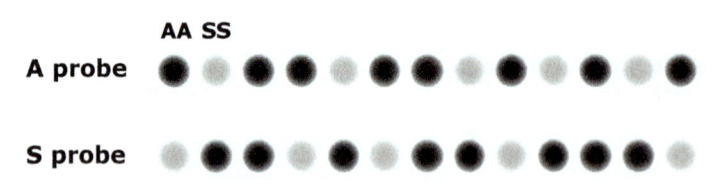

   AA SS
   A probe ● ● ● ● ● ● ● ● ● ● ● ●

   S probe ● ● ● ● ● ● ● ● ● ● ● ●

   A probe is complementary to the normal allele. The S probe is complementary to the mutant allele. AA and SS are homozygous controls.

   ▲ Figure 5–2.0B Specific Identification of the Sickle Cell Mutation in a Series of Samples

- **Fluorescence in situ hybridization (FISH):** May be used to confirm suspected deletions that cause contiguous gene deletion syndromes (see Figure 4–6.0E in Chapter 4).
- **Gel electrophoresis:** Can be used to discriminate between alleles when the mutation changes the size of a fragment:
  - Moderate expansions of triplet repeats (e.g., Huntington disease, Fragile X syndrome premutation) can be amplified by PCR separated by electrophoresis.
  - Larger expansions (e.g., Fragile X syndrome full mutation, myotonic dystrophy) and deletions of 1–30 kb require a combination of restriction enzyme digestion and Southern blot.

3 Indirect Testing

- In cases in which it is not practical to identify a precise mutation, it is possible to track the mutant allele in families using the principle of linkage. If a polymorphic marker and a gene are in close proximity, it is unlikely that the alleles at each will be rearranged by recombination.
- There are three main types of polymorphic markers:
  1. **Single nucleotide polymorphisms (SNPs):**
     - The most prevalent marker
     - More useful for genome-wide studies of multifactorial disorders
  2. **Restriction fragment length polymorphisms (RFLPs):**
     - A subset of SNPs in which the nucleotide change results in the gain or loss of a restriction site, thus changing the distance (fragment length) between two nonpolymorphic sites (Figure 5-3.0A)
     - Allows discrimination between the two alleles in a heterozygote and the establishment of linkage between the polymorphic marker and the phenotype (and the mutant allele)
     - The segregation of allele B with the phenotype is illustrated in the figure
     - The black bar in the upper portion of the figure presents the position of the probe used in the Southern blot

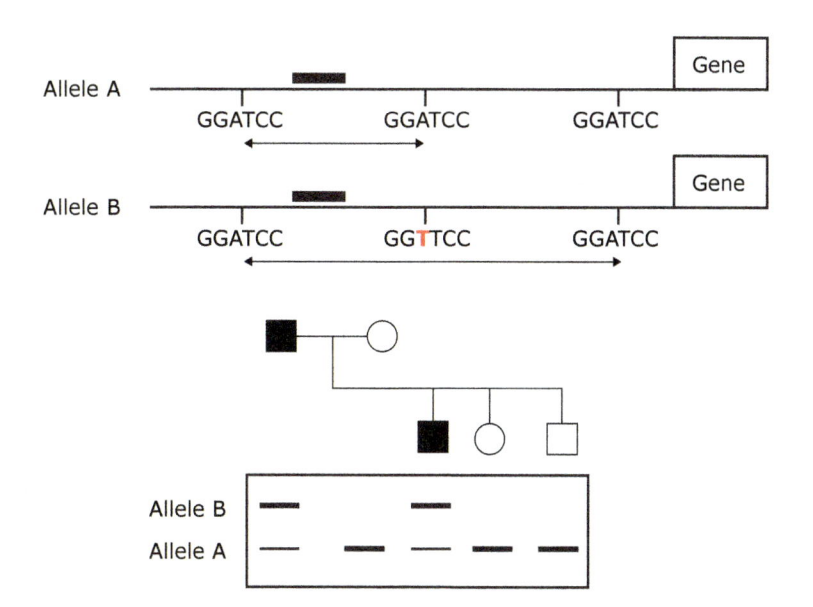

▲ **Figure 5-3.0A** Use of RFLP to Track a Mutant Allele

> **! Important Concept**
>
> Polymorphic variation in the genome is ancient. Over half of all sequence variation predates human migration from Africa. The oldest disease-causing mutations are no more than 2,000–4,000 years old. Almost all of those resulting in dominant phenotypes occurred in the past few generations.

3. Short tandem repeat polymorphisms (STRPs):

— Useful because the greater number of alleles generated by moderate repeat instability (Figure 5–3.0B) means that it is more likely that any one individual is heterozygous for the polymorphic marker—this characteristic makes STRPs informative in analysis.

— In Figure 5–3.0C, the smaller allele in the individual indicated by the arrow was inherited with the mutation from her mother. Individual III-1 is seen to be unaffected and inherited the other allele from his mother.

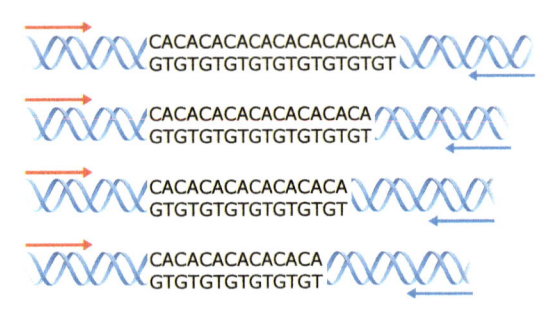

Position of PCR primers in flanking DNA indicated by arrows

▲ **Figure 5–3.0B** Variation in the Number of Repeats Generates Different-Size Alleles

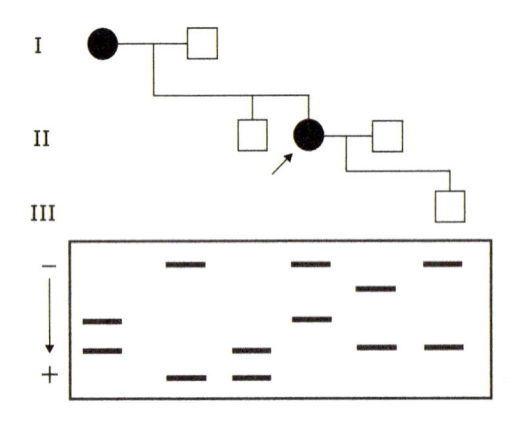

▲ **Figure 5–3.0C** Segregation of STRP Alleles With Normal and Mutant Gene Alleles

4 Gene Identification

- The genes mutated in single gene disorders can be identified utilizing one of four main methods (Table 5-4.0).

Table 5-4.0 Methods of Gene Identification

Method	Information Required	Example
Candidate gene analysis	Biological information	Hemoglobin genes
Positional cloning	Uses only genetic information—linkage and recombination	*CFTR*, dystrophin, huntingtin, thousands more
Breakpoint analysis	Genes disrupted by chromosomal translocations	*NSD1* (Sotos syndrome)
Exome sequencing	Uses only sequence information—no linkage, no biology	*MLL2* (Kabuki syndrome)

4.1 Candidate Gene Analysis

- In cases in which there is sufficient biological information, genes are identified by knowing the identity of the affected protein (e.g., globin genes for thalassemias).

4.2 Positional Cloning

- Identifies location of genes involved in disease using the power of linkage. Any two genes or markers (e.g., RFLPs or STRPs) that are seen to co-segregate through generations are more often than not linked.

- There is at least one recombination event per chromosome pair for each meiosis (Chapter 2). The closer together two genes or markers are, the less likely they are to be separated by recombination (Figures 5–4.2A and 5–4.2B).

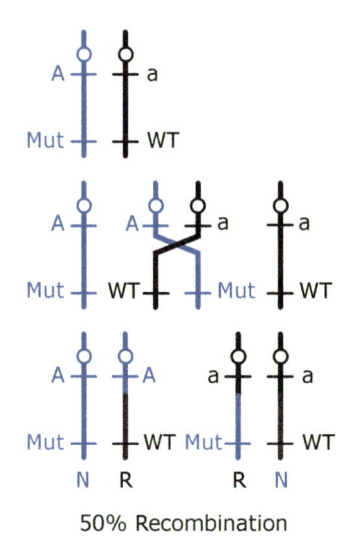

A marker and gene far apart on a chromosome will always show 50% recombination because there is enough space that a cross-over will always occur between them. Note that because two of the four chromatids are involved, two gametes are recombinant and two are not.

▲ Figure 5–4.2A 50% Recombination

- By comparing the outcomes of all meioses available for study (i.e., parents and children in families in which a phenotype is segregating), it is possible to estimate the distance between a gene and a marker. The number of recombination events identified out of the number of opportunities (meioses) expressed as a percentage is equal to the genetic distance (in centimorgans, cM) between two points on a chromosome. In Figure 5–4.2C, marker allele 2 appears to track with the phenotype and 2 of 10 meioses are seen to be recombinant (2/10 = 20% = 20 cM) having inherited allele 2, but not the phenotype. Across the genome, 1 cM equates to approximately 1 Mb, but there may be substantial variation.

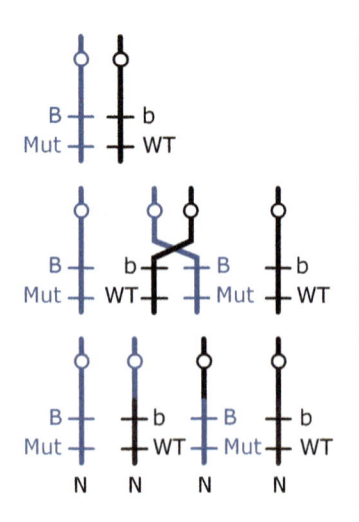

▲ **Figure 5–4.2B** No Recombination When Marker Is Close to Gene

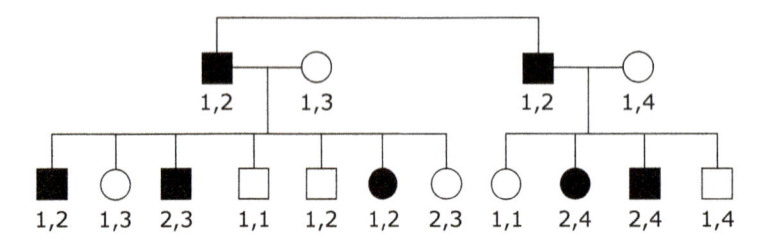

Identification of recombinant individuals provides an estimate of genetic distance between marker and disease locus.

▲ **Figure 5–4.2C** Linkage Analysis Using an STRP Marker

- These principles are utilized in linkage analysis to identify the region of the genome where a disease gene is likely located.
- In a typical study (Figure 5–4.2D), DNA from dozens of affected individuals and their first-degree relatives would be typed for ~400 STRP markers spread evenly across the genome.
- Analysis of this data (by computer) yields a log of odds (lod) score for each marker. This score serves as a measure of proximity to the disease gene:
  - An lod score ≥ 3 is interpreted as evidence in favor of linkage between two loci, and a score ≤ 2 is taken as evidence against linkage.
  - The more individuals who are available for study, the finer the estimate of location.
- Inspection of genome databases identifies genes within a candidate region that can then be sequenced in affected individuals to identify mutations.
- Only when mutations have been discovered, shown to segregate with phenotype, and proved to affect gene function can it be stated that the disease gene has been identified.

Gene Identification Strategy

```
[DNA from affected individuals     →    [Genome-wide marker
 and first-degree relatives]              panel-linkage analysis to
                                          identify chromosomal
                                          location]
                                                    ↓
[Sequence candidate genes          ←    [Database analysis to
 in affected individuals]                 identify candidate genes]
```

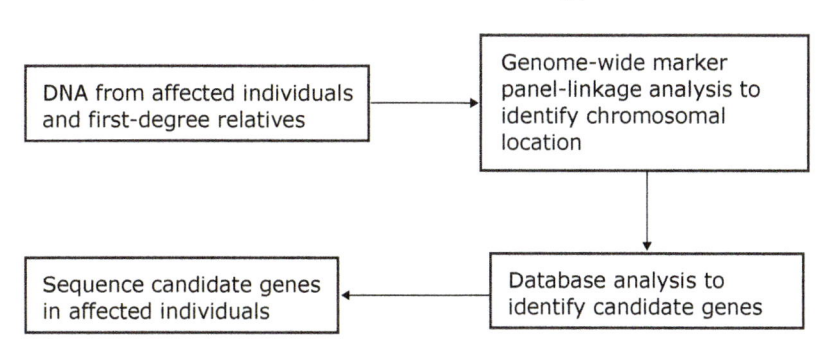

▲ Figure 5-4.2D Algorithm for Identification of Disease Genes by Positional Cloning

4.3 Breakpoint Analysis

- Translocation breakpoints may prove helpful in identifying disease genes when the number of informative meioses is limiting.

4.4 Exome Sequencing

- The availability of high-throughput sequencing technologies allows identification of mutations purely from sequence analysis.

- Exome sequencing is of particular use when most affected cases arise from spontaneous mutations (i.e., no affected relatives) or the mode of inheritance is unclear.

CHAPTER 6   Population Genetics

1 Overview

- The study of genetic variation in a population is called population genetics.
- Population genetics is used to evaluate the roles of evolutionary factors, such as natural selection, genetic drift, and gene flow in changing gene frequencies in human populations.

1.1 Genotype Frequencies

- The genotype frequency is the proportion of a given genotype at a specific locus in the population.
- Frequency (f) for the genotype is represented as follows:
  - Homozygous for one allele = f(AA)
  - Heterozygous = f(Aa)
  - Homozygous for the alternative allele = f(aa)
- Because these three alternatives are the only possible genotypes for the population, it naturally follows that:

$$f(AA) + f(Aa) + f(aa) = 1$$

- If a population was assayed for the presence of a particular genetic polymorphism at a specific locus, and it was determined that 48/100 individuals possessed the AA genotype, 44/100 possessed the Aa genotype, and 8/100 possessed the aa genotype, then their genotype frequencies would be expressed as:
  - AA = 0.48
  - Aa = 0.44
  - aa = 0.08

1.2 Allele Frequencies

- The allele frequency is the actual number of alleles at that locus on the chromosomes. To continue with the example given above:
  - The AA genotype has two copies of the A allele.
  - The Aa genotype has one copy each of the A allele and a allele.
  - The aa genotype has two copies of the a allele.
- Therefore, to calculate the allele frequency of the A allele in the population cited above, we would take the number of AA individuals (48) and realize that they had two copies (2 × 48); take the number of Aa individuals (44) and realize that they had one copy; and because the number of chromosomes in a diploid population of 100 people would be 200 for that chromosome, the formula becomes:

$$\frac{(2 \times 48) + 44}{200} = 0.7$$

- It follows that the allele frequency for "a" becomes 1 − 0.7 = 0.3 because the two allele frequencies added together must always equal 1.

USMLE® Key Concepts

For Step 1, you must be able to:

▶ Explain the meaning of allele frequency and genotype frequency.

▶ Estimate genotype frequencies and allele frequencies in recessive, dominant, and sex-linked diseases using the Hardy-Weinberg equation.

▶ Describe the roles of mutation, natural selection, genetic drift, gene flow, and consanguinity in population genetics.

2 Hardy-Weinberg Equilibrium

- In large populations that are mating at random (with respect to a given allele), there should be a constant and predictable relationship between genotype frequencies and allele frequencies.
- This relationship is expressed as the Hardy-Weinberg equilibrium, and if one knows the inheritance pattern of a specific disease, and the frequency of that disease, the equation can be used to calculate the frequency of alleles in that population:
  - p = frequency of the normal allele
  - q = frequency of the disease allele
  - p^2 = frequency of genotype AA
  - $2pq$ = frequency of the heterozygous genotype
  - q^2 = frequency of genotype aa
- So the Hardy-Weinberg equation results are:

$$p^2 + 2pq + q^2 = 1$$

2.1 Determining Genotype Frequencies for Autosomal Recessive Diseases

- In a population in which 1% of the individuals have a recessive disease, what percentage of individuals are asymptomatic carriers of the disease?
- In an autosomal recessive disease, asymptomatic carriers will be heterozygotes. Thus, the question is really asking for $f(Aa) = 2pq$.
- To answer this question, we start with the information we have, the frequency of diseased individuals: $f(aa) = q^2$.
- Calculating $f(a)$ or q:
  - $q^2 = 0.01$
  - $q = 0.1$
- Because $q = 0.1$, we can determine p and thus $f(A)$:
  - $p + q = 1$
  - $p = f(A) = 0.9$
- Using the last portion of the Hardy-Weinberg equation, we can calculate $f(Aa)$ or $2pq$:

$$2pq = 2(0.9)(0.1) = 0.18$$

- Thus, 18% of the population are carriers of the disease.
- For most recessive phenotypes of clinical significance, the population incidence is much less than 1% (e.g., cystic fibrosis, the most common lethal recessive disease in Caucasian populations, affects 1/2,500 live births). Therefore, q will be small (0.02 for cystic fibrosis) and so $p \sim 1$ and $2pq \sim 2q$.

2.2 Genetic Variables Affecting Hardy-Weinberg Equilibrium

- In its original form, the Hardy-Weinberg equilibrium works only for populations in which only two alleles are present at a locus. The equilibrium can be expanded to include multiple other alleles, but for practical purposes, the frequencies of all mutant alleles can be summed to equal q.
- Additionally, in order for the equation to function properly, several additional assumptions must hold true. Specifically:
  - There must be no new mutations.
  - There can be no selection pressure for or against alleles.
  - There can be no genetic drift.
  - There can be no gene flow in or out of the population.
- All of these conditions change the genotype, and thus the allele frequencies, and disturb the Hardy-Weinberg equilibrium.
- In large populations, the rate of new mutations balances negative selection.

2.2.1 New Mutations

- Spontaneous mutations will alter allele frequencies and upset the equilibrium.
  - For example, if new mutations in a gene occurred frequently, the frequency of the q allele would be ever increasing.
  - The odds of someone having the q allele would be dependent not only on their inherited genotype, but on mutations incurred within their parents' germline and their own development.
- In practice, the mutation rate is too low to make a difference for the more frequently occurring recessive phenotypes.

2.2.2 Selection Pressure

- Evolutionary selection for or against alleles can alter both the genotype and allele frequencies.

Negative Selection

- In the case of negative selection, if individuals with the disease (q^2) die before reproducing or are less able to reproduce, the allele frequency (q) will steadily decline.
- However, for every 2 mutant alleles lost, 2 are passed on to carriers. In a Punnett square, AA = p^2, 2Aa = 2pq, and aa = q^2

Heterozygote Advantage

- If there is a positive survival advantage for heterozygote carriers compared to normal individuals, referred to as a "heterozygote advantage," then the allele frequency (q) may increase.

Important Concept

A significant proportion of autosomal dominant and X-linked disorders are the result of a new mutation.

Connection to Microbiology

Individuals who are heterozygous for the sickle cell trait are resistant to *Plasmodium falciparum* malaria and this trait gives these individuals a selective advantage over normal homozygotes in areas where malaria is endemic. The selective advantage explains how this deleterious allele (lethal in the homozygous condition) can persist in populations at high frequency (up to 25% of people in parts of West Africa are heterozygous for the sickle allele). Carriers of thalassemia and G6PD mutations are also more resistant to malaria.

2.2.3 Genetic Drift

- Within a small population, allele frequencies can change by random chance.
  - For example, in a heterozygote cross, the probability of having a homozygous child (aa) is 25%.
  - However, if a heterozygote cross results in four children, three of whom are homozygous recessive (aa), then the allele frequency of a, which is represented as f(a), increases.
- The effect of genetic drift is minimal in large populations, but can have a significant impact on allele frequency in small populations.

2.2.4 Gene Flow

- In a given population, migration of one group of people into or out of that population may change allele frequencies, especially if a particular allele is more or less prevalent in the migrating population.
- Through time, gene flow within a population tends to make the people that make up that population more similar genetically to one another.
- As with genetic drift, the effect of gene flow is more pronounced in small populations.

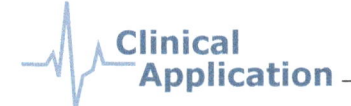

Clinical Application

Founder Effect

When a group of people move from one geographic area to another, they are taking a sample of all alleles in their original population. By chance, not all alleles will be at the same frequency in the migrants as they are in the original population. Therefore, phenotypes resulting from alleles at high frequency in the migrants will be more common in their new population as that population grows compared to the original population. This characteristic is termed the founder effect and is also seen in populations that survive from a drastic reduction in numbers (e.g., after a famine). The phenomenon applies to both recessive and dominant phenotypes. The Amish and Mennonite populations in North America are important examples of founder effect. A number of phenotypes are also seen at higher frequency in the Ashkenazi (e.g., Tay Sachs disease), but this tendency is probably due to more than just the founder effect.

2.2.5 Consanguinity

- A consanguineous union occurs between mating individuals descended from a common ancestor.
- Such unions are more likely to produce offspring with recessive diseases because of the likelihood of shared disease-causing mutations.
- Statistically speaking:
  - Siblings share 1/2 of their alleles
  - First cousins share 1/8 of their alleles
  - Second cousins share 1/32 of their alleles

Clinical Application

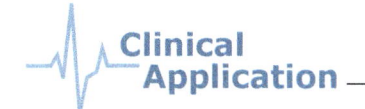

Using the Hardy-Weinberg Equilibrium

The affected individual in the pedigree (Figure 6-2.2) has cystic fibrosis.

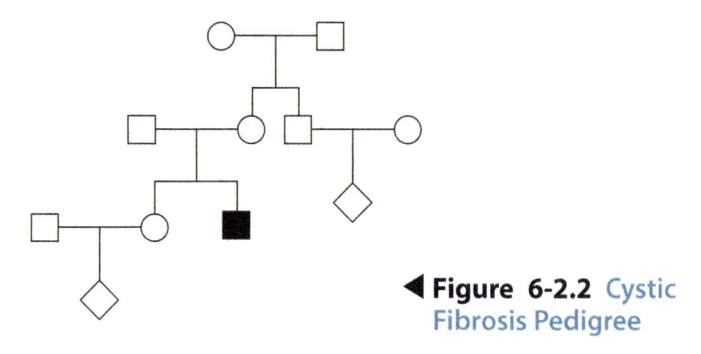

Figure 6-2.2 Cystic Fibrosis Pedigree

Question 1: If the incidence of CF in the population is 1/2,500, what is the chance that the child of the affected boy's sister will also have CF?

Answer: For the fetus to have CF, both parents must be carriers. The mother's risk of being a carrier is determined by her relationship to her brother. Since both of their parents MUST be carriers, and she is not affected, then her risk of being a carrier is 2/3 (Chapter 1). In the absence of a family history of CF, the fetus' father's risk is determined by the frequency of mutations in the population. Taking the population incidence = 1/2,500 = q^2, q = $\sqrt{(1/2,500)}$ = 1/50 and the carrier frequency (2q) = 1/25. The chance both parents have passed the mutation to the fetus (if they are both carriers) is 1/4. Therefore, the risk to the fetus is:

(2/3)(1/25)(1/4) = 1/150

Question 2: What is the chance the affected boy's uncle will have a child with CF?

Answer: Again, for the fetus to have CF, both parents must be carriers. The father's risk is determined by his relationship to his nephew. Since his sister MUST be a carrier, one of their parents MUST be a carrier, so his chance of being a carrier is 1/2. His wife's chance of being a carrier is the population risk (as before) = 1/25. Therefore, the risk to the fetus is:

(1/2)(1/25)(1/4) = 1/200

Question 3: Using the same pedigree (Figure 6-2.2), if the incidence of phenylketonuria (PKU) in the population is 1/10,000, what is the chance that the child of the affected boy's sister will also have PKU? What is the chance the affected boy's uncle will have a child with PKU?

Answers: The risks of direct relatives of the affected boy do not change—they are independent of the allele frequency in the population. The carrier frequency in the population is again calculated from the population incidence: 1/10,000 = q^2, so q = $\sqrt{(1/10,000)}$ = 1/100 and 2q = 1/50. So the calculations are:

Sister's child: (2/3)(1/50)(1/4) = 1/300

Uncle's child: (1/2)(1/50)(1/4) = 1/400

2.3 Determining Genotype Frequencies for Autosomal Dominant and X-linked Diseases

- Because of the significant new mutation rate for dominant and X-linked diseases, the Hardy-Weinberg equilibrium has limited utility in these cases.
- Theoretically, for dominant phenotypes of clinical significance, all affected individuals are described by 2pq (~2q), and for X-linked recessive pheneotypes, affected individuals are defined by q (not q^2 because males are hemizygous) and carriers by 2q.

> **Important Concept**
>
> - 20%–100% of individuals (varies with phenotype) with an autosomal dominant phenotype have a *de novo* mutation.
> - ⅓ of males with an X-linked phenotype have a *de novo* mutation (in the absence of family history of the phenotype).

CHAPTER 7 Genetics of Multifactorial Diseases

1 Overview

- Unlike single-gene defects that are discussed in previous chapters, most common human diseases are multifactorial: they have a genetic component, but they do not conform to mendelian inheritance patterns because they have complex polygenic and environmental etiologies.

2 Multifactorial Inheritance

- When there are multiple contributions (genetic and environmental) to the production of disease, the individual factors are referred to as risk factors and the sum of their contributions is an individual's liability for a disease.
- The distribution for these multifactorial diseases tends to follow a normal or bell-shaped curve.
- Blood pressure is an example of a multifactorial trait. There is a genetic component to the correlation between the blood pressures of parents and children. However, environmental influences, such as diet and stress, also play a significant role.

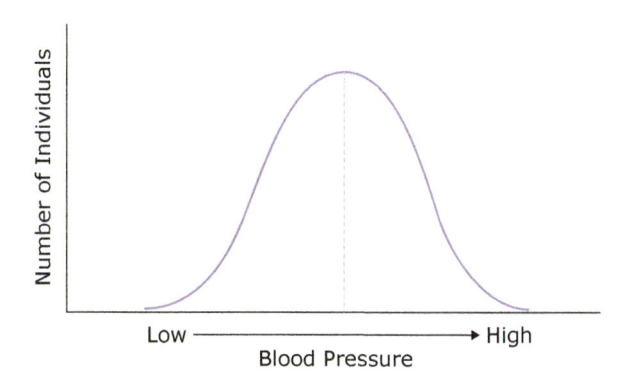

▲ **Figure 7–2.0** Multifactorial Inheritance

USMLE® Key Concepts

For Step 1, you must be able to:

▶ Describe the risk factors and liabilities for most common multifactorial diseases.

▶ Explain the relationship between liability threshold and recurrence risk.

▶ Describe how multifactorial disease recurrence risk is altered by the severity of disease in affected family members, and the prevalence of disease in the population.

▶ Interpret the findings from twin and adoption studies concerning trait heritability.

2.1 Threshold Model

- The multifactorial trait itself may not be a continuous spectrum:
  - In some cases, the patient either has the disease or does not (e.g., lung cancer).
  - The diagnosis of the disease is set by diagnostic criteria, and in these cases, disease occurs when a certain liability threshold has been achieved. In other words, for some individuals who have a few of the alleles, or have environmental stimuli that would cause the disease, there is little chance of disease.
  - Once some threshold for accumulated genetic and environmental factors is crossed, however, disease results.
- For some diseases, the thresholds for males and females are different:
  - If the male threshold is lower than the female threshold, then the prevalence of the disease is higher in males than in females.
  - The factors contributing to disease and the individual liability are usually determined empirically along with the recurrence risks.
    — As an example, infantile pyloric stenosis has a higher liability threshold in females than in males (Figure 7–7.2).

2.2 Recurrence Risk for Multifactorial Diseases

- The analysis of recurrence risks for single gene disorders is quite straightforward if one can construct a Punnett Square using the genotypes of the parents in a particular family, as shown in Chapter 1.
- In multifactorial diseases, the process is much more complex:
  - Recurrence risks for multifactorial diseases must be determined empirically by direct observation of data in the population.
  - Recurrence risk increases as the number of affected relatives increases. A family with a large number of affected members must be higher on the liability curve, with larger numbers of genetic and environmental risk factors.
  - Recurrence risk increases as the severity of the disease expression in the proband increases, again indicating the family's relatively higher liability.
  - Recurrence risk increases if the affected individual is a member of the less commonly affected gender.
  - Recurrence risk increases as the prevalence of the disease increases in a population.
  - Recurrence risk decreases rapidly for remotely related individuals.

! **Important Concept**

Variation in a gene can contribute to a multifactorial disease. If studied in isolation, however, each single gene still segregates according to mendelian principles. Multifactorial disease then can be viewed as the result of the accumulation of low penetrance mutations at a number of unlinked genes. The segregation of more than one or two genes implies that the risk alleles must be common in the population (common disease-common variant hypothesis).

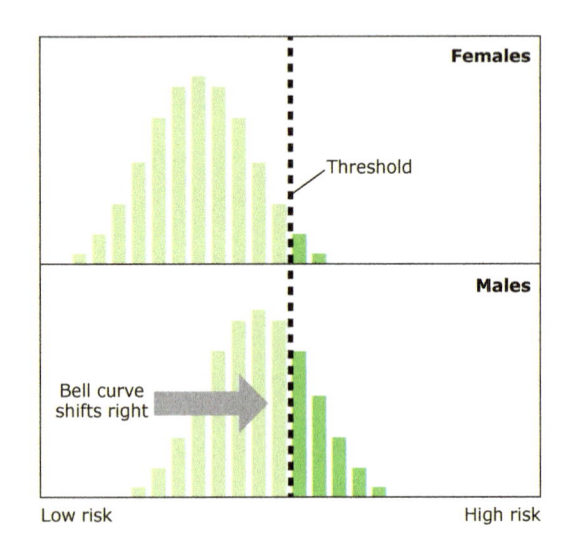

▲ Figure 7–2.2 Recurrence Risk

2.3 Heritability

- Heritability is defined as the proportion of the total variance of a trait that is caused by genetic variation.
- This determination can be a major challenge in the complexity of the human genome and society, but two forms of studies are most frequently used: twin studies and adoption studies.

2.3.1 Twin Studies

- If a trait were purely genetically determined, we would anticipate that monozygotic twins (formed from a cleaved embryo and therefore genetically "identical" in the absence of mutational change) would share that trait 100% of the time: there would be 100% concordance.
- In dizygotic twins, effectively siblings with 50% of their genes shared, there should be 50% concordance (they would share the trait 50% of the time).
- For a trait that is purely determined by the environment, we would expect the same concordance in monozygotic and dizygotic twins, as long as the pairs were raised together.

2.3.2 Adoption Studies

- If a biological parent has a genetic trait, but the child is adopted by parents who are phenotypically normal, another measurement can be made of the relative roles of genetics versus the environment.
- For example, if non-schizophrenic adoptive parents raise the children of a schizophrenic biological parent, 8%–10% of the children will develop schizophrenia. If non-schizophrenic adoptive parents raise the biological offspring of non-schizophrenic parents, only 1% of those children will develop the disease. This phenomenon provides evidence that there is at least some genetic component to that disease.

2.4 Familial Versus Sporadic Incidence

- Familial cases of genetic disease involve changes in germline DNA, which are inherited through generations.
- Sporadic somatic mutations in tumor suppressor genes and proto-oncogenes play a key role in common non-inherited cancers, such as breast and colon cancer, and mutations in these same genes in the germline cause inherited cancers.

3 Identification of Genes Involved in Multifactorial Disease

- Methods similar to those used to identify the mutation in single gene disorders have also been employed to identify the mutations involved in multifactorial disease.
- Techniques relying on linkage have had limited success due to the large number of low penetrance alleles involved.
- More recently, the identification of 6 million single nucleotide polymorphisms (SNPs) spread across the genome has facilitated large-scale case-control studies—genome-wide association studies (GWAS)—which are much more powerful.
- Copy number variation (CNV) also plays a significant role in multifactorial disease, often affecting gene expression rather than coding sequence.

Biochemistry-Genetics Index

Key:
bold: primary reference
t: table reference
f: figure reference

A

a/a3 (complex IV) BIC5-4
A-DNA BIC14-14
ABCD1 gene BIC10-7
abetalipoproteinemia BIC5-13, BIC9-17
absorptive phase BIC3-1
acanthocytosis BIC5-13
acceptor arm BIC17-8
acetaminophen BIC5-10
acetoacetate BIC10-8
acetone BIC10-8
acetyl-CoA carboxylase BIC8-5
acetyl-CoA BIC4-2
Acetyl-CoA, Important Sources of BIC4-1*f*
acid maltase BIC11-10
acquired homocysteinemia BIC13-11
actinomycin D BIC16-13
activation BIC1-5, BIC1-6, BIC1-7
activation of FFAs BIC10-2
active site BIC1-4
Acute Intermittent Porphyria (AIP) vs. Porphyria Cutanea Tarda (PCT) BIC13-19*f*
acyclovir BIC15-11
acyl carrier protein (ACP) BIC8-6
adenine BIC14-5
adenosine deaminase BIC14-2
adenosine deaminase deficiency BIC14-2
adenoviruses BIC19-2, BIC19-5
adipic acids BIC10-7
ADP Ribosylation BIC17-9, BIC17-9*f*
affinity BIC1-4, BIC1-5
AIP BIC13-16, BIC13-19
ALA dehydrase BIC13-18
alanine BIC13-2
Alanine Cycles, Cori and BIC11-8*f*
alanine transaminase (B6) BIC11-6
alcohol BIC3-2
alcohol, INH BIC13-16
Alcoholism and Gluconeogenesis BIC11-11*f*
aldolase BIC6-9
aldolase B BIC6-13
aldolase B deficiency BIC6-14
aldose reductase BIC6-13, BIC6-15
aldose sugar BIC6-13
Algorithm for Identification of Disease Genes by Positional Cloning GEN5-7*f*
Alignment of Nonhomologous Repeats GEN3-7*f*
alkaptonuria BIC13-7, BIC13-8
allopurinol BIC14-4, BIC14-5, BIC14-14
allopurinol febuxostat BIC14-2
Allosteric Regulation of Isocitrate Dehydrogenase BIC4-3*f*
alloxanthine BIC14-6
α-1,4 BIC8-2
α-1,4 glucosidase BIC11-4
α-1,6 BIC8-2
α-1,6 glucosidase BIC11-3
α-amanitin BIC16-13
α-galactosidase A BIC13-15
α-ketoglutarate DH BIC4-2, BIC4-3
α-KG DH BIC5-3*t*
α-oxidation of fatty acids BIC10-5
α subunit BIC2-4
α-tocopherol BIC5-13
Alport syndrome BIC17-21
ALT (alanine transaminase) BIC12-3
alternative splicing BIC16-10
amino acid degradation BIC13-6
amino acid metabolism BIC13-1
Amino Acid Precursors of Neurotransmitters BIC13-13*f*
amino acids BIC13-2
amino acids, aromatic BIC13-2
Amino Acids, Classification of BIC13-2*f*
Amino Acids, Degradation of Glucogenic BIC13-6*f*
Amino Acids, Degradation of Ketogenic BIC13-6*f*
Amino Acids, Essential BIC13-4*t*
amino acids, ionized/charged BIC13-2
Amino Acids, Metabolism of Branched Chain BIC13-9*f*
amino acids, nonpolar/aliphatic BIC13-2
amino acids, polar/uncharged BIC13-2
amino acids, sulfur containing BIC13-2
Amino Acids, Synthesis of Nonessential BIC13-5*f*
aminoacyl-tRNA synthetases BIC17-8
aminoglycosides BIC17-11
aminopeptidases BIC12-2
ammonia detoxification BIC12-1
Ammonia, Detoxification of BIC12-5*f*
AMP-activated kinase BIC8-5
AMP-dependent kinase BIC6-7
amylase BIC9-2
amylases BIC6-3
amylopectin BIC6-3
amylose BIC6-3
anaerobic glycolysis BIC5-6
Andersen disease BIC8-4
Andersen, type 4 BIC11-10
Angelman Syndrome GEN4-8*f*
anthracyclines BIC5-7*t*
Anticipation in a Pedigree Segregrating Huntington Disease GEN3-8*f*
anticodon arm BIC17-8
anticodons BIC17-2
antimalarials BIC8-9
antimycin A BIC5-7
antinuclear antibodies (ANAs) BIC16-9
antioxidant vitamins BIC5-13
antiparallel BIC14-13
AP endonuclease BIC15-12
apoA-1 BIC9-10
apoB-48 BIC9-3
apoB-100 BIC9-5
apoC-II BIC9-7
apoE BIC9-7, BIC9-9
apoenzyme BIC1-4
apoE receptors BIC9-9
arginase BIC12-6
arginase deficiency BIC12-8
arginine BIC12-6, BIC13-2
arginine therapy BIC12-7
argininosuccinate BIC12-6
argininosuccinate lyase BIC12-6
argininosuccinate lyase deficiency BIC12-8
argininosuccinate synthetase BIC12-6
argininosuccinate synthetase deficiency BIC12-8
Argonaute BIC16-12

Index

aromatic amino acid hydroxlases BIC13-8
array technologies BIC18-11
Arsenate and Phosphate, Similarities Between BIC6-12f
arsenate, AsO_4^{3-} BIC6-12
arsenic poisoning BIC6-12
arsenite, AsO_3^{2-} BIC6-12
arylsulfatase A BIC13-15
A-site BIC17-6
ASO probes BIC18-5, BIC18-10
asparagine BIC13-2
aspartate BIC13-2
aspirin BIC5-8
aspirin toxicity BIC5-9
Aspirin Toxicity Unfolds, Chain of Events as BIC5-9f
AST (aspartate transaminase) BIC12-3
ATM BIC15-12
atovaquone BIC5-7
ATP BIC3-1, BIC3-3
ATP-Coupled Reactions BIC1-2f
ATP, Fate of Key Intermediates in Presence of ↑ BIC4-5f
ATP Generation in the Glucagon World BIC3-5f
ATP Generation in the Insulin World BIC3-3f
atractyloside BIC5-7
atrophic gastritis type A BIC13-12
Autosomal Dominant Pedigree GEN1-3f
Autosomal Recessive Pedigree GEN1-4f
avidin BIC7-5
azathioprine BIC14-4
azide BIC5-7

B

B-DNA BIC14-14
B6 BIC13-16
B6 deficiency BIC13-17
B12 BIC13-10
B12 Deficiencies, Folate vs. BIC13-12t
B12 deficiency BIC10-5
bacterial promoters BIC16-4
barbiturates BIC5-7
base pairing BIC14-13
Base Pairing and Chargaff Rule BIC14-13f
basic helix-loop-helix (bHLH) BIC16-16
basic leucine zipper (bZIP) domains BIC16-16
Basic Mendelian Terminology GEN1-2t
basophilic stippling BIC13-18
beriberi, dry BIC4-7
beriberi, wet BIC4-7
β-carotene BIC5-13
β-keto-thiolase BIC10-4, BIC10-9
β-hydroxybutyrate BIC10-8
β-OH-butyrate dehydrogenase BIC10-8
β-oxidation BIC3-5
β-oxidation of even C-chain saturated fatty acids BIC10-4
β-oxidation of fatty acids BIC10-2
β-Oxidation of Palmitoyl-CoA (C16:0) BIC10-4f
βγ subunits BIC2-4
β-hydroxyacyl dehydrogenase BIC10-4
β-hydroxy-butyrate dehydrogenase BIC10-9
BH_4 BIC13-7, BIC13-5, BIC13-8
bidirectional BIC15-3
bile acids synthesis BIC9-14
Bile Salts BIC9-14f
bile sequestering resins BIC9-14
bilirubin BIC13-20

Bilirubin Metabolism and Jaundice BIC13-20f
biotin BIC7-4, BIC13-10
biotin deficiency BIC7-5
bite cells BIC8-9
1,3-bisphosphoglycerate (1,3-BPG) BIC6-10
Blotting Techniques BIC18-4, BIC18-4t
blunt ends BIC18-2
2,3-BPG BIC6-11
BPG mutase BIC6-11
branched chain amino acids catabolism BIC13-9
branched chain fatty acids BIC10-5
branched chain α-ketoacid dehydrogenase deficiency BIC13-9
branching enzyme BIC8-2
branching enzyme deficiency BIC8-4
BRCA1 BIC15-12
BRCA2 BIC15-12
broadly specific probes BIC18-5

C

caffeine BIC14-5
cAMP phosphodiesterases BIC2-3
cAMP response element binding protein (CREB) BIC16-17
canagliflozin BIC6-7
cap binding complex (CBC) BIC16-7
cap site BIC16-5
carbamoyl P BIC12-6
carbamoyl phosphate BIC12-6
carbamoyl phosphate synthetase II BIC14-8
carbohydrates BIC3-2
carboxin BIC5-7
carnitine acyltransferases (CAT) BIC10-3
carnitine deficiency BIC10-6
carnitine palmitoyltransferase II deficiency BIC10-6
Carnitine Shuttle BIC10-2, BIC10-3, BIC10-3f
carotenoids BIC5-13
catalase BIC5-12
catalysts BIC1-3
cataracts BIC6-14
CAT box BIC16-3
70 CAT box BIC16-3
CAT I BIC10-3
CAT II BIC10-3
CCl_4 BIC5-10
Cdc6 BIC15-4
cDNA or expression library BIC19-2
Cdt1 BIC15-4
Cell Cycle BIC15-2f
cell cycle concepts BIC15-2
cellulose BIC6-3
ceramide BIC13-14
ceramide trihexoside BIC13-15
cerebrohepatorenal syndrome BIC10-7
cerebroside sulfate BIC13-15
CGD BIC5-11f
chain terminators BIC15-11
Chain Terminators Used in HIV, Two BIC15-11f
Changes in Gene Expression, Effects of BIC1-7f
chaperones BIC17-15
Chargaff rule BIC14-13
Chargaff Rule, Base Pairing and BIC14-13f
chenodeoxycholic acid BIC9-14
cherry red spot BIC13-15
chief cells BIC12-2
chimera BIC19-6
chloramphenicol BIC17-10, BIC17-12

cholecystokinin BIC9-2
cholesterol BIC9-12
cholesterol ester transfer protein (CETP) BIC9-10
cholesterol esters BIC9-6
Cholesterol Synthesis BIC9-12f
cholestyramine BIC9-3, BIC9-14
cholic acid BIC9-14
chromatin BIC16-14
chromatin,10 nm BIC16-14
chromatin,30 nm BIC16-14
Chromatin Structure BIC16-14, BIC16-14f
chronic alcoholism and hypoglycemia BIC11-11
chronic granulomatous disease BIC5-11
Chylomicron and VLDL Catabolism BIC9-8f
Chylomicron and VLDL Remnants, Liver Uptake of BIC9-9f
chylomicron remnants BIC9-9
chylomicrons BIC9-3
Chylomicrons, Synthesis of BIC9-4f
chymotrypsinogen BIC12-2
Circumventing Glycolysis Irreversible Steps BIC11-5t
citrate BIC8-5
citrate lyase BIC8-5
Citrate Shuttle BIC8-5, BIC8-5f
citrulline BIC12-6
citrullinemia BIC12-8
classification BIC13-2
clinical relevance BIC11-8
cloning applications BIC19-4
Cloning Strategy BIC19-3f
cloverleaf structure BIC17-8
CN− BIC5-7
codons BIC17-1
Codon Table BIC17-2f
coenzyme BIC1-4
coenzyme Q (ubiquinone) BIC5-4
cofactor BIC1-4
colesevelam BIC9-14
colestipol BIC9-14
colipase BIC9-2
Collagen Disorders BIC17-21t
collagen BIC17-20
Common Damage Mechanism From Hypoxia BIC5-6f
competitive inhibition BIC1-5, BIC1-6
competitive inhibitor BIC1-7
competitive inhibitors BIC1-8
Competitive vs. Noncompetitive Inhibition BIC1-8t
complementary BIC14-13
complex I BIC5-4
Consequences of DNA Mutation GEN3-1t
35 consensus sequence BIC16-3
control of glycogen phosphorylase BIC11-4
control of glycogen synthase BIC8-3
Conversion of Fructose-1,6bisP to DHAP and GAP BIC6-9f
coproporphyrinogen III BIC13-16
CoQ BIC9-12
Cori and Alanine Cycles BIC11-8f
Cori, type III BIC11-10
cortisol BIC2-4
CO BIC5-7
co-transcriptional capping of RNA BIC16-7
co-trimoxazole BIC5-11
Coupling of ETC BIC5-5
CpG sites BIC16-15
CPSF (cleavage and poly(A) specificity factor) BIC16-6
creatine BIC13-13
creatine kinases BIC13-13

Creatine Synthesis, Role, and Degradation BIC13-13f
creatinine BIC13-13
CREB BIC2-4
CstF (cleavage stimulation factor) BIC16-6
cystathionine BIC13-10
cystathionine β-synthase BIC13-10
cystathionine β-synthase deficiency BIC13-11
cysteine BIC13-2
cystic fibrosis BIC9-3
Cystic Fibrosis, PCR in Direction Mutation
  Testing of BIC18-17f
Cystic Fibrosis Pedigree GEN6-5f
cytarabine BIC15-11
Cytarabine BIC15-11f
cytochrome b_5 BIC8-6
cytochrome c BIC5-4
cytochrome oxidase BIC5-4
cytochromes b/c1 (complex III) BIC5-4
Cytoplasmic P-Bodies, RNA Interference
  Pathway in BIC16-12f
cytosine BIC14-10

D

D-ALA dehydratase BIC13-16
D-ALA synthase BIC13-16
D Loop BIC17-8
dapagliflozin BIC6-7
daunorubicin BIC5-7
de novo pyrimidine synthesis BIC14-8
de novo synthesis of cholesterol BIC9-12
De Novo Synthesis of Purine Nucleotides BIC14-4f
de novo synthesis of purines BIC14-4
De Novo Synthesis of Purines and Pyrimidines,
  Comparison of BIC14-1t
De Novo Synthesis of Pyrimidines BIC14-8f
De Vivo disease BIC6-7
deacetylases BIC16-15
deaminases BIC14-2
debranching enzyme BIC11-3
deficiency of B6, B12, or folate BIC13-11
degenerate BIC17-1
Degradation of Sphingolipids and Selected
  Sphingolipidoses BIC13-15f
7-dehydrocholesterol reductase deficiency BIC9-13
dehydrogenases BIC3-3
Dehydrogenases (DH), Important BIC5-3t
deletions BIC17-4
δ-aminolevulinic acid (D-ALA) BIC13-16
ΔG BIC1-1, BIC1-2
ΔG‡ BIC1-1, BIC1-3
ΔG Values and Reaction Characteristics BIC1-1t
deoxythymidine kinase BIC14-3
desensitization BIC1-5, BIC1-6
detoxification of amino acid nitrogen BIC12-3
Detoxification of Ammonia BIC12-5f
dextrinoses BIC11-8
DHCR7 gene BIC9-13
DHF reductase BIC14-8
DHF reductase inhibitors BIC14-9
diabetes and hyperlipidemia BIC9-7
diabetes as a cause of acquired hyperlipidemia BIC9-16
dicarboxylic acid BIC10-5
dicarboxylic acidemia BIC10-7
Dideoxy Chain Termination Sequencing (Sanger Method)
  BIC18-18f

Index

dideoxyribonucleoside triphosphate BIC18-18
Dietary Carbohydrates, Digestion of Major BIC6-3f
dietary fuels BIC3-2
dietary niacin deficiency BIC4-6
dietary protein digestion and absorption BIC12-2
Dietary Sugars Across Cell Membranes,
  Transport of BIC6-5f
dihydrorhodamine flow cytometry BIC5-11
dihydroxyacetone phosphate (DHAP) BIC6-9
2,4 dinetrophenol (2-4 DNP) BIC5-8
diphtheria exotoxins BIC17-9
DNA 2 nuclease BIC15-7
DNA Coils, Supercoils, and Role of
  Topoisomerases BIC15-5f
DNA Damage and Specific Recognition
  Endonucleases BIC15-12t
DNA double helix BIC14-13
DNA Double Helix, The BIC14-14t
DNA Editing: High-Fidelity DNA Synthesis BIC15-10f
DNA Enhancer and Silencer Regions, Interaction of Specific
  Transcription Factors With BIC16-16f, BIC16-17t
DNA gyrase BIC15-5
DNA helicases BIC15-4
DNA ligases BIC15-7
DNA methylation BIC16-15
DNA Mutation, Consequences of GEN3-1t
DNA or RNA Probes, ss Labeled BIC18-5f
DNA polymerase inhibitors BIC15-11
DNA polymerases BIC15-5
DNA Polymerases in Eukaryotes BIC15-6t
DNA Polymerases in Prokaryotes BIC15-6t
DNA polymorphisms BIC18-6
DNA primase complex BIC15-6
DNA proofreading BIC15-10
DNA repair BIC15-12
DNA Repair, Steps in BIC15-12f
DNA Replication BIC15-1, BIC15-3f
DNA topoisomerase I BIC15-5
DNA topoisomerase II BIC15-5
DNA, Unwinding Parent BIC15-4f
DNA_A protein BIC15-3
dolichol phosphate BIC9-12
Dot Blot Analysis BIC18-10f
dot/slot blots BIC18-10
down-regulation BIC1-5, BIC1-6
Down Syndrome GEN2-6f
doxorubicin BIC5-7t

E

EcoRI Restriction Map BIC18-3f
Ehlers-Danlos type 4 BIC17-21
Electron Shuttles: Glycerol-3 Phosphate Shuttle BIC5-3f
Electron Shuttles: Malate Aspartate Shuttle BIC5-2f
electron transport chain (ETC) BIC3-3
Electron Transport Chain BIC5-1, BIC5-4f
Electron Transport Chain, Krebs Cycle BIC4-2f
Electron Transport Chain, Overview of BIC5-1f
Elongation BIC17-12f
Elongation (continued) BIC17-13f
endergonic reactions BIC1-2
endergonic BIC1-1
endonuclease 1 BIC15-7
endonucleases BIC14-12, BIC18-2
endoplasmic reticulum (ER) BIC17-17

Energy Activation, Effects of Enzyme on BIC1-3f
energy of activation BIC1-1, BIC1-3
Energy of Reaction BIC1-1, BIC1-1f
enhancer BIC16-16
enoyl-CoA hydratase BIC10-4
enteropeptidase BIC12-2
Enzyme, Branching BIC8-2f
Enzyme Deficiencies, Urea Cycle BIC12-8f
enzyme kinetics BIC1-4
epigenetic modifications BIC16-14
equilibrium BIC1-1
ERK (extracellular signal regulated kinase) BIC2-2
ESE (exonic splicing enhancer site) BIC16-10
E-site BIC17-6
essential fructosuria BIC6-14
ESS (exonic splicing silencer sites) BIC16-10
esterases BIC9-2
ETC (electron transport chain) BIC3-5
etoposide BIC15-5
euchromatin BIC16-14
Eukaryotes, Capping the hnRNA in BIC16-7f
eukaryotic promoters BIC16-4
eukaryotic ribosome BIC17-5
eukaryotic RNA polymerase BIC16-11
Eukaryotic RNA Polymerases, Roles of BIC16-13t
exergonic BIC1-1t
exonic splicing enhancer site (ESE) BIC16-10
exonic splicing silencer sites (ESS) BIC16-10
exon skipping BIC16-10
exonuclease activity, 3' → 5' BIC15-10
exonucleases BIC14-12
extracellular signal regulated kinase (ERK) BIC2-2
ezetimibe BIC9-16

F

F_1 BIC5-5
Fabry BIC13-15
$FADH_2$ BIC3-3, BIC5-4
farnesyl PP_1 BIC9-12
familial apoC-II deficiency, type I_b BIC9-15
familial combined hyperlipidemia, type II_b BIC9-15
familial dysbetalipoproteinemia, type III BIC9-15
familial hypercholesterolemia BIC9-15
familial hypercholesterolemia, type IIa BIC9-15
familial hyperchylomicronemia BIC9-16
familial hyperchylomicronemia, type Ia BIC9-15
Familial Hyperlipidemias, Fredrickson
  Classification of BIC9-15t
familial hypertriglyceridemia, type IV BIC9-15
familial mixed hyperlipidemia, type V BIC9-15
familial ALS BIC5-11
Fanconi-Bickel syndrome BIC6-7
Fanconi syndrome BIC11-9
Fate of Key Intermediates in Presence of ↑ ATP BIC4-5f
fat malabsorption BIC5-13, BIC9-3
fatty acid Synsthase complex BIC8-6
Fatty Acid Synthesis BIC3-4, BIC8-1, BIC8-5, BIC8-6f,
Fatty Acids, Activation of BIC10-2f
fatty acyl-CoA dehydrogenase BIC10-4
fatty acyl-CoA DH BIC5-3
fatty acyl-CoA synthetase BIC10-2
fatty streaks BIC9-10
fava beans BIC8-9
favism BIC8-9

febuxostat BIC14-6
Fenton reaction BIC5-10, BIC5-11
ferrochelatase BIC13-18
fertilized ovum microinjection BIC19-5
FH_4 BIC13-5
fibrates BIC9-16
FISH Showing Deletion on Chromosome 15 (long arrow) Versus Normal (arrowhead) GEN4-8f
5-fluorouracil (5-FU) BIC14-10
5-FU, flucytosine BIC14-8
flucytosine BIC14-10
FMN (flavin mononucleotide) BIC5-4
F_o BIC5-5
F_o, F1 ATP synthase BIC5-5
folate and B12 deficiencies BIC13-11
Folate vs. B12 Deficiencies BIC13-12t
Forensic Application, Repetitive Sequences and RFLPs: BIC18-9f
Fragile X Syndrome GEN3-9f
frameshift BIC17-4
Fredrickson classification BIC9-15
Fredrickson Classification of Familial Hyperlipidemias BIC9-15t
fructokinase BIC6-8, BIC6-13
fructokinase deficiency BIC6-14
fructose BIC6-1, BIC6-3, BIC6-8
fructose-1,6bisP BIC6-9
fructose-1,6-bisphosphatase BIC11-5, BIC11-6, BIC11-7
fructose-1P BIC6-8
fructose-2,6bisP BIC6-9
fructose-6-phosphate BIC6-9
Fructose Metabolism BIC6-13f
Fuel Used by Brain During Fasting, Pattern of BIC10-9f

G

G_0 BIC15-2
G_1 BIC15-2
G_2 BIC15-2
G_6PD deficiency BIC5-11
G_6PD Deficiency in RBCs BIC8-9f
gal-1P uridyltransferase deficiency BIC6-14
galactitol BIC6-13
galactocerebrosidase BIC13-15
galactocerebrosides BIC13-14
galactokinase BIC6-8, BIC6-13
galactokinase deficiency BIC6-14
galactose BIC6-1, BIC6-3, BIC6-8
galactose-1P BIC6-8
galactose-1P uridyl transferase BIC6-13
galactose epimerase deficiency BIC6-14
Galactose Metabolism BIC6-13f
galactosemia type 1 BIC6-14
galactosemia type 2 BIC6-14
galactosemia type 3 BIC6-14
gallbladder disease BIC9-3
γ-carboxylation BIC17-20
Gametogenesis, Parent of Origin Imprints and GEN4-5f
ganciclovir BIC15-11
gangliosides BIC13-14
gap phases BIC15-2
gastrin BIC12-2
Gaucher BIC13-15
Gaucher cells BIC13-15
GC-rich hairpin loop BIC16-5

Gene Cluster on Chromosome 15 Deleted in PWS and AS GEN4-8f
gene expression profiling BIC18-11
gene expression: transcription and control BIC16-1
gene expression: translation BIC17-1
Gene Identification, Methods of GEN5-5f
general transcription BIC16-16
general transcription factors (TFs) BIC16-3
Generic Transaminase Reaction and Examples BIC12-3f
Gene Structure BIC16-2, BIC16-2f
gene therapy BIC19-4
Genetic Code is Unambiguous but Degenerate, The BIC17-1f
genetic code, the BIC17-1
Genetic Deficiencies in Fructose and Galactose Metabolism, Comparison Between BIC6-14t
genomic DNA BIC19-1
genomic library BIC19-2
globoid cell leukodystrophy BIC13-15
glucagon, epinephrine, G-protein coupled receptors BIC2-3
glucagon world BIC3-1, BIC3-5
Glucagon World, ATP Generation in the BIC3-5f
Glucagon World, High ATP in the BIC3-5f
glucocerebrosidase BIC13-15
glucocerebrosides BIC13-14
Glucogenic and Ketogenic Amino Acids BIC11-5f
glucokinase BIC6-8
Glucokinase Regulation by GKRP BIC6-8f
glucokinase regulatory protein (GKRP) BIC6-8
gluconeogenesis BIC3-5
gluconeogenesis and glycogenolysis BIC11-1
Gluconeogenesis in Hepatocytes BIC11-6f
glucose BIC6-1, BIC6-3, BIC6-8
glucose-6P BIC6-8, BIC6-9
glucose-6-phosphatase BIC11-5, BIC11-6
glucose-6-phosphatase deficiency BIC11-8
glucose-6-phosphatase (G6Pase) BIC11-7
glucose-6-phosphate dehydrogenase deficiency BIC5-12, BIC8-9
Glucose Uptake, Effect of Exercise on BIC6-7f
GLUT Distribution in Humans BIC6-6f
GLUT family BIC6-6
GLUT1 BIC6-6
GLUT1 deficiency BIC6-7
GLUT2 BIC6-6
GLUT3 BIC6-6
GLUT4 BIC6-6
GLUT4 and diabetes BIC6-7
GLUT4 and exercise BIC6-7
GLUT5 BIC6-6
glutamate BIC13-2
Glutamate Dehydrogenase BIC12-4, BIC12-4f
Glutamate Synthetase BIC12-4f
glutaminase BIC12-5
glutamine BIC13-2
glutamine synthetase BIC12-4
glutamyl phosphoribosyl amidotransferase BIC14-4
Glutathione in Detoxification of H_2O_2 and Associated Diseases, Role of BIC5-12f
glutathione peroxidase (selenium) BIC5-12, BIC8-9
glutathione reductase BIC5-12, BIC8-9
glyceraldehyde-3P dehydrogenase BIC6-10
Glyceraldehyde-3 Phosphate Dehydrogenase and LDH BIC6-10f
glyceraldehyde-3 phosphate DH BIC5-3

Index

glyceraldehyde-3 phosphate (GAP) BIC6-9
glycerol-3P BIC9-5
glycerol-3P dehydrogenase BIC9-5, BIC11-6
glycerol-3P DH BIC5-3
glycerol-3 phosphate DH BIC5-3
glycerol-3 phosphate shuttle BIC5-2
glycerol kinase BIC9-5
glycerol phenylbutyrate BIC12-7
glycine BIC9-14, BIC13-2, BIC14-1
glycochenodeoxycholic acid BIC9-14
glycocholic acid BIC9-14
Glycogen and Fatty Acid Synthesis BIC8-1f
glycogenin BIC8-2
glycogenolysis BIC3-5
Glycogenoses BIC11-10t
glycogen phosphorylase BIC11-3
Glycogen Phosphorylase and Debranching Enzyme, Actions of BIC11-3f
Glycogen Phosphorylase, Hormonal Control of BIC11-4f
glycogen storage diseases BIC11-8
glycogen storage disease type 0 BIC8-4
glycogen synthase BIC8-2
glycogen synthase deficiency BIC8-4
Glycogen Synthase, Hormonal Control of BIC8-3f
Glycogen Synthesis BIC3-4, BIC8-1, BIC8-2, BIC8-3f
glycolysis BIC3-3, BIC6-8
Glycolysis in RBCs BIC6-11f
Glycolysis Irreversible Steps, Circumventing BIC11-5f
Glycolysis, Overview of BIC6-2f
Glycolysis vs. Gluconeogenesis BIC11-7f
glycosylation BIC17-18
GM_2 BIC13-15
Golgi complex BIC17-18
Goodpasture disease BIC17-21
gout BIC14-3, BIC14-6
Gout, Causes of BIC14-7f
G-proteins BIC2-4
GRB2 BIC2-2
G_s-Coupled Receptors BIC2-3f
guanine BIC14-5
gums BIC6-3
GYS1 BIC8-4
GYS2 BIC8-4
GYS2 Mutations, Effects of BIC8-4f

H

H_1 BIC16-14
H_{2A} BIC16-14
H_{2B} BIC16-14
H_3 BIC16-14
H_4 BIC16-14
Hartnup disease BIC4-6
HDL BIC9-10
heat-stable DNA polymerase BIC18-13
Heinz bodies BIC8-9
heme degradation BIC13-20
heme-iron BIC5-4
Heme Synthesis BIC13-16, BIC13-16f
hemochromatosis BIC5-11
hemolytic anemia BIC6-12
hemolytic uremic syndrome BIC17-7
Hemophilia GEN3-5f
Hepatic and Muscle Glycogen, Fate of BIC11-4f
hepatic lipases BIC9-10

Hepatic Triglycerides, Synthesis of BIC9-5f
Hepatocyte Metabolism During Fasting BIC11-2f
hereditary fructose intolerance BIC6-14
hereditary nonpolyposis colorectal cancer (HNPCC) BIC15-10
Hers, type VI BIC11-10
heterochromatin BIC16-14
heterogeneous nuclear (hn)RNA BIC16-11
Heterozygous Point Mutation: Sanger Method (left) and Chain-Terminator Sequencing (right) GEN5-1f
hexokinase BIC6-13
hexokinases BIC6-8
hexosaminidase A BIC13-15
Hexose-Monophosphate Shunt BIC8-7, BIC8-7f
HGPRT deficiency BIC14-3
High ATP in the Glucagon World BIC3-5f
High ATP in the Insulin World BIC3-4f
high-energy-level substrate BIC6-10
histidine BIC13-2
histone acetylases BIC16-15
histone methylation BIC16-15
HIV viral load: RT-PCR BIC18-15
HIV Viral Load Using RT-PCR, Determining BIC18-16f
HMG-CoA lyase BIC10-8
HMG CoA-reductase BIC9-12
HMG-CoA synthase BIC10-8
$hMLH_1$ BIC15-10
$hMSH_2$ BIC15-10
hnRNA (heterogeneous RNA) BIC16-7
holoenzyme BIC1-4
Holoprosencephaly BIC16-18, BIC16-18f
homocysteine BIC13-10
homocysteine methyltransferase BIC13-10
homocysteinemia BIC13-11
homocystinuria BIC13-11
homogentisate BIC13-7
homogentisate oxidase BIC13-7
Hormonal Control of Glycogen Phosphorylase BIC11-4f
hormone response element (HRE) BIC2-4
hormone sensitive lipase (HSL) BIC3-5, BIC10-1
HOX BIC16-17
Huntington Disease, Anticipation in a Pedigree Segregating GEN3-8f
hydrogen (H) bonds BIC14-13
hydrogen peroxide: H_2O_2 BIC5-10
hydroxyacyl-CoA DH BIC5-3
hydroxyl radical: •OH BIC5-10
hydroxyurea BIC14-8, BIC14-9
hyperlipidemias BIC9-15
hypoxanthine BIC14-4, BIC14-5
Hypoxanthine (I), Wobble Hypothesis and Role of BIC17-2f
Hypoxia, Common Damage Mechanism From BIC5-6f
hypoxia BIC5-6

I

I cell disease BIC17-18
IDL BIC9-10
IDL, LDL, and HDL, Relationship Between BIC9-11f
Ile BIC13-9
IMP dehydrogenase BIC14-4
importins BIC17-17
inactivation BIC1-5, BIC1-6, BIC1-7
Indomethacin BIC14-6

inducers BIC16-16
induction BIC1-5, BIC1-6, BIC1-7
inflammation BIC5-11
in-frame BIC17-4
Inhibitors, Effects of BIC1-7f
inhibitors of ETC BIC5-7
Inhibitors of ETC, Site of Action of Selected BIC5-7t
Initiation Complex, Formation of BIC17-11f
initiation BIC15-3
initiator tRNA BIC17-11
inosine BIC14-4
inosine monophosphate BIC14-4
insertions BIC17-4
insoluble fibers BIC6-3
Insulin and Glucagon Control of Lipid Metabolism BIC10-3f
insulin receptor BIC2-2
Insulin Receptor Signaling BIC2-2f
insulin world BIC3-1, BIC3-3
Insulin World, ATP Generation in the BIC3-3f
Insulin World, High ATP in the BIC3-4f
Interaction of Specific Transcription Factors With DNA Enhancer and Silencer Regions BIC16-16f, BIC16-17t
Intracellular Lipids by HSL, Mobilization of BIC10-1f
intronic splicing enhancer site (ISE) BIC16-10
intronic splicing silencer sites (ISS) BIC16-10
Intron Removal by Spliceosome BIC16-9f
introns BIC16-5
intron splicing BIC16-8
iron-sulfur centers (FeS) BIC5-4
ironotecan topotecan BIC15-5
ISE (intronic splicing enhancer site) BIC16-10
Isocitrate Dehydrogenase, Allosteric Regulation of BIC4-3f
isocitrate DH BIC4-2, BIC4-3, BIC5-3
isoleucine BIC13-2, BIC13-10
isomaltase BIC6-3
isomerase BIC6-9
isoprenes BIC9-12
ISS (intronic splicing silencer sites) BIC16-10

J

JAK-STAT BIC16-17

K

KDEL sequence BIC17-18
ketoacidosis BIC10-10
Ketogenesis BIC10-8, BIC10-8f
ketogenic diet BIC6-7
ketogenic diets BIC10-11
Ketogenolysis BIC10-8, BIC10-9, BIC10-9f
ketone bodies BIC10-1
ketones BIC3-5
ketose sugar BIC6-13
Key Sugar Positions BIC14-11f
Klein-Waardenburg syndrome BIC16-18
Klinefelter Syndrome GEN2-7f
K_M BIC1-1, BIC1-4, BIC1-5
knockout animal BIC19-5
Korsakoff syndrome BIC4-7
Kozak consensus sequence BIC16-5
Krabbe BIC13-15
Krebs cycle BIC3-3, BIC3-5
Krebs Cycle/Electron Transport Chain BIC4-2f
Krebs cycle intermediates BIC4-4

Krebs Cycle Intermediates, Important Sources of BIC4-4f
Krebs cycle (Tricarboxylic Acid cycle) BIC4-1
kwashiorkor BIC13-4

L

lactase BIC6-3
lactase deficiency BIC6-4
lactate dehydrogenase (LDH) BIC6-10
lactate DH BIC5-3
lactic acidosis BIC5-10
lactose BIC6-3
lagging strand BIC15-6
lanosterol BIC9-12
lariat BIC16-8
LCAT (lecithin cholesterol acyltransferase) BIC9-10
LDH BIC11-6
LDL receptors BIC9-10
lead BIC13-16
Lead Intoxication, Effects of BIC13-18f
lead poisoning BIC13-16, BIC13-18
leader peptide BIC16-5
Leading and Lagging Strand, Synthesis of BIC15-8f
leading strand BIC15-6
Leber hereditary optic neuropathy BIC5-10t
lecithin cholesterol acyltransferase (LCAT) BIC9-10
lentiviruses BIC19-5
Lesch-Nyhan syndrome BIC14-3
Leu BIC13-9
leucine BIC13-2
leukodystrophy BIC10-7
lignin BIC6-3
Lineweaver-Burk Plot BIC1-4, BIC1-6, BIC1-6f
Lineweaver-Burk Plot, Mechanisms Changing V_{max} or K_M on BIC1-6f
linezolid BIC17-11
Linkage Analysis Using an STRP Marker GEN5-6f
linker DNA BIC16-14
linoleic acid (ω-6) BIC9-1
linolenic acid (ω-3) BIC9-1
lipase BIC9-2
Lipid Absorption, Central Role of CCK in BIC9-2f
lipid catabolism BIC10-1
lipid digestion BIC9-1
Lipid Metabolism, Insulin and Glucagon Control of BIC10-3f
lipids BIC3-2
lipoprotein lipase (LPL) BIC3-4, BIC9-7
lipoprotein metabolism BIC9-1, BIC9-3
Lipoproteins and Roles BIC9-11t
liposomes BIC19-2
lutein BIC5-13
Lynch syndrome BIC15-10
lysine BIC13-2
lysophospholipids BIC9-2
lysosomal α-1,4 glucosidase deficiency BIC11-10

M

M phase BIC15-2
macrolides clindamycin BIC17-12
malate-aspartate shuttle BIC5-2
malate dehydrogenase BIC11-5
Malate DH BIC4-2f, BIC4-3, BIC5-3t
maleylacetoacetate BIC13-7
malic enzyme BIC8-5

Index

malonyl-CoA BIC8-5, BIC10-3
maltase BIC6-3, BIC11-4
MAPK BIC2-2
maple syrup urine disease BIC13-9
marasmus BIC13-4
Marfan Syndrome GEN3-2f
Marfan Syndrome, Variable Expressivity in GEN1-8f
Maternal Age Effect GEN2-5f
Maternally Imprinted, Paternally Expressed Gene, Pedigree for Mutation in GEN4-6f
MCAD deficiency BIC10-7
McArdle disease BIC10-6, BIC11-9
McArdle, type V BIC11-10
MCM (mini-chromosome maintenance) BIC15-4
Mechanisms Changing V_{max} or K_M on Lineweaver-Burk Plot BIC1-6f
Mechanisms Changing V_{max} or K_M on Michaelis-Menten Graph BIC1-5f
megaloblastic anemia BIC14-9, BIC13-11, BIC13-12
Meiosis GEN2-2f
MEK (mitogen/exrracellular signal regulated kinease) BIC2-2
MELAS (mitochondrial encephalomyopathy, lactic acidosis, stroke-like episodes) BIC5-10
Mendelian Disorders GEN1-6t
Menke disease or EDS type IX BIC17-21
mercaptopurine BIC14-4
MERRF (myoclonic epilepsy, ragged red fiber disease) BIC5-10
messenger (m)RNA BIC16-11
Metabolism, Comparison Between Genetic Deficiencies in Fructose and Galactose BIC6-14t
Metabolism, Fructose BIC6-13f
Metabolism, Galactose BIC6-13f
Metabolism of Branched Chain Amino Acids BIC13-9f
metachromatic leukodystrophy BIC13-15
methionine BIC13-2, BIC13-10
methionine synthase BIC13-10
Methods of Gene Identification GEN5-5f
methotrexate BIC14-8, BIC14-9
7-methylguanosine BIC16-7
methylmalonic acid BIC10-5, BIC13-12
methylmalonic aciduria BIC13-11
methylmalonyl-CoA BIC13-10
methylmalonyl-CoA mutase BIC10-5, BIC13-10
methylmercury BIC5-7
methylxanthines BIC14-5
mevalonate BIC9-12
Mg^{2+} BIC6-8
Michaelis-Menten Graph BIC1-4, BIC1-4f
Michaelis-Menten Graph, Mechanisms Changing V_{max} or K_M on BIC1-5f
microRNAs (miRNAs) BIC16-12
microsatellites BIC18-9
microsomal triglyceride transfer protein (MTP) BIC9-17
mini-chromosome maintenance (MCM) BIC15-4
minisatellites BIC18-9
mipomersen BIC9-16
mismatch repair BIC15-10
mismatch repair endonucleases BIC15-10, BIC15-12
mismatches BIC15-10
missense mutations, conservative BIC17-3
missense mutations, nonconservative BIC17-3
Mitochondrial Diseases, Selected BIC5-10t
mitochondrial disorders BIC5-10

mitochondrial encephalomyopathy BIC5-10
Mitochondrial Inheritance Pedigree GEN1-7f
Mitochondrial Mutations, Heteroplasmy of GEN1-7f
mitochondrial targeting signal BIC17-17
mitogen/extracellular signal related kinase (MEK) BIC2-2
Mitosis GEN2-1f
molecular technologies BIC18-1
molybdenum (Mo) BIC14-6
2-monoacylglycerol BIC9-2
MPTP BIC5-7
mRNA guanylyltransferase BIC16-7
MTP (microsomal tryglceride transfer protein) BIC9-17
mucilages BIC6-3
Multifactorial Inheritance GEN7-1f
muscle glycogen phosphorylase deficiency BIC11-9
Mutant Allele, Use of RFLP to Track a GEN5-3f
Mutation Mechanism Algorithm GEN3-4f
mutations BIC17-3
Mutations Following Insertion of Nucleotides, In-Frame vs. Frameshift BIC17-4f
Mutations in Selected Diseases, Important BIC17-4t
Mutations, Point BIC17-3f
myeloperoxidase BIC5-11
myeloperoxidase deficiency BIC5-11
myoclonic epilepsy BIC5-10
Myopathic Carnitine Deficiency vs. McArdle Disease BIC10-6t
myristoyl-CoA BIC10-4

N

N-acetylglucosamine-1-phosphotransferase BIC17-18
N-acetylglutamate (NAG) BIC12-6
N-Acetylglutamate (NAG) Production BIC12-6f
N-terminal hydrophobic signal sequence BIC17-17
NADH BIC3-3, BIC5-4
NADPH BIC8-5, BIC8-7
NADPH oxidase BIC5-11
NADPH oxidase deficiency BIC5-11
NAG synthetase deficiency BIC12-8
NBT test BIC5-11
neural tube defects BIC13-12
Neurotransmitters, Amino Acid Precursors of BIC13-13f
NF-γ BIC16-3
NF-κβ BIC16-17
niacin BIC4-6
Niemann-Pick BIC13-15
nitric oxide: NO BIC5-10
nitric oxide synthase BIC13-8
noncompetitive inhibition BIC1-5, BIC1-6
noncompetitive inhibitor BIC1-7
noncompetitive inhibitors BIC1-8
Nondisjunction in Meiosis I (left) and Meiosis II (right) GEN2-4f
Nondisjunction of Sex Chromosomes GEN2-8t
Nonhomologous Repeats, Alignment of GEN3-7f
"Nonrandom" Inactivation GEN4-4t
nonsense mutations BIC17-3
non-spontaneous reaction BIC1-1
No Recombination When Marker Is Close to Gene GEN5-6f
Normal Male Karyotype GEN2-3f
Northern Blot of Creatine Kinase MM and MB mRNA in Various Tissues BIC18-11f
Northern blots BIC18-11
Northern blotting techniques BIC18-4

NRTIs (nucleoside reverse transcriptase inhibitors) BIC15-11
nuclear localization sequences (NLS) BIC17-17
nuclear pore complex BIC16-7
nuclear pore complexes BIC17-17
nucleases BIC14-12
Nucleases on a DNA Strand, Action of BIC14-13f
nucleoside reverse transcriptase inhibitors (NRTIs) BIC15-11
nucleosides BIC14-11
nucleosome BIC16-14
5'-nucleotidase inhibition BIC13-18
Nucleotides BIC14-1, BIC14-11, BIC14-11f

O

obesity BIC6-4
ochronosis BIC13-8
odd C-chain fatty acids BIC13-10
Odd C-Chain Fatty Acids, Terminal Oxidation of BIC10-5f
Okazaki fragments BIC15-6
oligomycins BIC5-7t
ω-oxidation BIC10-7
ω-oxidation of fatty acids BIC10-5
ORI BIC15-3
ornithine BIC12-6
ornithine transcarbamoylase (OTC) BIC12-6
ornithine translocase BIC12-6
orotate phosphoribosyltransferase BIC14-9
orotate PRTase BIC14-8
orotic acid BIC12-8, BIC14-8, BIC14-10
orotic aciduria BIC14-8, BIC14-9
Orotic Aciduria and Megaloblastic Anemia, Differential Diagnosis of BIC14-9f
orotic aciduria BIC14-9
orotidylic acid decarboxylase BIC14-8
orotidylic acid decarboxylase deficiency BIC14-9
Osteogenesis Imperfecta BIC17-21, GEN3-2f
oxidation of odd C-chain fatty acids BIC10-5
oxidation of unsaturated fatty acids BIC10-5
oxidative phosphorylation BIC3-3
oxidized LDL BIC9-10
oxido-reduction steps BIC5-4

P

P-bodies BIC16-12
P-site BIC17-6
palindromes BIC14-12, BIC18-2
Palindromes and Restriction Enzymes, Examples of BIC18-2f
palmitoyl-CoA BIC10-4
Palmitoyl-CoA (C16:0), β-Oxidation of BIC10-4f
pancreatic insufficiency BIC5-13, BIC9-3
pantothenate BIC4-8
pantothenic acid (vitamin B5) BIC8-6
Parent of Origin Imprints and Gametogenesis GEN4-5f
parietal cells BIC12-2
Paternally Imprinted, Maternally Expressed Gene, Pedigree for Mutation in GEN4-6f
Pathway and Clinical Relevance, Polyol BIC6-15f
Pathway, Purine Salvage BIC14-2f
Pathway, Pyrimidine Salvage BIC14-3f
Pathways Occurring in the Liver, Summary of BIC3-6t
PAX3 BIC16-17
PAX3 gene BIC16-18
PBL deaminase (HMB synthase) BIC13-16

PCR for HIV Provirus (cDNA) BIC18-15f
PCR in Direction Mutation Testing of Cystic Fibrosis BIC18-17f
PCR in direct mutation testing BIC18-17
PCR in HIV diagnosis BIC18-15
PCT BIC13-16
PDH Deficiency BIC7-3, BIC7-3f
PDPK1 BIC2-2
Pedigree for Mutation in Maternally Imprinted, Paternally Expressed Gene GEN4-6f
Pedigree for Mutation in Paternally Imprinted, Maternally Expressed Gene GEN4-6f
Pedigree Interpretation, Logic of GEN1-3f
pellagra BIC4-6
pentavalent arsenic BIC6-12
PEPCK BIC11-6
pepsin BIC12-2
Peptide Bond BIC17-10, BIC17-10f
peptidyltransferase BIC17-5, BIC17-10
Pericentric (left) and Paracentric (right) Inversions GEN2-10f
peroxisomal disorders BIC10-7
peroxisomal oxidation of fatty acids BIC10-5
peroxisomal targeting signals (PTS) BIC17-17
peroxisome proliferator activated receptors BIC16-17
peroxynitrite: ONOO− BIC5-10
PEX mutations BIC10-7
PFK-2 BIC6-9
phages BIC19-2
PH domain BIC2-2
Phe BIC13-7
Phe and Tyr Catabolism and Clinical Relevance BIC13-7f
Phenotypes for Expansion of Repeat Sequences GEN3-8f
phenylalanine BIC13-2
phenylalanine and tyrosine catabolism BIC13-7
phenylalanine hydroxylase BIC13-7
phenylketonuria BIC13-7
phenylketonuria (PKU) BIC13-7
phenylketonuria, tetrahydrobiopterin-deficient hyperphenylalaninemia BIC13-7
phosphodiester bonds BIC14-11
Phosphodiester Bonds (PDE) and Polarity BIC14-12f
phosphoenolpyruvate carboxykinase BIC11-5, BIC11-7
phosphoenolpyruvate (PEP) BIC6-11
Phosphofructokinase-1 (PFK-1) BIC6-9, BIC6-9f
phosphoglucomutase BIC6-13
2-phosphoglycerate BIC6-11
phosphoglycerate kinase BIC6-10
Phosphoglycerate Kinase (PGK) BIC6-10f
3-phosphoglycerate (3-PG) BIC6-10
phospholipase A_2 BIC9-2
phosphopantetheine BIC8-6
phosphoribosylpyrophosphate (PRPP) BIC14-4
phosphoribosyltransferases BIC14-2
phosphorylase kinase BIC11-4
Phosphorylation/Dephosphorylation, Effects of BIC1-7f
Phosphorylation Traps Dietary Sugars in Cells BIC6-8f
phosphotransferases BIC6-8
PI-3 kinase BIC2-2
PIP3 BIC2-2
PKB (protein kinase B) BIC2-2
plasmids BIC19-2
pleckstrin homology domains (PH domains) BIC2-2
PLP (pyridoxal phosphate) BIC13-5
point mutation BIC17-3

Index

Point Mutations BIC17-3f
Pol I BIC15-6
Pol II BIC15-6
Pol III BIC15-6
polyadenylate polymerase (PAP) BIC16-8
polyadenylation (poly(A) polymerase) signal BIC16-6
polyadenylation signal BIC16-5
poly(A) tail BIC16-5
poly(A) tail addition BIC16-8
Poly(A) Tail Addition in Eukaryotes BIC16-8f
Polymerase Chain Reaction BIC18-13, BIC18-14f
polymerases BIC14-11
Polyol Pathway and Clinical Relevance BIC6-15f
polyol (sorbitol) pathway BIC6-15
Pol α BIC15-6
Pol β BIC15-6
Pol δ BIC15-6
Pol ε BIC15-6
Pol γ BIC15-6
Pompe disease BIC11-4, BIC11-10
Pompe, type II BIC11-10
porphobilinogen BIC13-16
porphyria BIC13-19
Porphyria Cutanea Tarda (PCT), Acute Intermittent Porphyria (AIP) Versus BIC13-19f
Positional Cloning, Algorithm for Identification of Disease Genes by GEN5-7f
positive supercoils BIC15-5
postabsorptive phase BIC3-1, BIC3-5
potentiation BIC1-5f, BIC1-6
PP1 BIC2-3
PPARα BIC9-16
Prader-Willi Syndrome GEN4-8f
prenylation BIC17-20
pre-replication complex BIC15-3
primary biliary cirrhosis BIC7-3
primary hyperlipidemias BIC9-15
Primer Removal and Ligation BIC15-8f
probes BIC18-5
procarboxypeptidases BIC12-2
production of recombinant proteins BIC19-4
proelastase BIC12-2
Prokaryote and Eukaryote Transcription Units, Comparison of BIC16-5t
Prokaryotes and Eukaryotes, Upstream Promoter Elements in BIC16-4f
Prokaryotic and Eukaryotic ORI, Comparison of BIC15-4t
Prokaryotic and Eukaryotic Ribosomes BIC17-5f
Prokaryotic and Eukaryotic Transcription Units BIC16-6f
prokaryotic ribosome BIC17-5
prokaryotic RNA polymerase BIC16-11
proline BIC13-2
promoter BIC16-2
promoters BIC16-3
propionyl-CoA BIC13-10
pronionyl-CoA carboxylase BIC10-5, BIC13-10
prosthetic group BIC1-4
proteases BIC9-2
Proteasome Digestion BIC17-16f
protein catabolism BIC3-6
protein coding sequence BIC16-5
Protein Digestion BIC12-1, BIC12-2f
protein folding BIC17-15
protein phosphatase 2 BIC8-5
protein phosphatases BIC2-3

protein structures, primary structure BIC17-15
protein structures, secondary structure BIC17-15
protein structures, tertiary structure BIC17-15
protein structures, quaternary structure BIC17-15
protein targeting BIC17-17
proteins BIC3-2
proton ionophore BIC5-8
pseudomonas BIC17-9
Punnett Square for Autosomal Dominant Inheritance GEN1-3f
Punnett Square for Autosomal Recessive Inheritance GEN1-4f
Punnett Square for X-Linked Recessive Inheritance GEN1-5f
purine catabolism BIC14-6
purine nucleoside phosphorylases BIC14-2
Purine Nucleotides, De Novo Synthesis of BIC14-4f
Purine Salvage Pathway BIC14-2f
purines BIC14-1
Purine Structure BIC14-5f
purine structure BIC14-5
pyridoxal phosphate (PLP) BIC13-5, BIC13-17
pyrimethamine (PYR) BIC14-9
Pyrimidine Salvage Pathway BIC14-3f
Pyrimidine Structure BIC14-10, BIC14-10f
pyrimidine phosphorylase BIC14-3
pyrimidines BIC14-1
pyruvate BIC6-11
pyruvate carboxylase BIC7-1, BIC7-4, BIC11-6, BIC11-5, BIC8-5, BIC11-7
Pyruvate Carboxylase Deficiency BIC7-5, BIC7-5f
pyruvate carboxylase BIC7-4
Pyruvate Dehydrogenase BIC7-2, BIC7-2f
pyruvate dehydrogenase (PDH) BIC3-3
pyruvate DH BIC5-3
pyruvate, fates of BIC7-1
pyruvate kinase BIC6-11
pyruvate kinase deficiency BIC6-12
Pyruvate Kinase (PK), Control of BIC6-11
Pyruvate Metabolism BIC7-1, BIC7-1f
pyruvate translocase BIC8-5

Q

quinolones BIC15-5

R

Raf BIC2-2
ragged red fiber disease BIC5-10
Random X Inactivation Results in Mosaic Females GEN4-2f
RAS BIC2-2
rate of reaction BIC1-3
RBC Pyruvate Kinase Deficiency BIC6-12f
Reaction Characteristics, ΔG Values and BIC1-1t
Reciprocal Translocation GEN2-8f
Recombinant DNA Technology Concept BIC18-3f
recombinant DNA technology BIC19-1
Recombination, 50% GEN5-5f
Recurrence Risk GEN7-2f
Reduced Penetrance in an Autosomal Dominant Pedigree GEN1-8f
rel homology (RHD) BIC16-17
removal of RNA primers BIC15-7
reperfusion injury BIC5-10

Repetitive Sequences and RFLPs: Forensic
    Application BIC18-9f
repetitive sequences and RFLPs BIC18-9
repression BIC1-5f, BIC1-6, BIC1-7
repressors BIC16-16
respiratory burst BIC5-11
restriction endonucleases BIC14-12
restriction enzyme mapping BIC18-3
restriction enzymes BIC18-2
Restriction Fragment Length Polymorphisms:
    RFLP BIC18-6
restriction fragments BIC14-12, BIC18-2
retinoid and retinol receptors BIC16-17
retroviruses BIC19-2, BIC19-5
reverse cholesterol transport BIC9-10
reversible reaction BIC1-1
rhabdomyolysis BIC9-13
ρ-factor (rho) BIC16-5
ribavirin BIC14-4, BIC14-5
riboflavin BIC4-8
ribonucleotide reductase BIC14-8
ribose 5-phosphate BIC8-7
Ribose vs. Deoxyribose BIC14-11f
ribosomes BIC17-5
Ribosome/tRNA Binding Sites BIC17-6f
ribozyme BIC17-10
ricin BIC17-7
rifampin BIC16-11
rifamycins BIC16-11
RNA glycosylases BIC17-7
RNA-induced silencing complex (RISC) BIC16-12
RNA Interference Pathway in Cytoplasmic P-Bodies
    BIC16-12f
RNA interference (RNAi) BIC16-12
RNA primase BIC15-5
RNA processing BIC16-7
RNA silencing BIC16-12
RNA, types of BIC16-11
RNase H BIC15-7
RNase III Dicer BIC16-12
RNAP I BIC16-11
RNAP II BIC16-11
RNAP III BIC16-11
Robertsonian Translocation GEN2-9f
ROS and RNOS-Mediated Cellular Alterations BIC5-10f
ROS Generation and Disease Association BIC5-11f
rotenone BIC5-7
rRNAs BIC16-11

S

S-adenosyl methionine BIC13-10
S phase BIC15-2
26S proteasomes BIC17-15
salvage enzymes BIC14-2
Salvage Pathways for Purines and Pyrimidines,
    Comparison of BIC14-2t
salvage pathways BIC14-2
(Sanger Method), Dideoxy Chain Termination
    Sequencing BIC18-18f
Sanger Method (left) and Chain-Terminator Sequencing
    (right), Heterozygous Point Mutation: GEN5-1f
sarcoma (src) homology 2 domain BIC2-2
sarcoma (src) homology 3 domain BIC2-2

SCID (severe combined immunodeficiency
    syndrome) BIC14-2
scurvy BIC17-21
Sec61 proteins BIC17-17
Segregation of Alleles: Heterozygous Parents GEN1-2f
Segregation of Alleles: Homozygous Parents GEN1-2f
Segregation of Alleles: Punnett Square GEN1-2f
Segregation of STRP Alleles With Normal and
    Mutant Gene Alleles GEN5-4f
selenium BIC5-12
semiconservative BIC15-3
sensitization BIC1-5f, BIC1-6
sequencing DNA BIC18-18
serine BIC13-2
ser/thr kinase BIC2-2, BIC2-3
severe combined immunodeficiency syndrome
    (SCID) BIC14-2
SGLT1 BIC6-5
SGLT2 BIC6-5
SH2 BIC2-2
SH3 BIC2-2
SHH BIC16-17
Shiga toxin BIC17-7
Shine-Dalgarno sequence BIC16-5
Shunt, Hexose-Monophosphate BIC8-7f
Sickle Cell Mutation in a Series of Samples,
    Specific Identification of the GEN5-2f
sideroblastic anemia BIC13-18
σ-70 BIC16-3
sigmoid BIC1-8
signal peptidase BIC17-17
signal recognition particles (SRP) BIC17-17
signal transduction BIC2-1
silencer BIC16-16
silencing BIC1-5f, BIC1-6
silent mutations BIC17-3
Similarities Between Arsenate and Phosphate BIC6-12f
single gene probes BIC18-5
single-stranded DNA binding proteins (SSBPs) BIC15-4
SLC6A19 chromosome 5) deficiency BIC4-6
small interfering RNAs (siRNAs) BIC16-12
small nuclear RNAs (snRNAs) BIC16-8
small nuclear (sn)RNA BIC16-11
Smith-Lemli-Optiz syndrome BIC9-13
SNAP proteins BIC17-18
SNARE proteins BIC17-18
SNRNPs (small nuclear ribonucleoproteins) BIC16-8
snurps BIC16-8
SOD Enzymes and Their Location, Three BIC5-12t
sodium-dependent glucose uptake BIC6-5
soluble fibers BIC6-3
sonic hedgehog gene (*SHH*) BIC16-18
sorbitol dehydrogenase BIC6-15
SOS BIC2-2
sources of NADH and $FADH_2$ BIC5-2
Sources of pyruvate BIC7-1
Southern Blot Analysis of RFLPs BIC18-7f
southern blot analysis of RFLPs BIC18-7
Southern blotting techniques BIC18-4
Southwestern blotting techniques BIC18-4
Specific Identification of the Sickle Cell Mutation in a
    Series of Samples GEN5-2f
specific transcription factor BIC16-16
specific transcription factors BIC16-16
sphingolipidoses BIC13-14

Index

sphingolipids BIC13–14
Sphingolipids and Selected Sphingolipidoses, Degradation of BIC13–15f
Sphingolipids, Synthesis of Major BIC13–14f
sphingomyelinase BIC13–15
sphingomyelins BIC13–14
sphingosine BIC13–14
splice acceptor site BIC16–5, BIC16–8
splice donor site BIC16–5, BIC16–8
spliceosome BIC16–5, BIC16–8
Spliceosome, Intron Removal by BIC16–9f
Splicing, Alternative BIC16–10f
splicing factors BIC16–10
splicing repressor proteins BIC16–10
spontaneous reaction BIC1–1
squalene BIC9–12
SR-B1 receptors BIC9–10
Src homology 3 domain BIC2–2
Src homology 2 domain BIC2–2
SRP receptor BIC17–17
ss Labeled DNA or RNA Probes BIC18–5f
starches BIC6–3
statins BIC5–7, BIC9–13
stem cell transgenesis BIC19–6
steroid receptors BIC16–17
sticky ends BIC18–2
stop codons, 3 BIC17–1
streptogramins BIC17–12
stroke-like episodes BIC5–10
STRP Alleles With Normal and Mutant Gene Alleles, Segregation of GEN5–4f
Structure of A and B DNA BIC14–14f
subacute combined degeneration of the spinal cord BIC13–11
suberic (8C) acids BIC10–7
substitutions BIC17–3
substrate-level phosphorylation BIC4–3, BIC5–6, BIC6–1, BIC6–10, BIC6–11
substrates for gluconeogenesis BIC11–5
succimer, oral BIC13–18
Succinate DH (complex II of ETC) BIC4–2f
succinate DH BIC4–3, BIC5–3
succinate thiokinase BIC4–2, BIC4–3
succinyl-CoA BIC10–5, BIC13–10, BIC13–16
succinyl-CoA: acetoacetate CoA-transferase BIC10–9
sucrase BIC6–3
sucrose BIC6–3
sulfonamides BIC8–9
Summary of Pathways Occurring in the Liver BIC3–6t
superoxide dismutase (SOD) BIC5–11, BIC5–12
superoxide: O_2 BIC5–10
Svedberg unit BIC17–5
Synthesis is Complementary and Antiparallel to Template BIC14–13f
synthetase 1 (CPS 1) BIC12–6
systemic carnitine deficiency BIC10–6

T

T ψ C loop BIC17–8
Targeting Proteins to Their Appropriate Locations BIC17–19f
Tarui, type VII BIC11–10
TATA binding protein (TBP) BIC16–3
10 TATA box (Pribnow) BIC16–3
25 TATA box (Hogness) BIC16–3
taurine BIC9–14
taurocheno deoxycholic acid BIC9–14
taurocholic acid BIC9–14
Tay-Sachs BIC13–15
telomerase BIC15–9
telomeres BIC15–9
template BIC16–2
tendon xanthoma BIC9–16
teniposide BIC15–5
Ter protein BIC15–9
TERC: Telomerase RNA component BIC15–9
Terminal Oxidation of Odd C-Chain Fatty Acids BIC10–5f
Termination BIC17–14f
Terminations BIC15–9f
terminator BIC16–2
terminators BIC16–6
TERT: Telomerase reverse transcriptase BIC15–9
tetracyclines BIC17–12
Tetrahydrobiopterin (BH_4) BIC13–5
Tetrahydrobiopterin (BH_4) as a Cofactor, Roles of BIC13–8f
tetrahydrobiopterin deficiency BIC13–8
tetrahydrofolate (FH_4) BIC13–5
TFIIB BIC16–3
35 TFIIB recognition element (BRE) BIC16–3
TFIID BIC16–3
TFIIH BIC16–4
theophylline BIC14–5
therapeutic protein expression BIC19–1
thermodynamics BIC1–1
thermogenin BIC5–8
THF (N^5-methyltetrahydrofolate) BIC13–10
thiamine BIC7–2
Thiamine Deficiency BIC8–8, BIC8–8f
thiamine BIC4–7
thioguanine BIC14–4
thiokinase BIC9–3
thiolase BIC10–8
thiophorase BIC10–9
threonine BIC13–2, BIC13–10
thymidine phosphorylase BIC14–3
thymidylate synthase BIC14–8
thymidylate synthase inhibitors BIC14–10
thymine BIC14–10
transamination reactions BIC12–3
Transcription Factors and Binding Sites in Promoters BIC16–3t
transcription start +1 BIC16–3
transcription units BIC16–4
Transfer RNA Cloverleaf Structure BIC17–8f
transfer RNA (tRNA) BIC17–8
Transgenic Animals BIC19–5, BIC19–6f
transition BIC17–3
transition state BIC1–3
transketolase BIC4–7
Translation Factors BIC17–9, BIC17–9t
translocation BIC17–12
translocon BIC17–17
transcription start BIC16–3
transmembrane domains BIC2–3
7 transmembrane domains BIC2–3
transversion BIC17–3
Triglycerides, Fatty Acids, and Cholesterol Esters, Structure of BIC9–6f

triglycerides BIC9-6
trimethoprim pyrimethamine BIC14-8
trimethoprim (TMP) BIC14-9
triose kinase BIC6-13
Trisomy Rescue, Uniparental Disomy Follows from GEN4-7f
trivalent arsenic BIC6-12
tRNAs BIC16-11
trypsin BIC12-2
trypsinogen BIC12-2
tryptophan BIC13-2
Turner Syndrome GEN2-7f
Tus protein BIC15-9
type V hyperlipidemia BIC9-16
Tyr BIC13-7
tyrosine BIC13-2
tyrosine kinase BIC2-2

U

ubiquitin ligases BIC17-15
ubiquitination BIC17-15
UDP-glucose BIC8-2
UDP-glucose/galactose epimerase BIC6-13
UMP synthase BIC14-8
unambiguous BIC17-1
uncouplers of ETC BIC5-8
uncoupling protein 1 (UCP1) BIC5-8
Uniparental Disomy Follows from Trisomy Rescue GEN4-7f
unwinding BIC15-4
upregulation BIC1-5, BIC1-6
Upstream open reading frames (uORF) BIC16-5
uracil BIC14-10
Uracil glycosylase BIC15-12
urea BIC12-6
Urea Cycle BIC3-6, BIC12-6, BIC12-6f
Urea Cycle Enzyme Deficiencies BIC12-7, BIC12-8f
urea structure BIC12-6
uric acid BIC14-2, BIC14-3, BIC14-6
Uric Acid, Breakdown of Purines to BIC14-6f
uridine/cytidine kinase BIC14-3
Uroporphyrinogen decarboxylase BIC13-16
uroporphyrinogen III BIC13-16
Use of RFLP to Track a Mutant Allele GEN5-3f
UTP BIC8-2
3'UTR BIC16-5
5'UTR BIC16-5
UV excinuclease BIC15-12

V

Val BIC13-9
valine BIC13-2, BIC13-10
Variable number of tandem repeats (VNTRs) BIC18-9
Variation in the Number of Repeats Generates Different-Size Alleles GEN5-4f
vectors BIC19-2
Vectors, Use of Expression BIC19-4f
verotoxin BIC17-7
very-long-chain fatty acids BIC10-5
viral vectors BIC19-4
Viral Vectors in Human Gene Therapy BIC19-5t
vitamin A BIC5-13
vitamin B12 BIC13-10
Vitamin B6 Deficiency, Effects of BIC13-17f
vitamin C BIC5-13
vitamin D receptors (VDR) BIC16-17
vitamin E and clotting BIC5-13
Vitamins, Role of Antioxidant BIC5-13f
VLDL BIC9-5
VLDL remnants BIC9-9
V_{max} BIC1-1, BIC1-4, BIC1-5
VOMIT Pathway, The BIC13-10, BIC13-10f
Von Gierke disease BIC10-7, BIC11-8
Von Gierke, type I BIC11-10

W

Wernicke encephalopathy BIC4-7
Western Blot and HIV Testing BIC18-12f
Western blot BIC18-12
Western blotting techniques BIC18-4
Wilson disease BIC5-11f
wobble BIC17-2
Wobble Hypothesis and Role of Hypoxanthine (I) BIC17-2f

X

xanthelasma BIC9-16
xanthine oxidase BIC5-10, BIC14-2, BIC14-6
X-Autosome Translocation GEN4-4f
X-Linked Dominant Pedigree GEN1-6f
X-Linked Recessive Pedigree GEN1-5f

Z

Z-DNA BIC14-14
zeaxanthin BIC5-13
zebra bodies BIC13-15
Zellweger syndrome BIC10-7
zinc fingers BIC2-4, BIC16-16

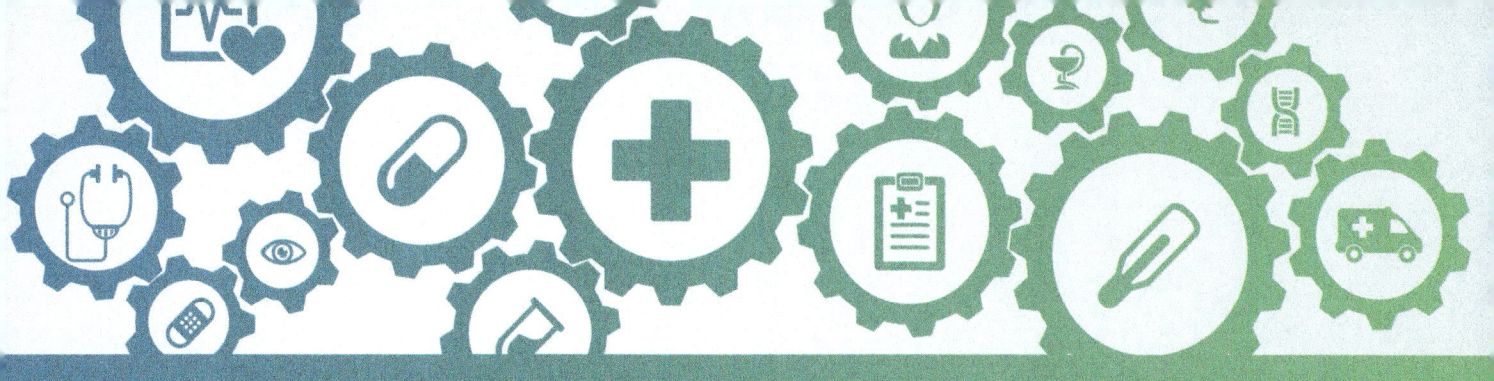

Integrated Cases with
Dr. Lionel Raymon for USMLE® Step 1

Interactive case-based review for Step 1 to help you achieve your goals

Integrated Cases with Dr. Lionel Raymon provides an interactive and engaging approach to Basic Sciences to help students pull all the concepts together—and maximize your performance on the exam. Dr. Raymon is well versed in Biochemistry, Pharmacology and Pathology. He possesses a strong understanding of Microbiology, Immunology and Pathophysiology, allowing him to synthesize basic science concepts for the USMLE® Step 1 exam.

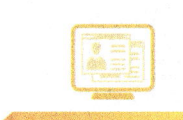

30 hours of unique Live Online case-based review over six days

Student-driven content that's unique to each session

Problem-based questions focused on high-yield concepts for Step 1

Exclusive student handouts for each course

Direct references to Becker's Step 1 lecture notes.

Maximize your performance on the exam!

To enroll in an Integrated Cases Course with Dr. Lionel Raymon, please visit **becker.com/usmle**

Stay Connected:

USMLE is a registered trademark of the National Board of Medical Examiners and this trademark owner does not sponsor, endorse or support Becker Professional Education in any manner.

© 2016 DeVry/Becker Educational Development Corp. All rights reserved.

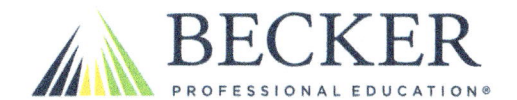

BECKER
PROFESSIONAL EDUCATION®

Becker | *Think Like a Doctor*

QMD — Advanced USMLE® Question Bank

GuideMD — Advanced Interactive Learning

Becker's QMD provides over 2,100 exam-relevant practice questions that allow you to identify your strengths and learning needs, acclimate yourself to the format of the exam and develop your critical thinking skills.

Becker's GuideMD brings topics to life by combining curriculum with interactive technology taking advantage of over 200 hours of multimedia instruction from esteemed faculty including - video introductions, animation, graphics and audio lectures.

Becker's QMD features:

- A unique personal dashboard displaying all user activities to easily monitor and track progress, review tests taken, and to retake any tests.
- Full, detailed rationales for each question, including details on why the answers are incorrect.
- Customized blocks to help students master challenging subjects while improving their performance.

Becker's GuideMD features:

- Advanced search allowing students to set criteria to search the complete Step 1 curriculum program.
- Playback functionality providing seamless play of audio and all annotations, starting from the page selected by the user.
- Full color illustration, embedded motion graphics and animations to demonstrate complex concepts.

If you are interested in more information or in purchasing GuideMD and QMD, visit
www.becker.com/usmle

BECKER PROFESSIONAL EDUCATION®

Stay Connected:

USMLE® is a registered trademark of the National Board of Medical Examiners and this trademark owner does not sponsor, endorse or support Becker Professional Education in any manner.

© 2016 DeVry/Becker Educational Development Corp. All rights reserved.

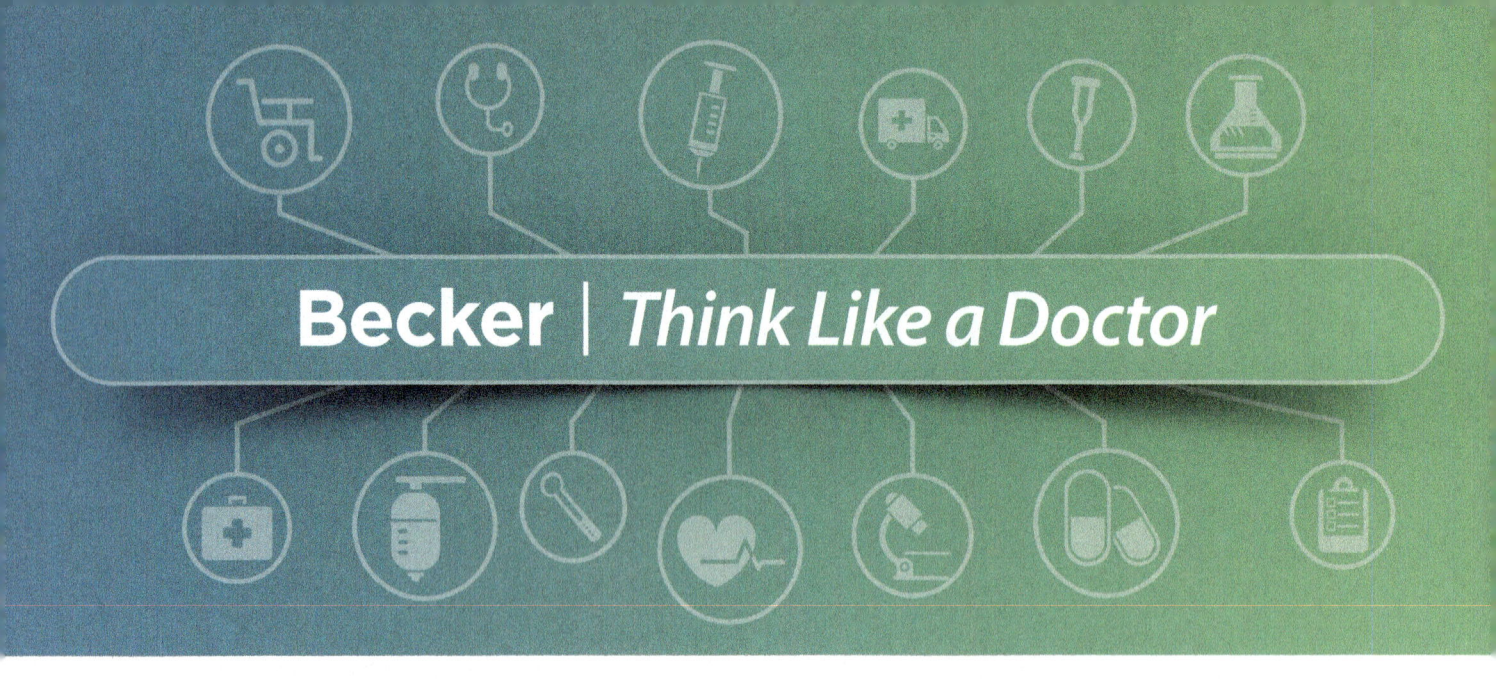

Becker | *Think Like a Doctor*

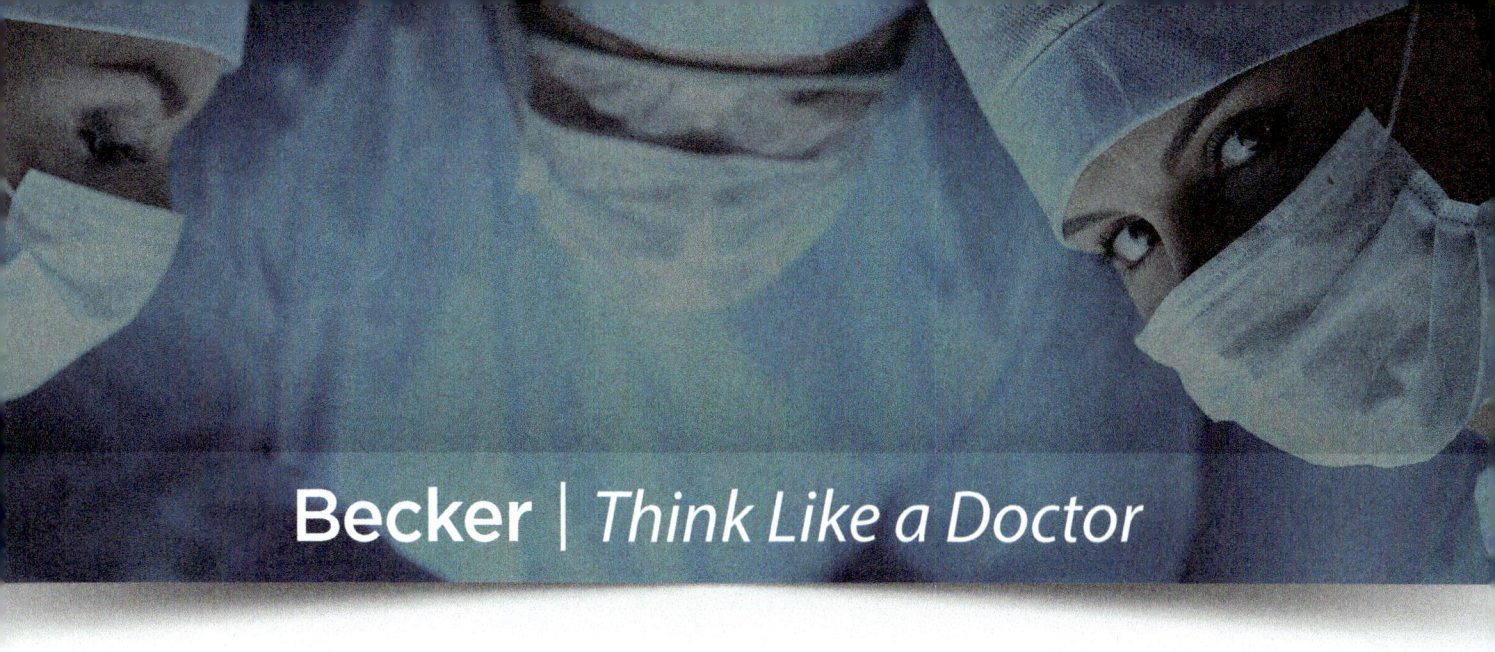

USMLE® Step 2 CK Live Online

Becker Professional Education's Step 2 CK Live Online Review course provides you with the tools you need to help you succeed on exam day. It's the ideal combination of structure and expert Clinical Science instruction along with flexibility and accessibility.

Here's what you receive:

- Over 100 hours of live online lectures over 4-weeks by our expert faculty held on evenings and weekends.

- Full set of Clinical Knowledge hardcopy textbooks and eBooks featuring our exam-relevant curriculum.

- Clinical examples to illustrate your understanding of high-yield topics.

- Optional Question package inclusive of UWorld 90-day Question Bank.

- 1 NBME Exam with Assessment to assess your progress and help you focus your remaining study time.

- Test Taking Workshop to learn strategies on how to best approach the exam.

- Access to a Becker Medical Advisor to help guide your Step 2 CK studies and exam preparation.

Visit **becker.com/usmle** if you are interested in enrolling in Becker's Step 2 CK live online course.

BECKER PROFESSIONAL EDUCATION®

USMLE® is a registered trademark of the National Board of Medical Examiners and this trademark owner does not sponsor, endorse or support Becker Professional Education in any manner.

© 2016 DeVry/Becker Educational Development Corp. All rights reserved.

Stay Connected:

CPSIA information can be obtained
at www.ICGtesting.com
Printed in the USA
LVOW02s0718101216
516683LV00002B/6/P